Post-traumatic Stress Disorder

Post-traumatic Stress Disorder: Diagnosis, Management and Treatment

Edited by

David Nutt DM MRCP FRCPsych
Professor of Psychopharmacology
School of Medical Sciences
University of Bristol
Bristol
UK

Jonathan RT Davidson MD
Professor of Psychiatry
Department of Psychiatry and Behavioral Sciences and
Director, Anxiety and Traumatic Stress Program
Duke University Medical Center
Durham, North Carolina
USA

Joseph Zohar MD
Professor of Psychiatry
Sackler Medical School
Tel Aviv University and
Director, Division of Psychiatry
The Chaim Sheba Medical Center
Israel

First published in the United Kingdom in 2000 by

Martin Dunitz Ltd
The Livery House
7–9 Pratt Street
London NW1 0AE

A CIP record for this book is available from the British Library.

ISBN 1-85317-926-4

Distributed in the United States by:
Blackwell Science Inc.
Commerce Place, 350 Main Street
Malden MA 02148, USA
Tel: 1-800-215-1000

Distributed in Canada by:
Login Brothers Book Company
324 Salteaux Crescent
Winnipeg, Manitoba R3J 3T2
Canada
Tel: 1-204-224-4068

Distributed in Brazil by:
Ernesto Reichmann Distribuidora de Livros, Ltda
Rua Coronel Marques 335, Tatuape 03440-000
Sao Paulo,
Brazil

Composition by Tek-Art, Croydon, Surrey
Printed and bound in Spain by Grafos, S.A.

CONTENTS

Contributors

Lisa Amaya-Jackson PhD
Program in Childhood & Adolescent Anxiety Disorders
Departments of Psychiatry and Psychology: Social and Health Sciences
Duke University Medical Center
Durham, North Carolina
USA

J Douglas Bremner MD
Assistant Professor of Psychiatry
Department of Psychiatry
Yale University School of Medicine
New Haven, Connecticut
USA

E Jane Costello PhD
Professor, Developmental Epidemiology Program
Department of Psychiatry and Behavioral Sciences
Duke University Medical Center
Durham, North Carolina
USA

Nick J Coupland MBChB MRCPsych
Assistant Professor
Department of Psychiatry
University of Alberta
Edmonton, Alberta
Canada

Jonathan RT Davidson MD
Professor of Psychiatry
Department of Psychiatry and Behavioral Sciences and Director, Anxiety and Traumatic Stress Program
Duke University Medical Center
Durham, North Carolina
USA

Martin Deahl OSt J TD MA MPhil MB BS FRCPsych
Consultant and Senior Lecturer in Psychological Medicine
St Bartholomew's and Royal London School of Medicine and Dentistry
Queen Mary and Westfield College
London
UK

Lori Ebert PhD
Research Clinical Psychologist
Research Triangle Institute
Research Triangle Park, North Carolina
USA

John A Fairbank PhD
Associate Professor
Developmental Epidemiology Program
Department of Psychiatry and Behavioral Sciences
Duke University Medical Center
Durham, North Carolina
USA

Norah Feeny PhD
Center for the Treatment and Study of Anxiety
Department of Psychiatry
University of Pennsylvania
Philadelphia, Pennsylvania
USA

Edna Foa PhD
Center for the Treatment and Study of Anxiety
Department of Psychiatry
University of Pennsylvania
Philadelphia, Pennsylvania
USA

Berthold PR Gersons MD PhD
Department of Psychiatry
Amsterdam Medical Centre
Amsterdam
The Netherlands

Selby Jacobs MD MPH
Professor of Psychiatry
Department of Psychiatry
Yale University School of Medicine
New Haven, Connecticut
USA

Debra Kaminer MA
MRC Research Unit on Anxiety and Stress Disorders
Department of Psychiatry
University of Stellenbosch
Cape Town
South Africa

Stanislav V Kasl PhD
Professor of Epidemiology
Yale University School of Medicine
Department of Psychiatry
New Haven, Connecticut
USA

Geoffrey van der Linden MB
MRC Research Unit on Anxiety and Stress Disorders
University of Stellenbosch
Cape Town
South Africa

Alexander C McFarlane MB BS (Hons) MD Dip.Psychother.FRANZCP
Head, Department of Psychiatry
University of Adelaide
Director of Clinical Services
North Western Adelaide Mental Health Services and
The Queen Elizabeth Hospital
Adelaide SA
Australia

Paul K Maciejewski PhD
Biostatistician, Department of Psychiatry
Yale University School of Medicine
New Haven, Connecticut
USA

Andrea L Malizia BA MBBS MRCPsych
Psychopharmacology Unit
School of Medical Sciences
University of Bristol and
Section of Neuroimaging
Institute of Psychiatry
London
UK

John S March MD MPH
Programs in Pediatric Anxiety Disorders and
Psychopharmacology
Department of Psychiatry
Duke University Medical Center
Durham, North Carolina
USA

Meena Narayan MD
Assistant Professor of Psychiatry
Department of Psychiatry
Yale University School of Medicine
New Haven, Connecticut
USA

David Nutt DM MRCP FRCPsych
Professor of Psychopharmacology
School of Medical Sciences
University of Bristol
Bristol
UK

Holly G Prigerson PhD
Assistant Professor of Psychiatry
Department of Psychiatry
Yale University School of Medicine
New Haven, Connecticut
USA

Barbara O Rothbaum PhD
Associate Professor in Psychiatry and
Director, Trauma and Anxiety Recovery Program
Department of Psychiatry and Behavioral Sciences
Emory University School of Medicine
Emory Clinic
Atlanta, Georgia
USA

Soraya Seedat MB
MRC Research Unit on Anxiety and Stress Disorders
Department of Psychiatry
University of Stellenbosch
Cape Town
South Africa

Arieh Y Shalev MD
Professor of Psychiatry and
Head, Department of Psychiatry
Hadassah University Hospital
Jerusalem
Israel

M Katherine Shear MD
Professor of Psychiatry
Department of Psychiatry
University of Pittsburgh School of Medicine
Pittsburgh, Pennsylvania
USA

Gabriel K Silverman BA
Department of Psychiatry
Yale University School of Medicine
New Haven, Connecticut
USA

Dan J Stein MB
Director of Research
MRC Research Unit on Anxiety and Stress Disorders
Department of Psychiatry
University of Stellenbosch
Cape Town
South Africa

Rachel Yehuda PhD
Professor of Psychiatry
Mount Sinai School of Medicine and
Bronx Veterans Affairs Hospital
New York City, New York
USA

Joseph Zohar MD
Professor of Psychiatry
Sackler Medical School
Tel Aviv University and
Director, Division of Psychiatry
The Chaim Sheba Medical Center
Israel

PREFACE

For many years, post-traumatic stress disorder (PTSD) has been the Cinderella diagnosis in the anxiety disorders. The reasons for this are many and varied and include the fact that many mental health professionals are concerned about diagnoses which need provoking incidents for their genesis. Another issue is the relationship between childhood trauma and later PTSD. We think that many therapists have been in effect treating consequences of PTSD without really understanding the origins.

Another important problem has been the question mark over treatment. Until recently, there has been no drug treatment licenced for the indication of PTSD and the (admittedly relatively few) clinical trials that have been done in this disorder with antidepressants and anxiolytics, have been rather unpromising. Paradoxically, there has been, in the public perception, a view that PTSD is eminently treatable by the simple intervention of debriefing or counselling. However, this approach has not been shown to be anything like as effective when subject to proper clinical trials. It is therefore not surprising when professionals are confronted with such a complicated and seemingly unintelligible syndrome, they tend to shy away from it.

Post-traumatic Stress Disorder we hope will begin to cut through some of the confusion and allow psychiatrists, psychologists and other mental health professionals to begin to understand that there is a significant degree of evidence on which they can base their understanding and treatment of this common and disabling disorder.

We have brought together a series of experts in all the fields relevant to an understanding of PTSD. This book examines the epidemiology and diagnosis of the disorder, emphasizing its prevalence and cost to the individual as well as to society and its role in different societies, different age groups and following grief. In addition, we cover the difficult issues of making a diagnosis and also the impact that hearing of trauma can have on the therapist. A number of chapters deal with our emerging understanding of the biological basis of this disorder. Here we have concentrated on human studies that have made significant advances in the past decade. The clear and growing understanding of endocrine abnormalities in PTSD are described and a theory of their pathogenesis and the way they relate to the persistence of the disorder is described. The extensive neurochemical literature on stress reactivity and sensitivity is outlined in a way which allows the reader to make an easy transition from preclinical to clinical insights. Finally, the growing ability to use neuroimaging to explore the brain basis of psychiatric disorders is discussed and some of the fascinating, if not yet conclusive, insights into brain abnormalities in PTSD is described. The last section of the book looks critically at the way in which PTSD should be treated. One chapter is dedicated to the very controversial issue of debriefing which is now seen as a right by many individuals, particularly those in caring professions such as police and hospital service. The controversial nature of its efficacy and value are critically outlined.

The other psychological treatments, particularly cognitive behavioural therapy, is reviewed in detail and the clear efficacy of this approach revealed. Finally, there is a full overview of the whole range of drug treatment which has been tried, it shows how much progress has been made in the past decade culminating in a number of positive clinical trials for new antidepressants, such as the SSRIs.

The last chapter of the volume pulls together our current knowledge of PTSD with an emphasis on where the field must go. New ideas for treatment approaches and potential research avenue which could address key questions in aetiology and treatment are outlined.

We have tried to produce a book which is readable, informative and also clinically helpful. We trust that we have succeeded and hope that by pulling all current knowledge together in one volume we will improve the diagnosis and treatment of this difficult and disabling condition.

David J Nutt
Jonathan RT Davidson
Joseph Zohar
2000

1

Post-traumatic stress disorder: diagnosis, history and life course

Arieh Y Shalev

What is post-traumatic stress disorder?

Post-traumatic stress disorder (PTSD) is an anxiety disorder, currently defined by the coexistence of three clusters of symptoms (re-experiencing, avoidance and hyperarousal), persisting for at least 1 month, in survivors of a traumatic event.[1] Unlike most other mental disorders, the diagnostic criteria for PTSD specify an aetiological factor, namely the traumatic event. The diagnosis of PTSD, therefore, includes both an observation of current symptoms and an attribution of such symptoms to a specific event or series of events. Such attribution, however, is not only historical, but rather relies on multiple appearances of reminders of the traumatic event in the patient's current symptoms through intrusive and distressful re-experiencing of the traumatic event *and* fearful avoidance of its reminders (both mental and real). For individuals so affected, therefore, the traumatic event is repeatedly and painfully relived. The image of men and women condemned to forever relive a traumatic event has captivated human imagination, and was immortalized in ancient legends, such as in that of Lot's wife, petrified into a column of salt as she looked backward to the chaos of Sodom. More recent expressions depict combat soldiers, for whom 'the war does not end when the shooting stops'[2] or holocaust survivors, living a 'concentration camp syndrome' for years after liberation.[3]

Yet the definition of PTSD goes beyond being reminded of a traumatic event to include pervasive restrictions to one's daily life along with persistent tension, restlessness and irritability (Box 1.1). PTSD, therefore, is a complex consequence of exposure to extreme events, which encompasses trauma-related symptoms, anxiety symptoms and symptoms otherwise found in depressive disorders. PTSD is also thought to be the final pathological outcome of all types of traumatic events, including the most horrifying and protracted (for example, concentration camp experiences, prolonged child abuse) and the very short and frequent ones (for example, road traffic

Box 1.1. DSM-IV diagnostic criteria for post-traumatic stress disorder (PTSD).

A. **The person has been exposed to a traumatic event in which both of the following were present.**
   (1) the person experienced, witnessed, or was confronted with an event or events that involved actual or threatened death or serious injury, or a threat to the physical integrity of self or others
   (2) the person's response involved intense fear, helplessness, or horror

B. **The traumatic event is persistently reexperienced in one (or more) of the following ways.**
   (1) recurrent and intrusive distressing recollections of the event, including images, thoughts and perceptions
   (2) recurrent distressing dreams of the event
   (3) acting or feeling as if the traumatic event were recurring
   (4) intense psychological distress at exposure to internal or external cues that symbolize or resemble an aspect of the traumatic event
   (5) physiological reactivity on exposure to internal or external cues that symbolize or resemble an aspect of the traumatic event

C. **Avoidance of stimuli associated with the trauma and numbing of general responsiveness (not present before the trauma), as indicated by three (or more) of the following:**
   (1) efforts to avoid thoughts, feelings, or conversations associated with the trauma
   (2) efforts to avoid activities, places, or people that arouse recollections of the trauma
   (3) inability to recall an important aspect of the trauma
   (4) markedly diminished interest or participation in significant activities
   (5) feeling of detachment or estrangement from others
   (6) restricted range of affect (e.g., unable to have loving feelings)
   (7) sense of a foreshortened future (e.g., does not expect to have a career, marriage, children or a normal life span)

D. **Persistent symptoms of increased arousal (not present before the trauma) as indicated by two (or more) of the following.**
   (1) difficulty falling or staying asleep
   (2) irritability or outbursts of anger
   (3) difficulty concentrating
   (4) hypervigilance
   (5) exaggerated startle response

E. **Duration of the disturbance (symptoms in criteria B, C and D) is more than 1 month.**

F. **The disturbance causes clinically significant distress or impairment in social occupational or other important areas of functioning**

accidents). Given the disorder's occurrence across traumatic events, PTSD is thought to result from a common element to all such events, currently referred to as 'stress'. Stress, accordingly, activates a complex biopsychological response which, in some individuals, leads to a chronic mental disorder. The occurrence of PTSD in a limited number of survivors further suggests that exposure to a traumatic event is not sufficient to cause the disorder.

Instead, the traumatic event is currently viewed as 'triggering' a reaction, to which prior and posterior (post-event) factors contribute at least as much.[4,5] Far beyond exposure to stressful events, therefore, the aetiology of PTSD is multifactorial and complex.[6]

PTSD was introduced into a formal classification of mental disorders in 1980.[7] Received with widespread scepticism, the disorder has won a central place in the current discourse on mental disorders. Among the many reasons for such 'success' are:

1. Extended focus of modern psychiatry on non-psychotic disorders and their impact on individuals' autonomy and wellbeing.
2. Increased social awareness regarding human rights, violence, disasters and their consequences.
3. A recent emphasis of the neurobehavioural sciences on brain plasticity and gene expression, and the paradigmatic role of traumatic events as triggering such reactions.

As other disorders born of the Diagnostic and Statistical Manual of Mental Disorders (DSM), the definition of PTSD is essentially phenomenological, that is, based on the co-occurrence of specific symptoms in an individual for a certain time. Admittedly, DSM-III opted for firstly creating reliability (that is, agreement between observers), and did so by positing specific symptoms as 'diagnostic criteria, to be present if the disorder is to be properly diagnosed'. It was hoped that by enhancing reliability the recognition of mental disorders would be improved and systematic research into their prevalence, causes and underlying mechanisms thereby enabled. In the case of PTSD, such hopes were largely fulfilled, as attested by an ever-growing number of empirical studies of this disorder. Yet the DSM-III and the subsequent DSM-IV and International Classification of Diseases, Tenth Edition (ICD-10) do not and did not posit a pathogenic or pathophysiological mechanism (such as, in the case of traumatic stress disorders, a 'neurotic conflict', 'fear conditioning', or 'shattered cognitive assumptions)'.[8–10]

A question often asked by observing clinicians is: 'He (or she) has all the required symptoms to meet a diagnosis of PTSD, but does he (or she) really suffer from PTSD?' As restated in a recent paper,[11] the answer to this question is an unqualified yes, as there is no other 'gold standard' to ascertain the presence of disorder (p. 1678). There are, however, numerous rating scales, and several structured interviews, which add a continuous 'severity' dimension to the categorical diagnosis regarding the presence or absence of PTSD. Some of these instruments will be described below.

In this chapter, therefore, the discussion regarding the diagnosis of PTSD is not concerned with the disorder's 'truthfulness' but rather with the 'effectiveness' of having clustered together this group of symptoms – effectiveness in helping clinicians and researchers correctly identify diseased individuals among trauma survivors. The disorder is also discussed in terms of its boundaries, that is, its relationship with co-occurring, 'comorbid' mental disorders and with normal responses to a traumatic event, and the logic of subdividing PTSD into subcategories (that is, acute stress disorder, acute PTSD, chronic PTSD, delayed-onset PTSD). We shall also present arguments for and against assuming a 'complex PTSD' or a trauma-related personality disorder. As a starter we briefly examine the history of PTSD, report findings related to the syndrome's reliability and construct validity and discuss the changes introduced into the definition of PTSD over time. A historical review of trauma-related disorders before 1980 is beyond the scope of this chapter, yet has been dealt with extensively in the literature.[12–16]

A brief history

Traumatic syndromes resembling PTSD have been repeatedly described and harshly debated during the twentieth century. Rescuers of survivors of ship explosions in Toulon in 1907 and 1911, for example, exhibited 'recapitulation of the scene, terrifying dreams, diffuse anxiety, fatigue, and various minor phobias' (cited in Trimble,[12] p. 247). A debate concerning the nature and the therapy of 'shell shock' raged during most of World War I. Subsequently, the burden of compensation for war-induced neurotic illness resulted in restrictive administrative decisions, such as *not* to compensate financially for battle shock during World War II in the United Kingdom, or to use the name 'battle fatigue' in the United States army in order not to imply pathology.[14]

Yet descriptions across generations of clinicians are very similar. For example, for 'operational fatigue' the following symptoms were noted:[14]

> Irritability, fatigue, difficulties falling asleep, startle reaction, depression, tremor and evidences of sympathetic over-reactivity, difficulties in concentration and mental confusion, preoccupation with combat experiences, nightmares and battle dreams, phobias, personality changes, and increased alcoholism. (p. 210)

Traumatic neurosis[8] similarly consisted of the following problems:

> Fixation on the trauma, typical dream life, contraction of general level of functioning, irritability and proclivity to explosive aggressive reactions. (p. 86)

These and other descriptions clearly resemble those used nowadays to define PTSD in DSM-IV and ICD-10.

Despite knowledge gained during the two world wars, the introduction of PTSD into DSM-III was driven by social and humanitarian forces, within and outside the psychiatric community.[15,16] DSM-II, in vogue between 1968 and 1980, did not include a diagnostic category of stress-related disorders. Yet the need for such a diagnostic category was increasingly felt by those concerned with Vietnam veterans following the defeat in 1973. The Vietnam Veterans Working Group (VVWG) was formed in 1974. This group was supported by both professional and humanitarian organizations, including, for example, the American Orthopsychiatric Association and the National Council of Churches. The VVWG drew the attention of the American Psychiatric Association (APA) Task Force on Nomenclature (the DSM-III Task Force) to the need for stress-related syndromes to be recognized. It further compiled 724 observations of psychologically disabled Vietnam veterans, and provided a tentative description of a syndrome closely resembling Kardiner's[8] description of traumatic neuroses in World War I veterans. These and other observations were submitted to a Committee of Reactive Disorders, especially appointed by the APA task force. The decision to include PTSD in DSM-III was obtained in 1978 and included 'consensus' rather than 'empirically validated' diagnostic criteria.[17]

Empirical findings have helped refine the diagnostic criteria for PTSD between DSM-III and the current DSM-IV. Mainly the definition of a traumatic event has changed (see below). DSM-IV includes a minimum duration of 1 month for the disorder to be formally diagnosed. Survivor guilt, which appeared in DSM-III, was omitted. Increased physiological reaction to reminders of the trauma was moved from the 'hyperarousal' (D) to the 'intrusion' (B) criterion. Box 1.1 presents DSM-IV diagnostic criteria for PTSD.

The syndrome

DSM-IV diagnostic criteria differ from those originally included in DSM-III in several points. First, DSM-IV definition of a traumatic event does not require an outstanding stressor that 'would evoke significant symptoms of distress in almost everyone', as in DSM-III. Milder and frequent stresses, such as road traffic accidents or assaultive violence, have, in fact, been shown to induce prolonged PTSD symptoms.[18,19] Exposure to traumatic events, therefore, is not perceived as rare, and indeed would occur quite frequently. Table 1.1 summarizes the likelihood of being exposed to a traumatic event, as recorded in several studies of civilian adults in the United States. In studies using DSM-IV criteria,[20,21] the probability of experiencing a traumatic event during one's life is indeed very high, reaching 97% of male adults in the United States.

Secondly, traumatic events in DSM-IV include instances of witnessing trauma to others (such as witnessing an execution or being involved in rescue operations). The element of being under direct threat, therefore, is not required any more: suffice it to be 'confronted' with an event. Thirdly, the definition of the 'event' now includes an intense reaction, involving intense fear, helplessness or horror. The definition of traumatic events in IDC-10, however, is more conservative and consists of: 'event or situation (either short or long-lasting) of an exceptionally threatening or catastrophic nature, which is likely to cause pervasive distress in almost anyone'.

Table 1.1 Likelihood of exposure to traumatic events in the general population

Study	Population (*n*)	Lifetime exposure rate		Notes
		Male	Female	
Kessler et al 1995[35]	General population USA (5877)	61%	51%	Any trauma
Breslau et al 1991[19]	Young adults (age=21–30) USA (1007)	43%	37%	Any trauma
Norris et al 1992[57]	Adults, USA (1000)	74%	65%	Ten selected events
Stein et al 1997[21]	Adults, Canada (1000)	81%	74%	List of traumatic events
Breslau et al 1998[20]	Adults, USA (2181)	97%	87%	Extensive list of 19 events
Resnick et al 1993[66]	Female, USA (4008)	–	69%	Any trauma

Internal consistency and stability

All PTSD symptoms may be present shortly after exposure to a traumatic event.[22] Symptoms of intrusion and re-experiencing are often found in trauma survivors (for example, holocaust survivors) who otherwise are not disabled by an overt mental disorder. Avoidance alone may characterize other trauma survivors, in the form of specific phobias, reluctance to evoke or discuss specific memories or avoidance of places or situations. Irritability and insomnia are also seen among survivors. Yet, how robust and stable is the co-occurrence of these three categories of symptoms? Studies have examined the construct validity of PTSD in various samples of trauma survivors[17,23,24] and found it to be good, and to generally match the subdivision into three clusters of symptoms. Despite somewhat fluctuating individual trajectories, symptom severity, in cohorts of chronic PTSD patients, remains stable over time.[25]

The data show, however, that the avoidance criterion (C) is *not* met by some trauma survivors, who otherwise express most PTSD symptoms. An important reason for this is the requirement for *three* avoidance symptoms in order meet the 'C' criterion.[25] This has led to studies of 'partial PTSD' – a subsyndromal condition, which is often as frequent as PTSD in the general population,[26] and may be as stable as PTSD across time.[27,28]

A closer look at the C criterion also shows that only three of its seven items (items 1–3) are directly related to avoiding the traumatic event, whereas the other four items ('diminished interest', 'detachment and estrangement', 'restricted range of affect' and 'sense of foreshortened future') are not. The latter are linked with the concept of 'psychological numbing', brought to PTSD from studies of traumatic loss.[29,30] For example:[30]

> After the first emotional reactions and physical responses there may be a period of comparative denial and numbing. Then an oscillatory period commonly emerges in which there are impulsive ideas or images, attacks of emotions, or compulsive behavior alternating with continued denial, numbing and other indications of efforts to ward off the implications of the new information.
>
> (p. 789)

Importantly, these four symptoms also overlap with those seen in depression – a disorder that often co-occurs with PTSD.

PTSD criterion D includes several expressions attributed to 'increased arousal' as well as exaggerated startle. Increased response to sudden auditory stimuli has been linked with post-traumatic morbidity throughout history. 'Stragglers', who ceased to function as soldiers following the Civil War combats, were described as 'trembling, staring into the middle distance and jumping at any loud noise'.[31] Following World War I 'auditory hypersensitiveness' has been recognized as a central feature of traumatic neuroses (Kardiner,[8] p. 95). Startle reaction was among the frequent symptoms seen in airmen with 'operational fatigue' (14 p. 210). Exaggerated startle has been reported by up to 88% of PTSD patients.[32]

The course of PTSD

PTSD symptoms are expressed by most trauma survivors shortly after exposure. PTSD symptoms were found in 94% of rape victims 1 week following trauma.[33] In a study of civilian survivors of traumatic events in Israel, 39% had diagnosable PTSD 1 month following trauma, 17% had PTSD 4 months after trauma and only 10% had PTSD 1 year following trauma.[22,34] Recovery from early PTSD has been estimated, in an epidemiological study, to involve 60% of those initially expressing the disorder.[35] In the National Vietnam Veterans Readjustment Study, the difference between lifetime and current prevalence of PTSD (30% and 15.2%) suggests an overall 50% recovery or remission rate of those once diagnosed as suffering from the disorder.[36] Similar recovery rates were obtained in prospective studies (Table 1.2) . Most cases of spontaneous recovery occur within a year from the traumatic event, whereas no further recovery has been found to occur after expressing the disorder for 6 years.[35] Recovery from prolonged PTSD, however, may be incomplete, with some individuals expressing subsyndromal forms of the disorder[34] and being vulnerable to relapse upon re-exposure.[37]

Given the frequent expression of PTSD symptoms by trauma survivors shortly after a traumatic event, and their subsequent disappearance in those who do not develop PTSD, predicting PTSD from early symptoms is particularly difficult. Such early symptoms are, in fact, *sensitive* predictors of the disorder: very few individuals develop PTSD without expressing PTSD symptoms during the first weeks that follow a traumatic event.[34] Yet early symptoms are *non-specific* predictors, in that most individuals who express such symptoms will still recover. The clinician's dilemma, therefore, is to identify, among those who express high levels of distressful symptoms at the early aftermath of exposure, those who are more likely to remain symptomatic.

Some clinical attributes can help – such as the occurrence of dissociative symptoms (for example, detachment, time distortion, feeling 'on automatic pilot', out of the body experience) during the traumatic event or shortly afterwards.[4] The early occurrence of depression,[38] or the presence of elevated autonomic (for example heart rate) responses to the traumatic event, may also predict the subsequent development of PTSD.[39] Yet other risk factors must be considered as well, such as past history of mental illness and previous traumatic experiences. Most importantly, factors occurring at the aftermath of traumatic events (such as relocation, physical

Table 1.2 Percentage of trauma survivors with PTSD and recovery rates in prospective studies

Study	Event/sample size	1 month	2–5 months	6–12 months	1–3 years	3–6 years	Recovered
Solomon 1993[2]	Israeli veterans *n*=238	100	–	59	47	42	58%
Feinstein and Dolan, 1991[58]	MVA *n*=48	25	–	14.6	–	–	42%
Perry et al 1992[59]	Burn victims *n*=51	–	35	>32	>28	–	
Blanchard et al 1997[45]	MVA *n*=132	39	31	12	–	–	66%
Shalev et al 1997[22]	Misc. civil. *n*=236	30	17	–	10	–	66%

pain, separation from relatives and other 'secondary stressors') contribute significantly to the occurrence and the persistence of PTSD. Amongst the latter, the survivor's cognitive appraisal of his or her responses may have a major role in mediating chronicity,[40] hence the recently reported success of cognitive behavioural treatment in preventing PTSD.[41,42] A recent study of physiological response to startle in early trauma survivors shows, in fact, that the elevated responses which are typical of chronic PTSD do not exist 1 week after trauma, but rather develop within 4 months of expressing the disorder.[43] The early aftermath of traumatic events may offer a window of opportunity for preventing both psychological and biological components of PTSD.

Severity and comorbidity

In its chronic form PTSD is a debilitating disorder, associated with significant disability and distress. These will be dealt with in other chapters of this book. The severity of PTSD symptoms in individual patients is subject to fluctuations.[25] These may be due to the effect of ongoing life pressures, and to exposure to reminders of the traumatic event. In general, patients with chronic PTSD are believed to be very sensitive to ongoing environmental stressors, and to react readily by increased distress, anger, isolation and use of medication or alcohol. For the clinician, this feature of PTSD suggests that the environment within which chronic PTSD patients live (for example, stable family, good working environment) may significantly affect the expression of PTSD symptoms and patient's response to treatment interventions.

PTSD often co-occurs with other mental disorders, particularly with major depression, anxiety disorders and substance abuse. The US National Comorbidity survey, for example,[35] shows that 88.3% of men and 79% of women with PTSD experience at least one other mental disorder. Depression is experienced by about one-half of all PTSD subjects (48.5% in women and 47.9% in men). Anxiety disorders are seen in more than one-third, drug and alcohol abuse

Table 1.3 Prevalence and co-occurrence of post-traumatic stress disorder (PTSD) and depression

Author	Population	*n*	PTSD (%)	Depression (%)	Overlap (% of PTSD)
Shore et al 1989[60]	Community sample: Mt St Helen disaster	274	3	NA	51.3
Green et al 1990[61]	Vietnam veterans	200	29	15	34.5
Engdahl et al 1991[62]	World War II prisoners of war	62	29	25.8	61
McFarlane and Papay 1992[63]	Fire fighters	398	18	10	51
North et al 1994[64]	Survivors of mass shooting	136	26	10.2	30.1
Kessler et al 1995[35]	Population sample	5877	7.8	17.9	48.2
Bleich et al 1997[65]	Israeli war veterans	60	87	50	56

by a third of all women and half of all men. Table 1.3 summarizes the results of studies in which the association between PTSD and major depression was examined. As can be seen, the association between PTSD and depression is very frequent. Importantly, depression can be seen in trauma survivors at the early aftermath of traumatic events, in which case it increases the likelihood of developing chronic PTSD.[38]

Boundaries and subtypes

Acute stress disorder

In an attempt better to differentiate the early and normal responses to traumatic events from 'pathological' ones, DSM-IV has proposed a new diagnostic category, the acute stress disorder (ASD, Box 1.2). ASD includes most symptoms of PTSD *and* additional symptoms related to dissociation (numbing, reduction of awareness to one's surroundings, derealization, depersonalization, and dissociative amnesia). Three dissociation symptoms must be present in order to meet criteria for ASD. ASD can be diagnosed immediately after the traumatic event, and should occur within 4 weeks of the traumatic event. ASD has been critically evaluated.[44] It was found to be a sensitive predictor of subsequent PTSD (as are most other parameters of early distress).

Box 1.2. Symptom criteria for acute stress disorder.

A. As in PTSD: Box 1.1

B. Either while experiencing or after experiencing the distressing event, the individual has three (or more) of the following dissociative symptoms:

   1 a subjective sense of numbing, detachment, or absence of emotional responsiveness
   2 a reduction in awareness of his or her surroundings (e.g., 'being in a daze')
   3 derealization
   4 depersonalization
   5 dissociative amnesia (i.e., inability to recall an important aspect of the trauma)

C. The traumatic event is persistently reexperienced in at least one of the following ways:

   recurrent images, thoughts, dreams, illusions, flashback episodes, or a sense of reliving the experience; or distress on exposure to reminders of the traumatic event.

D. Marked avoidance of stimuli that arouse recollections of the trauma (e.g., thoughts, feelings, conversations, activities, places, people).

E. Marked symptoms of anxiety or increased arousal (e.g., difficulty sleeping, irritability, poor concentration, hypervigilance, exaggerated startle response, motor restlessness).

F. The disturbance causes clinically significant distress or impairment in social, occupational, or other important areas of functioning or impairs the individual's ability to pursue some necessary task, such as obtaining necessary assistance or mobilizing personal resources by telling family members about the traumatic experience.

G. The disturbance lasts for a minimum of 2 days and a maximum of 4 weeks and occurs within 4 weeks of the traumatic event.

Dissociation symptoms, however, were not found significantly to improve predictions made from other early symptoms. Moreover, numerous trauma survivors who do not show dissociation symptoms, and who do not qualify for the diagnosis of ASD, develop PTSD. For these reasons ASD has been recently criticized as being of little value.[11] Clinicians may wish to use this diagnostic category with great caution and, specifically, not to exclude individuals without ASD, and who are otherwise distressed, from receiving treatment. Interestingly, ICD-10 defines an acute response to stress as starting at the time of the traumatic events and lasting for up to 2 or 3 days. This is a totally different syndrome, which may or may not be self-limited, and may or may not predict long-term outcome.

Acute PTSD and chronic PTSD

Another controversial matter is the subdivision of PTSD into acute (duration of symptoms less than 3 months) and chronic (duration of symptoms exceeds 3 months) subtypes. The two subtypes are identical, and indeed the full syndrome has been found 1 month, 4 months and 1 year following trauma.[34,45] Two points are subject to criticism. First, a 'chronic' condition is inferred after 3 months of expressing PTSD symptoms, whereas prospective studies show that more than a half of those showing symptoms of PTSD 3 months following trauma will recover within the next year. Secondly, acute PTSD (that is, between 1 and 3 months) currently has no distinct clinical usefulness (no specific therapy or management). The advice to clinicians is, therefore, to identify and eventually treat all subjects who show high levels of PTSD symptoms, anxiety or depression in the weeks following trauma, without paying much attention to the current subdivisions.

Delayed-onset PTSD

This condition consists of delayed appearance of full PTSD syndrome more than 6 months after a traumatic event. Such delayed appearance has been linked with seeking compensation and malingering. Yet, one sometimes encounters individuals who have been coping well with the consequences of a traumatic event, and who developed PTSD at a distance from the traumatic event, often as a result of another event. A systematic study of 150 combat veterans with delayed PTSD (first referral to treatment between 6 months and 6 years following trauma[46]) has shown, however, that 90% of these individuals had been symptomatic prior to seeking help. Some 40% of the cases were identified as 'delayed referral', that is, subjects who suffered without seeking help; 33% had subsyndromal PTSD since the traumatic event; 13% had reactivated previously recovered PTSDs and 4% had been given other psychiatric diagnoses before being identified as suffering from PTSD. Delayed-onset PTSD is, therefore, an exception which poses puzzling clinical problems.

Trauma-induced personality changes

Some individuals show a particularly severe form of PTSD, associated with profound personality changes. The degree to which traumatic events can affect personality structures has been the subject of a heated debate, which ended by not including in the DSM-IV the diagnostic category of 'disorders of stress not otherwise specified' (DESNOS, DSM-IV draft criteria, 1991). DESNOS was found to be consistently associated with PTSD, and therefore was not granted an independent status. Interestingly, ICD-10[47] recognized enduring personality changes resulting from exposure to 'catastrophic stress' such as concentration camp experiences, torture or hostage situation. Traumatic personality changes must be present for at least 2 years and include the following symptoms: permanent hostile or distressful attitude towards the world, social withdrawal, feeling of emptiness, enduring feeling of being 'on edge' and estrangement (a permanent feeling of being changed or being different from others).

Clearly, the discussion of trauma-induced personality change is hampered by several attributes of the current view of mental disorders. Indeed, the boundary between 'personality' and the very chronic mental disorders is not well traced. Moreover, PTSD symptoms of pervasive avoidance, irritability, increased stimulus responsivity and restriction to one's life are very likely to be perceived, by the patient and by the family, as changes to his or her 'personality'. Indeed, one of the most frequent complaints of PTSD patients is 'I am not the same'. Finally, the impression of an association between PTSD and profound personality changes may result from clustering, in many trauma clinics, of treatment-resistant PTSD patients or patients whose PTSD is particularly complex and whose life circumstances are particularly unfavourable. Understandably, childhood trauma, and particularly prolonged exposure to abuse and neglect, are causes of severe developmental difficulties, which often present as personality disorders.

Measuring PTSD

Making a diagnosis

A DSM-IV-derived instrument for making the diagnosis of PTSD (and other Axis I disorders) is the Structured Clinical Interview for DSM-IV disorders (SCID-IV[48]). The SCID yields categorical diagnoses and does not evaluate symptom severity. The SCID must be administered by trained clinicians and relies on clinical judgement and experience.

The Clinician Administered PTSD Scale (CAPS[49]) is a structured clinical interview dedicated to PTSD. The CAPS quantifies PTSD symptoms' frequency and intensity, and therefore yields a continuous measure of symptom severity as well as dichotomous diagnosis of PTSD. As with the SCID, the administration of the CAPS requires clinical skills, judgement and experience.

Complementing these clinical interviews, the Posttraumatic Diagnostic Scale (PTDS[50]) is a self-report measure of post-traumatic stress disorder that yields both a diagnosis of PTSD and a measure of PTSD symptom severity. The instrument's items follow DSM-IV diagnostic criteria for PTSD. The PTSD also addresses the nature of the stressful event, the duration of the disturbance and the resulting impairment. The instrument has been validated against the SCID and was found to have good sensitivity and specificity.

Assessing symptom severity

The Impact of Events Scale (IES[51,52]) is the oldest and the most widely used self-report rating scale of trauma-related symptoms. The current version of the IES evaluates the three symptom domains of PTSD: intrusion, avoidance and hyperarousal. The IES is fairly sensitive to change in symptom severity. The instrument's subscales (intrusion, avoidance and hyperarousal) can be scored separately.

The Davidson Trauma Scale (DTS[53]), a 17-item clinician-administered scale, is a self-report instrument that measures both the frequency and severity of each DSM-IV PTSD symptom. The DTS has been shown to have good predictive properties for response to treatment and is sensitive to treatment effect.

The Mississippi Scale for Posttraumatic Stress Disorder (MISS[54,55]) is a 35-item self-report questionnaire that focuses on symptomatology found specifically after trauma. The MISS has been used in numerous epidemiological studies of PTSD from which a cut-off score has been derived to define 'caseness' (the presence or absence) of PTSD. The usefulness of the MISS in clinical studies may be limited, as similar results can be obtained by shorter instruments.

An example of a short instrument, the Davidson's eight-item Treatment Outcome PTSD scale (TOP-8[53]) examines eight PTSD symptoms that have been shown to respond well to treatment interventions. The eight items belong to all three symptom clusters for PTSD, and have been shown to detect drug/placebo differences better than the original scale.

Finally, global measures of improvement, such as the Clinical Global Impression (CGI[56]), capture and quantify a global impression by the clinician regarding both severity and improvement in the patient's condition. Global instruments offer an advantage in evaluating clinical improvement in patients with PTSD and comorbid disorders.

Conclusion

The uniqueness of PTSD among mental disorders is that this condition develops after salient events, and therefore can be detected at an early stage and, to some extent, prevented. Despite its 'political' origins and despite the admixture of various symptoms in this man-made syndrome, PTSD has proved to be robust, persistent, reliably diagnosable and clearly linked with substantial distress and dysfunction. Indeed, similar constellations of symptoms have been described in diseased trauma survivors throughout. Biologically, the disorder has been associated with consistent, converging and replicable findings, particularly in the areas of startle physiology and neuroendocrinology and some recent brain-imaging studies. Several recent treatment studies, including pharmacology and psychological therapies, are quickly reversing a previous image of a hopeless condition. PTSD, therefore, is a story of success.

Yet, PTSD is also a matter of debate, mainly because the disorder is being used and abused in compensation claims, in ideological debates (for example the false memory debate) and in introducing magical yet not medical therapies. The main threat to the survival of this condition is, therefore, its misuse and overextension to include any and all illnesses that follow trauma. Intrinsic inconsistencies, however, do exist. First, the co-occurrence of PTSD and depression is a major area for future research – particularly when the contribution of early depression to chronic PTSD is considered. Secondly, the boundary with normal reactions to traumatic stress, particularly at the early aftermath of traumatic events, needs better definition. Finally, the complex causation of chronic PTSD, and particularly the role of post-event factors in maintaining the disorder, should make us rethink about the nature of the link between the triggering traumatic event and the subsequent psychological, biological and genomic events. PTSD, therefore, faces an exciting future as a subject of clinical and scientific investigation. PTSD is also likely to be at the centre of future debates concerning human nature, human resilience to stress and the role of culture in defining what is disordered and what is not.

References

1. American Psychiatric Association, *Diagnostic and Statistical Manual of Mental Disorders*, 4th edn (DSM-IV) (American Psychiatric Press: Washington, DC, 1994).
2. Solomon Z, *Combat Stress Reaction: The Enduring Toll of War* (Plenum: New York, 1993).
3. Eitinger L, *Concentration Camp Survivors in Norway and Israel* (Allen & Unwin: London, 1964).
4. Shalev AY, Peri T, Canneti L, Schreiber S, Predictors of PTSD in recent trauma survivors: a prospective study, *Am J Psychiatry* (1992) **153**:219–25.
5. King LA, King DW, Fairbank JA et al, Resilience-recovery factors in post-traumatic stress disorder among female and male Vietnam veterans: hardiness, postwar social support, and additional stressful life events, *J Pers Soc Psychol* (1998) 74:420–34
6. Yehuda R, McFarlane AC, Conflict between current knowledge about posttraumatic stress disorder and its original conceptual basis, *Am J Psychiatry* (1995) **152**:1705–13.
7. American Psychiatric Association, *Diagnostic and Statistical Manual of Mental Disorders*, 3rd edn (DSM-III) (American Psychiatric Press: Washington, DC, 1980).
8. Kardiner A, *The Traumatic Neuroses of War* (Hoeber: New York, 1941).
9. Pitman RK, Post-traumatic stress disorder, conditioning, and network theory, *Psychiatric Annals*, **18**:182–9.
10. Janoff Bulman R, The aftermath of victimization: rebuilding shattered assumptions. In: Figley CR, ed, *Trauma and its Wake, the Study and Treatment of Post-traumatic Stress Disorder* (Brunner-Mazel: New York, 1985) 15–36.
11. Marshall RD, Spitzer R, Liebowitz MR, Review and critique of the new DSM-IV diagnosis of acute stress disorder, *Am J Psychiatry* (1999) **156**:1677–85.
12. Trimble MR, *Post-traumatic Neurosis. From Railway Spine to the Whiplash* (John Wiley: Chichester, 1981).
13. Merskey H, Shell shock. In: Berrios EG, Freedman H, eds, *150 years of British Psychiatry* (Gaskell: London, 1991).
14. Grinker RR, Spiegel JP, *Men under Stress* (Backiston: Philadelphia, 1945).
15. Bloom SL, Our hearts and our hopes are turned to peace: origins of the International Society for Traumatic Stress. In: Shalev AY, Yehuda R, McFarlane AC, eds, *International Handbook of Human Response to Trauma* (Kluwer Academic/ Plenum: New York, 2000) 27–50.
16. Young A, An alternative history of traumatic stress. In: Shalev AY, Yehuda R, McFarlane AC, eds, *International Handbook of Human Response to Trauma* (Kluwer Academic/Plenum: New York, 2000).
17. Keane TM, Symptomatology of Vietnam veterans with posttraumatic stress disorder. In: Davidson JRT, Foa E, eds, *Posttraumatic Stress Disorder: DSM IV and Beyond* (American Psychiatric Press: Washington, DC, 1993) 99–111.
18. Breslau N, Davis GC, Posttraumatic stress disorder: the etiologic specificity of wartime stressors, *Am J Psychiatry* (1988) **144**:578–83.
19. Breslau N, Davis GC, Andreski P, Peterson E, Traumatic events and posttraumatic stress disorder in an urban population of young adults, *Arch Gen Psychiatry* (1991) **48**:216–22.
20. Breslau N, Kessler RC, Chilcoat HD et al, Trauma and posttraumatic stress disorder in the community: the 1996 Detroit Area Survey of Trauma, *Arch Gen Psychiatry* (1998) **55**:626–32.
21. Stein MB, Walker JR, Hazen AL, Forde DR, Full and partial posttraumatic stress disorder: findings from a community survey, *Am J Psychiatry* (1997) **154**:1114–19.
22. Shalev AY, Freedman S, Brandes D et al, Predicting PTSD in civilian trauma survivors: prospective evaluation of self report and clinician administered instruments, *Br J Psychiatry* (1997) **170**:558–64.
23. Fawzi MC, Pham T, Lin L et al, The validity of posttraumatic stress disorder among Vietnamese refugees, *J Trauma Stress* (1997) **10**:101–8.
24. Kilpatrick DG, Resnick HS, Posttraumatic stress disorder associated with exposure to criminal victimization in clinical and community populations. In: Davidson JRT, Foa E, eds, *Posttraumatic Stress Disorder: DSM IV and Beyond* (American Psychiatric Press: Washington, DC, 1993) 113–43.
25. Niles BL, Newman E, Fisher LM, Obstacles to assessment of PTSD in longitudinal research. In: Shalev AY, Yehuda R, McFarlane AC, eds, *International Handbook of Human Response to Trauma* (Kluwer Academic/Plenum: New York, 2000) 213–22.

26. Stein MB, Walker JR, Hazen AL, Forde DR, Full and partial posttraumatic stress disorder: findings from a community survey, *Am J Psychiatry* (1997) **154**:1114–19.
27. Carlier IV, Lamberts RD, Fouwels AJ, Gersons BP, PTSD in relation to dissociation in traumatized police officers, *Am J Psychiatry* (1996) **153**:1325–8.
28. Carlier IV, Gersons BPR, Partial posttraumatic stress disorder (PTSD): the issue of psychological scars and the occurrence of PTSD symptoms, *J Nerv Ment Dis* (1995) **183**:107–9.
29. Lindemann E, Symptomatology and management of acute grief, *Am J Psychiatry* (1944) **101**:141–8.
30. Horowitz MJ, Stress response syndromes: character style and dynamic psychotherapy, *Arch Gen Psychiatry* (1974) **31**:768–81.
31. Marlowe DH, *Psychological and Psycho-social Consequences of Combat and Deployment with Special Emphasis on the Gulf War* (Rand: Santa Monica, CA, in press).
32. Davidson JRT, Kudler HS, Smith RD, Assessment and pharmacotherapy of posttraumatic stress disorder. In: Giller EL, ed, *Biological Assessment and Treatment of Posttraumatic Stress Disorder* (American Psychiatric Press: Washington, DC, 1990) 203–21.
33. Foa EB, Rothbaum BO, Riggs DS, Murdock TB, Treatment of posttraumatic stress disorder in rape victims: a comparison between cognitive-behavioral procedures and counseling, *J Consult Clin Psychol* (1991) **59**:715–23.
34. Freedman SA, Peri T, Brandes D, Shalev AY, Predictors of chronic PTSD – a prospective study, *Br J Psychiatry* (1999) **174**:353–9.
35. Kessler RC, Sonnega A, Bromet EJ et al, Posttraumatic stress disorder in the National Comorbidity Survey, *Arch Gen Psychiatry* (1995) **52**:1048–60.
36. Kulka RA, Schlenger WE, Fairbank JA et al, *Trauma and the Vietnam War Generation: Report of Findings from the National Vietnam Veterans Readjustment Study* (Brunner/Mazel: New York, 1990).
37. Solomon Z, Garb R, Bleich A, Grupper D, Reactivation of combat related posttraumatic stress disorder, *Am J Psychiatry* (1985) **144**: 51–5.
38. Shalev AY, Freedman S, Peri T et al, Prospective study of posttraumatic stress disorder and depression following trauma, *Am J Psychiatry* (1998) **155**:630–7.
39. Shalev AY, Sahar T, Freedman S et al, A prospective study of heart rate responses following trauma and the subsequent development of PTSD, *Arch Gen Psychiatry* (1998) **55**:553–9.
40. Ehlers A, Mayou RA, Bryant B, Psychological predictors of chronic posttraumatic stress disorder after motor vehicle accidents, *J Abnorm Psychol* (1998) **107**:508–19.
41. Bryant RA, Harvey AG, Dang ST et al, Treatment of acute stress disorder: a comparison of cognitive-behavioral therapy and supportive counseling, *J Consult Clin Psychol* (1998) **66**:862–6.
42. Bryant RA, Sackville T, Dang S et al, Treatment of acute stress disorder: an evaluation of cognitive behavioral therapy and supportive counseling techniques, *Am J Psychiatry* (1999) **156**:1780–6.
43. Shalev AY, Peri T, Brandes D et al, Auditory startle responses in trauma survivors with PTSD: a prospective study, *Am J Psychiatry* (2000)**157**:255–61.
44. Harvey AG, Bryant RA, The relationship between acute stress disorder and posttraumatic stress disorder: a prospective evaluation of motor vehicle accident survivors, *J Consult Clin Psychol* (1998) **66**:507–12.
45. Blanchard EB, Hickling EJ, Forneris CA et al, Prediction of remission of acute posttraumatic stress disorder in motor vehicle accident victims, *J Trauma Stress* (1997) **10**:215–34.
46. Solomon Z, Kotler M, Shalev A, Lin R, Delayed post-traumatic stress disorders, *Psychiatry (*1989) **52**:428–36.
47. World Health Organization, *The ICD 10 Classification of Mental and Behavioural Disorders: Diagnostic Criteria for Research* (WHO: Geneva, 1993).
48. Spitzer RL, Williams JBW, Gibbon M, First MB, Structured Clinical Interview for DSM-IV (SCID-IV). Biometric Research Department, New York State Psychiatric Institute, 1994.
49. Blake DD, Weathers FW, Nagy LM et al, A clinician rating scale for assessing current and lifetime PTSD: The CAPS-1, *Behav Therapist* (1990) **13**:187–8.
50. Foa EB, Cashman L, Jaycox L, Perry K, The validation of a self-report measure of posttraumatic stress disorder, the posttraumatic diagnostic scale, *Psychol Assessment* (1997) **9**:445–51.
51. Horowitz MJ, Wilner N, Alvarez W, Impact of event scale: a measure of subjective stress, *Psychosom Med (*1979) **41**:209–18.
52. Weiss DS, Marmar CR, The Impact of Events Scale – Revised. In: Wison JP, Keane TM, eds, *Assessing*

Psychological Trauma and PTSD (Guilford: New York, 1997) 399–411.

53. Davidson JR, Colket JT, The eight-item treatment-outcome post-traumatic stress disorder scale: a brief measure to assess treatment outcome in post-traumatic stress disorder, *Int Clin Pharmacol* (1997) 12:41–5.
54. Keane TM, Caddell JM, Taylor KL, Mississippi Scale for Combat-Related Posttraumatic Stress Disorder: three studies in reliability and validity, *J Consult Clin Psychol* (1988) **56**:85–90.
55. Vreven DL, Gudanowski DM, King LA, King DW, The civilian version of the Mississippi PTSD Scale: a psychometric evaluation, *J Trauma Stress* (1995) **8**:91–109.
56. Guy W, Clinical Global Impressions. *ECDEU Assessment Manual for Psychopharmacology* (ECDEU: National Institutes of Health, 1976) 218–22.
57. Norris FH, Epidemiology of trauma: frequency and impact of different potentially traumatic events on different demographic groups, *J Consult Clin Psychol* (1992) **60**:409–18.
58. Feinstein A, Dolan R, Predictors of post-traumatic stress disorder following physical trauma: an examination of the stressor criterion, *Psychol Med* (1991) **21**:85–91.
59. Perry S, Difede J, Musngi G et al, Predictors of posttraumatic stress disorder after burn injury, *Am J Psychiatry* (1992) **149**:931–5.
60. Shore JH, Vollmer WM, Tatum EL, Community patterns of posttraumatic stress disorders, *J Nerv Ment Dis* (1989) 177:681–5.
61. Green BL, Grace MC, Lindy JD et al, Risk factors for PTSD and other diagnoses in a general sample of Vietnam veterans, *Am J Psychiatry* (1990) 147:729–33.
62. Engdahl BE, Speed N, Eberly RE, Schwartz J, Comorbidity of psychiatric disorders and personality profiles of American World War II prisoners of war, *J Nerv Ment Dis* (1991) **179**:181–91.
63. McFarlane AC, Papay P, Multiple diagnoses in posttraumatic stress disorder in the victims of a natural disaster, *J Nerv Ment Dis* (1992) **180**:498–504.
64. North CS, Smith EM, Spitznagel EL, Posttraumatic stress disorder in survivors of a mass shooting, *Am J Psychiatry* (1994) **151**:82–8.
65. Bleich A, Koslowsky M, Dolev A, Lerer B, Post-traumatic stress disorder and depression. An analysis of comorbidity, *Br J Psychiatry* (1997) **170**:479–82.
66. Resnick HS, Kilpatrick DG, Dansky BS et al. Prevalence of civilian trauma and posttraumatic stress disorder in a representative national sample of women. *J Consult Clin Psychol* (1993) **61**:984–91.

2

Epidemiology of traumatic events and post-traumatic stress disorder

John A Fairbank, Lori Ebert and Elizabeth Jane Costello

Epidemiology is the study of patterns and correlates of disease onset and course in human populations. Psychiatric epidemiology includes studies of the prevalence of psychiatric disorders (i.e., how many people have specific disorders), the distribution of disorders among subgroups of populations, the relationship of a particular disorder to other disorders, and factors that affect the onset and course of a disorder.[1–5] In this chapter, we review current information on: (a) the frequency of exposure to traumatic events, (b) the prevalence of post-traumatic stress disorder (PTSD), (c) the comorbidity of PTSD with other mental and physical health problems, and (d) factors suspected to affect risk for exposure to traumatic experiences and for PTSD.

Epidemiologic research has documented that most people experience a potentially traumatic event at least once in their lives. Natural disasters, such as earthquakes, hurricanes and cyclones, floods, and tornadoes, cause traumatic stress on a massive scale worldwide. Green[6] cited a report by the International Federation of Red Cross and Red Crescent Societies that attests to the frequency, mortality and morbidity of natural and technological disasters globally. From 1967 to 1991, a total of 7766 disasters were reported throughout the world, killing over 7 million people and adversely affecting many times more.[6] In a single year, 1998, natural disasters killed more than 50 000 people throughout the world and destroyed US$65 billion worth of property and infrastructure.[7] Although natural disasters cause devastation in both high- and low-income countries, some 95% of disaster-related deaths in 1999 occurred in developing countries, where the poorest of the poor are the worst affected.[7]

Human-caused disasters also affect the lives of millions of people. For example, Zwi[8] listed 127 wars and more than *twenty million* war-related deaths in the world since World War II. Orner[9] reviewed the history of armed conflicts involving European countries since 1918 and counted over 60 instances of war between countries, civil wars, episodes of terrorism, or military interventions. Orner[9] noted that although there are no reliable estimates of the numbers of civilians and combatants directly or indirectly affected by these armed conflicts, the prevalence of war-related stressors is likely to be extremely high. The lethality and destruction of natural disasters and human-caused catastrophies in developed and developing countries suggests that PTSD among the general population is a major public health concern.

Research suggests that the traumatic effects of wars and disasters are not necessarily limited to those who directly experience these stressors. A recent epidemiologic study of adults in the United States has shown that the trauma most frequently reported as the precipitating event for PTSD was the unexpected death of a loved one.[10]

Epidemiologic studies have shown that some people will experience multiple traumatic events over their lifetime. Moreover, at least within the United States, research indicates that many of these experiences involve violence, specifically interpersonal violence, occurring outside the context of wars or natural disasters. In the National Comorbidity Study (NCS), the first nationally representative general population survey to assess traumatic stressor exposure and PTSD, 60.7% of men and 51.2% of women reported exposure to one or more potentially traumatic events.[11] Nearly twenty percent 19.7%) of the men and 11.4% of the women who participated in the NCS reported three or more potential traumas. Findings from a national survey of exposure to crime among adult women in the United States indicated that 12.7% reported a completed rape, 14.3% reported molestation or attempted sexual assaults, 10.3% had been physically assaulted, 13.4% reported the death of a close friend or relative by homicide, and 35.6% reported that at some time in their life they had been the victim of any type of crime.[12] Among women exposed to some type of crime, more than half (51.8%) reported that they had experienced more than one type of crime or multiple episodes of the same type of crime. The prospective epidemiologic research of Breslau et al[13] has provided evidence that past exposure to traumatic events confers increased risk for future exposure to such experiences.

Epidemiologic studies in the United States generally find higher rates of PTSD in women than in men.[11,14,15] These findings for PTSD are consistent with sex differences reported for other anxiety disorders and major depression.[16] This gender difference does not appear to be due to higher overall rates of exposure to potentially traumatic stressors among women. Data from community surveys in fact indicate that men are more likely than women to be exposed to potentially traumatic events.

At the same time, the types of traumatic events men and women experience may differ. For example in the NCS,[11] women were more likely than men to report having experienced rape, sexual molestation, and childhood physical abuse. Men were more likely to report witnessing death or injury, being involved in a natural disaster or life-threatening accident, physical attack, and combat exposure. Differences in the types of traumas men and women are exposed to may partially account for gender differences in rates of PTSD.

A recent epidemiological study, however, reported that the overall conditional risk of PTSD (that is, probability of PTSD among respondents exposed to a trauma) was approximately twofold higher in women than men, even after statistically adjusting for gender differences in the distribution of trauma types.[17] Note that these findings do not rule out the possibility that gender differences in the characteristics of stressors experienced within trauma type may contribute to higher rates of PTSD observed among women.

Exposure to trauma is also associated with age and a number of contextual risk factors, such as social deprivation, low education, urban residence, personality traits, childhood behaviour problems, family history of psychiatric and substance use problems, and preexisting major depression.[13–15,18,19] Breslau et al[14] found that 39% of a sample of urban young adults (21–30 years of age) had been exposed to traumatic events during their lifetimes. At 3- and 5-year follow-ups, the cumulative incidence of exposure to traumatic events increased for the overall sample.[13,20]

The prevalence of exposure to traumatic events has also been examined in samples of adolescents and young adults. A longitudinal study of adolescents and young adults recruited from publicly funded schools in the southeastern United States found that 15% of young persons 16–22 years of age reported exposure to at least one potentially traumatic event during their lifetime.[21] A study of 18-year-olds from a predominantly working-class community in the northeastern United States found that 43% experienced a potentially traumatic event during their lifetimes.[22] Witnessing injury to or death of others, hearing news of another's sudden death or accident, and personally experiencing a sudden injury or accident were the most commonly reported potentially traumatic experiences, with prevalences of 13%, 13%, and 10%, respectively. Physical assaults were reported by 7% of the sample, while more females (4%) than males (less than 1%) reported ever having been raped.

Epidemiologic studies have also shown that risk factors explain a significant amount of the variability in children's exposure to traumatic experiences. Empirically identified risk factors for abuse of children, for example, include younger age, female gender, and contextual variables such as the extent of the child's social isolation, and substance abuse and emotional problems in the child's family.[23] The likelihood of exposure to child abuse also appears to increase with the number of such risk factors. A survey of 644 18-year-old youths found that the prevalence of child maltreatment increased from 3% when no risk factors were present to 24% when four or more risk factors were present.[24]

Prevalence of PTSD

Estimates of the lifetime prevalence of PTSD from surveys of the general adult population have ranged from 1.0% to 12.3%. Using data from two sites in the Epidemiologic Catchment Area (ECA) program, Helzer et al[19] reported a lifetime PTSD prevalence of 1.0% among adults in the St Louis metropolitan area, and Davidson et al[25] estimated that 1.3% of adults in the Piedmont Region of North Carolina met diagnostic criteria for PTSD. In the NCS, lifetime prevalence of PTSD was 7.8% and current (30-day) prevalence was 2.3%.[11] Breslau and colleagues[10] have estimated the conditional risk of PTSD following exposure to any traumatic stressor as defined by the fourth edition of the *Diagnostic and Statistical Manual of Mental Disorders* (DSM-IV) at 9.2%. A number of factors have been postulated to account for the variations in PTSD prevalence estimates in these and other studies including differences in (a) diagnostic criteria, (b) the measurement approach used to ascertain exposure and assess PTSD, and (c) the demographic characteristics and representativeness of the study populations.[11]

Resnick et al[12] examined PTSD prevalence rates associated with different types of extreme events in a nationally representative community sample of women. The overall prevalence of PTSD was 12.3% lifetime and 4.6% within the past 6 months (current). Prevalence of lifetime and current PTSD varied by type of traumatic event. Women who reported interpersonal violence (physical or sexual assault, homicide of a close friend or relative) were more likely to meet criteria for lifetime (25.8%) and current (9.4%) PTSD than women who reported other stressors only (9.7% lifetime; 3.4% current). Norris[26] examined rates of PTSD in a community sample of 1000 men and women residing in four metropolitan areas in the southeastern United States. Respondents were asked if they had ever experienced an event in any of eight categories of potentially traumatic events: (1) robbery, (2) physical assault, (3) sexual assault, (4) tragic death, (5) motor vehicle crash, (6) combat, (7) fire, or (8) other disaster. Rates of current PTSD varied by type of exposure, and were highest for sexual assault (14%), physical assault (13%), and motor vehicle accident (12%).

Epidemiologic studies of PTSD have often assessed at-risk groups of survivors of specific types of traumas, such as veterans of armed conflicts;[27,28] internally displaced persons and refugees;[29] victims of a range of criminal acts, including sexual assault,[30] terrorist attacks,[31,32] and torture.[33] The prevalence of PTSD has been widely studied among American veterans of the Vietnam War. Findings from the 1989 National Vietnam Veterans Readjustment Study (NVVRS) indicated that 15.2% of men and 8.5% of women who served in Vietnam met criteria for diagnoses of current PTSD at the time of the study interviews.[18] By contrast, the current prevalence among a matched sample of military veterans who did not serve in Vietnam was 2.5% among men and 1.1% among women; for nonveterans, prevalence was 1.2% among men and 0.3% among women. Lifetime PTSD prevalence rates among Vietnam veterans were 30.9% for men and 26.9% for women. Findings from several major studies of PTSD in Vietnam veterans are quite consistent with these.[27,28] The PTSD prevalence estimates of the majority of studies lie within the 95% confidence interval of the NVVRS estimates (13.0–17.4%).

The prevalence of PTSD associated with forms of interpersonal violence other than combat has also been well studied. Kilpatrick and colleagues[34] assessed exposure to crime and PTSD symptoms in a community sample of women. Findings indicated that about three-quarters of the women had been exposed to criminal events, with 7.5% meeting criteria for current PTSD. Winfield and associates[35] analysed data from the North Carolina site of the ECA study and found that 7% of the women aged 18–44 had a history of sexual assault. A history of sexual assault was found to be a risk factor for a variety of psychiatric disorders, including PTSD. Current PTSD prevalence among those with a history of sexual assault was estimated to be 3.7% compared to less than 1% for those with no such history.

Epidemiologic studies assessing PTSD have also been conducted in the aftermath of a number of disasters including floods, earthquakes, tornadoes, and hurricanes or cyclones. For example, Green and her colleagues[36,37] have studied survivors of the Buffalo Creek dam collapse. This team reported that, 14 years after this event, 28% of the sample followed up longitudinally met the criteria for current PTSD. This represented a decrease from the 44% current prevalence estimated at 2 years post-exposure. In a similar vein, Smith et al[38] reported findings concerning the sequelae of an event in which a plane crashed into a hotel. From a sample of 46 hotel employees, only some ($n = 17$) of whom were at the site at the time of the crash, it was estimated that 29% of those on-site and 17% of those off-site developed PTSD following the event.

A report by Shore and colleagues[39] addressed PTSD in the population exposed to the Mount St Helens (MSH) volcanic eruption, as well as a control group that was unexposed to the effects of this natural disaster. Base lifetime prevalence rates were 3.6% in the MSH group and 2.6% in the control group. A study by McFarlane[40] assessed PTSD among a sample of 315 firefighters of an Australian brush fire. Prevalence rates of 32%, 27%, and 30% were obtained at 4, 11, and 29 months post-exposure, respectively.

The examples just described are from a maturing literature on PTSD prevalence that includes studies of the psychological impact of radiation leaks at Three-Mile Island[41] and Chernobyl,[42,43] earthquakes,[44] hurricanes and cyclones,[45,46] fires,[47] airplane crashes[48] and chronic exposure to community violence,[49] to name but a few. Clearly, the existing literature demonstrates that a variety of traumatic experiences precipitate PTSD reactions in at least a portion of exposed individuals.

Comorbidity of PTSD and other disorders

In psychiatric epidemiology, comorbidity generally refers to the simultaneous occurrence of two or more mental disorders in one individual.[50] Both clinical and community studies have demonstrated that most people who have PTSD meet the criteria for at least one other psychiatric disorder as well. In the St Louis ECA study,[19] almost 80% of persons with PTSD had a previous or concurrent psychiatric disorder, compared to about one-third of respondents with no post-traumatic stress symptoms. In the North Carolina ECA study,[25] 62% of individuals with PTSD had a lifetime comorbidity of a psychiatric illness as compared to only 15% of individuals who did not receive a PTSD diagnosis.

Similarly, in the study by Breslau et al[14] of urban young adults, 83% of persons with lifetime PTSD had at least one other lifetime psychiatric disorder. In the NCS, Kessler et al[11] reported that 79% of the women and 88% of the men with lifetime PTSD also met criteria for another lifetime psychiatric disorder. In contrast, 46% of women and 55% of men with disorders other than PTSD were found to have comorbid psychiatric disorders. The disorders most prevalent for men with lifetime PTSD were alcohol abuse or dependence (51.9%), major depressive episode (47.9%), conduct disorder (43.3%), and drug abuse and dependence (34.5%). The disorders most comorbid with lifetime PTSD among women were major depressive episode (48.5%), simple phobia (29.0%), social phobia (28.4%), and alcohol abuse/dependence (27.9%).

High lifetime prevalence of comorbid psychiatric disorders has also been found in studies of PTSD among individuals experiencing a specific type of trauma. In the NVVRS, Kulka et al[18] found that virtually all Vietnam veterans with PTSD met with the criteria for one or more other lifetime psychiatric disorders (including substance abuse). Three-quarters still met criteria for a co-occurring psychiatric disorder at some time during their lives even if alcohol disorders were excluded, and half were characterized by a current comorbid disorder. In men, the most prevalent comorbid disorders were alcohol abuse or dependence (75% lifetime, 20% current), generalized anxiety disorder (44% lifetime, 20% current), and major depression (20% lifetime, 16% current). Among women, the most frequently occurring were major depression (42% lifetime, 23% current), generalized anxiety disorder (38% lifetime, 20% current), and dysthymic disorder (33% lifetime).

McFarlane and Papay[51] investigated the comorbidity of PTSD, other anxiety disorders, and affective disorders in a community sample of firefighters, 42 months after exposure to a natural disaster. Among firefighters with PTSD, co-occuring major depressive disorder was assessed in 51%, generalized anxiety disorder in 39%, panic disorder in 33%, obsessive-compulsive disorder in 13%, and manic episode in 8%.

Epidemiologic studies[11,52–54] have also examined the temporal order of PTSD in relation to other disorders that are highly comorbid with PTSD. Kessler and colleagues[11] reported that PTSD was a primary disorder, in terms of having an earlier onset than all other comorbid disorders. In a sample of women, preexisting anxiety and PTSD were associated with increased risk for first-episode onset of major depression and alcohol abuse and dependence.[52] A history of PTSD has also been found to be associated with an increased risk of subsequent drug abuse and dependence[53] and subsequent symptoms of somatization disorder.[54]

There is a growing body of research describing the long-term effects of trauma exposure and PTSD on physical health and utilization of medical services. PTSD has been associated with more medical complaints, poorer health status, more visits to specialty mental health clinics and primary care physicians, greater functional impairment, and higher rates of cardiovascular, neurological, gastrointestinal and other explained and unexplained physical symptoms.[11,18,55–57] For example, in the NVVRS, Kulka et al[18] found that Vietnam veterans with PTSD reported more health problems and rated their health more poorly than did Vietnam-era veteran or nonveteran controls. Shalev and colleagues[57] found that Israeli veterans with PTSD reported more somatic symptoms than did matched controls, but that groups did not differ on laboratory test findings. This study and others have also shown a greater frequency of adverse health practices (for example, smoking, alcohol use) among persons with PTSD.[58]

Research has only begun to examine how exposure to trauma and PTSD relate to health care utilization, with initial reports indicating that PTSD is associated with increased use of mental health services. For example, the NVVRS found that male Vietnam veterans with PTSD reported more lifetime and current use of Veterans Administration (VA) health care services for physical and mental health problems than era veterans without PTSD.[18] Turning to studies that have focused on women in the general population, severely victimized women have been found to make physician visits twice as frequently as and have outpatient costs that are 2.5 times greater than those of nonvictims.[59] Similarly, Walker and colleagues[60] found that women with a history of childhood abuse and neglect had higher annual health care costs than women without such histories. Those women who reported histories of sexual abuse had median annual health care costs that were US$245 greater than those who reported no abuse, as well as having more emergency department visits.

Risk factors for PTSD

Epidemiologic studies are empirical sources of information about risk factors for PTSD: variables that are believed to be related to the probability of an individual developing this disorder. A number of studies have examined risk factors and predictors of PTSD in community samples and among individuals exposed to traumatic stressors. Suspected risk factors for PTSD among persons exposed to trauma include female gender, previous exposure to trauma including childhood abuse, neuroticism and preexisting anxiety or major depression.[11,14,17–19] For example, Kessler and colleagues[11] found that the lifetime prevalence of PTSD is highest among women, the previously married, and persons of lower socioeconomic status. Another study found that the probability of PTSD among those exposed to a trauma was approximately twofold higher in women than men, adjusting for gender differences in the distribution of trauma types.[17]

Research indicates that the characteristics or severity of the stressor can also influence risk for developing PTSD. In the North Carolina ECA study,[35] the prevalence of PTSD in victims of sexual assault who were physically injured during the assault (14.1%) was 22 times higher than the prevalence of PTSD in noninjured victims of sexual assault (0.64%). In studying those exposed to the Mount St Helens (MSH) eruption, Shore et al[61] found a strong dose–response relationship between proximity to the mountain and the contribution of exposure. The MSH study showed that the three MSH stress-related disorders (of which PTSD was one) increased in frequency with the victim's proximity to the eruption. First-year postdisaster onset rates of MSH stress-related disorders for males were 0.9%, 2.5%, and 11.1% in nonexposed controls, low-exposure populations, and high-exposure populations, respectively. Onset rates for females in these groups were 1.9%, 5.6%, and 20.9%, respectively. In his study of Australian firefighters, McFarlane[40,62] found that the relative contribution of background versus exposure factors changed over time, with the contributions of the stressor seeming to diminish progressively.

Risk factors for PTSD have been most frequently studied among military veterans. A number of these studies have separated risk factors into premilitary, military, and postmilitary factors.[18,63,64] Identified risk factors that predate military service include positive family history of psychiatric disorder and other types of family instability;[18,65] emotional or psychological disorder as a youth, such as enuresis[66] or conduct disorder/antisocial behavior;[18] previous trauma history, including sexual or physical abuse during childhood;[67,68] and immaturity at time of entry into armed conflict.[18] There is evidence[69] that poorer intellectual ability or a compromised neurodevelopmental history constitutes a neurocognitive risk factor for PTSD.

Among war-related factors, variables such as enlisted rank, having been drafted/conscripted into the military (versus volunteering), and receiving wounds in action have been shown to increase risk for PTSD.[18,19] Specific dimensions of war stressor exposure that have been found directly to affect PTSD are participation in or witnessing atrocities or abusive violence, perceptions of threat to personal safety, and day-to-day discomforts associated with living in a war zone (such as inadequate food, exposure to extremes of weather).[63,64] Participation in traditional combat activities (for example, firing a weapon, receiving incoming rounds) has an effect on PTSD, though recent research suggests that combat affects PTSD indirectly through perceptions of threat to personal safety.[63,64]

A host of postmilitary factors have been shown to affect PTSD in military veterans. These include social cognitive variables, such as perceived control, attributional style, and coping,[70,71] functional and structural social support variables including homecoming experiences, and stressful life events experienced postmilitary.[64,72] Similarly, studies of rape survivors have demonstrated a positive relationship between post-exposure social support and subsequent adjustment. A consistent finding in the literature concerning predictions of post-rape functioning has been the positive association between social support and adjustment, in terms of both immediate impact and latency of recovery.[73]

The bulk of the research evidence to date appears consistent with a model of PTSD that posits a role for pretrauma and post-exposure risk and protective factors (potentially including biological, psychological, and sociocultural factors), in addition to the nature and characteristics of the traumatic experience, per se[63] (Figure 2.1). It remains for further research to identify the specific contributions of factors within each of these major domains, as well as ways in which they may interact.

Conclusions

The relevance of epidemiologic studies lies largely in providing data for developing interventions and public policy planning. The studies discussed in this chapter suggest that PTSD is an important and continuing public health problem. Epidemiologic studies have demonstrated that although many kinds of extreme events can cause PTSD (for example, exposure to combat, criminal victimization, natural disasters), not all of those exposed will develop the disorder. Evidence suggests that exposure to potentially traumatic events may be more common than once thought, and that risk factors for PTSD include personal and biographical histories at the time of exposure to the extreme event, characteristics of the event itself, and characteristics of the post-exposure environment.

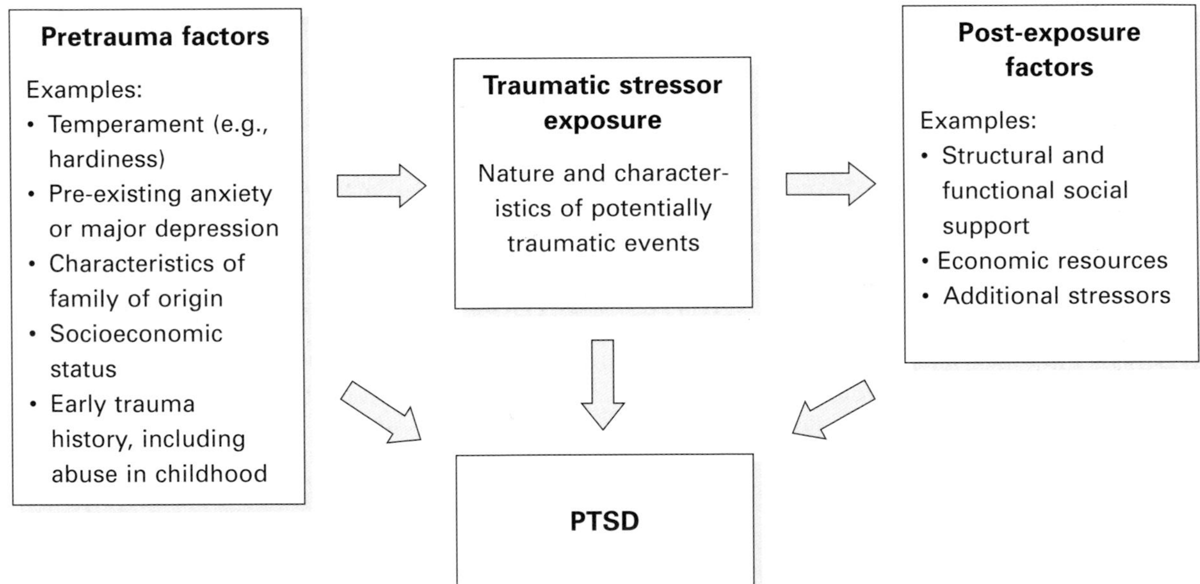

Figure 2.1 Schematic representation of factors postulated to affect the development of post-traumatic stress disorder.

References

1. Friedman GD, *Primer of Epidemiology*, 3rd edn (McGraw Hill: New York, 1987).
2. Kleimbaum DG, Kupper LL, Morganstein H, *Epidemiologic Research: Principles and Quantitative Methods* (Van Nostrand Reinhold: New York, 1982).
3. Mausner JS, Kramer S, *Mausner & Bahn: Epidemiology – and Introductory Text* (WB Saunders: Philadelphia, 1985).
4. Davidson JRT, Fairbank JA, The epidemiology of posttraumatic stress disorder. In: Davidson JRT, Foa EB, eds, *Posttraumatic Stress Disorder. DSM-IV and Beyond* (American Psychiatric Press: Washington, DC, 1993).
5. Fairbank JA, Schlenger WE, Saigh PA, Davidson JRT, An epidemiological profile of posttraumatic stress disorder: prevalence, comorbidity, and risk factors. In: Friedman MJ, Charney DS, Deutch AY, eds, *Neurobiological and Clinical Consequences of Stress: From Normal Adaptation to PTSD* (Lippincott-Raven: Philadelphia, 1995).
6 Green BL, Traumatic stress and disaster: mental health effects and factors influencing adaptation. In: Davidson JRT, McFarlane AC, eds, *International Review of Psychiatry*, vol 2, in press.
7. World Bank, Reducing 'preventable' costs of natural disasters vital for developing countries. World Bank News Release No. 2000/18915, February 2000.
8. Zwi AB, Militarism, militarization, health, and the third world, *Medicine and War* (1991) 7:262–8.
9. Orner RJ, Post-traumatic stress disorders and European war veterans, *Br J Clin Psychol* (1992) 31:387–403.
10. Breslau N, Kessler RC, Chilcoat HD et al, Traumatic and posttraumatic stress disorder in the community: the 1996 Detroit Area Survey of Trauma, *Arch Gen Psychiatry* (1998) **55**:626–31.
11. Kessler RC, Sonnega A, Bromet E et al, Posttraumatic stress disorder in the National Comorbidity Survey, *Arch Gen Psychiatry* (1995) **52**:1048–60.
12. Resnick HS, Kilpatrick DG, Dansky BS et al, Prevalence of civilian trauma and posttraumatic stress disorder in a representative national sample of women, *J Consult Clin Psychol* (1993) **61**:948–91.
13. Breslau N, Davis GC, Andreski P, Risk factors for PTSD-related traumatic events: a prospective analysis, *Am J Psychiatry* (1995) **152**:529–35.
14. Breslau N, Davis GC, Andreski P, Peterson EL, Traumatic events and posttraumatic stress disorder in an urban population of young adults, *Arch Gen Psychiatry* (1991) **48**:216–22.
15. Breslau N, Davis GC, Posttraumatic stress disorder in an urban population of young adults: risk factors for chronicity, *Am J Psychiatry* (1992) **149**:671–5.
16. Green BL, Traumatic stress and disaster: mental health effects and factors influencing adaptation. In Mak FL, Nadelsdon C, eds, *International Review of Psychiatry, Vol 2* (American Psychiatric Press: Washington, DC, 1996) 177–210.
17. Breslau N, Chilcoat HD, Kessler RC et al, Vulnerability to assaultive violence: further specification of the sex difference in post-traumatic stress disorder, *Psychol Med* (1995) **29**:813–21.
18. Kulka RA, Schlenger WE, Fairbank JA et al, *Trauma and the Vietnam War Generation: Report of Findings from the National Vietnam Veterans Readjustment Study* (Brunner/Mazel: New York, 1990).
19. Helzer JE, Robins LN, McEvoy L, Posttraumatic stress disorder in the general population: findings of the Epidemiologic Catchment Area survey, *N Engl J Med* (1987) **317**:1630–4.
20. Breslau N, Davis GC, Andreski P et al, Sex differences in the posttraumatic stress disorder, *Arch Gen Psychiatry* (1997) **54**:1044–8.
21. Cuffe SP, Addy CL, Garrison CZ et al, Prevalence of PTSD in a community sample of older adolescents, *J Am Acad Child Adolesc Psychiatry* (1998) **37**:147–54.
22. Giaconia RM, Reinherz HZ, Silverman AB et al, Traumas and posttraumatic stress disorder in a community population of older adolescents, *J Am Acad Child Adolesc Psychiatry* (1995) **34**:1369–80.
23. Leventhal JM, Epidemiology of sexual abuse of children: old problems, new directions, *Child Abuse Negl* (1998) **22**:481–91.
24. Brown J, Cohen P, Johnson JG, Salzinger S, A longitudinal analysis of risk factors for child maltreatment: findings of a 17-year prospective study of officially recorded and self-reported child abuse and neglect, *Child Abuse Negl* (1998) **22**:1065–78.
25. Davidson JRT, Hughes D, Blazer DG, George L K, Posttraumatic stress disorder in the community: an epidemiological study, *Psychol Med* (1991) **21**:713–21.

26. Norris FH, Epidemiology of trauma: frequency and impact of different potentially traumatic events on different demographic groups, *J Consult Clin Psychol* (1992) **60**:409–18.
27. Goldberg J, True WR, Eisen SA, Henderson WC, A twin study of the effects of the Vietnam War on posttraumatic stress disorder, *JAMA* (1990) **263**:1227–32.
28. Snow BR, Stellman JM, Stellman SD, Sommer JF, Posttraumatic stress disorder among American Legionnaires in relation to combat experience in Vietnam: associated and contributing factors, *Environ Res* (1988) **48**:175–92.
29. Steel Z, Silove DM, Bird K, Pathways from war trauma to posttraumatic stress symptoms among Tamil asylum seekers, refugees, and immigrants, *J Trauma Stress* (1999) **12**:421–35.
30. Saunders BE, Kilpatrick DG, Hanson RF et al, Prevalence, case characteristics, and long-term psychological correlates of child rape among women: a national survey, *Child Maltreatment* (1999) **4**:187–200.
31. Abenhaim L, Dab W, Salmi L, Study of civilian victims of terrorist attacks, *J Clin Epidemiol* (1992) **45**:103–9.
32. North CS, Nixon SJ, Shariat S et al, Psychiatric disorders among survivors of the Oklahoma City bombing, *JAMA* (1999) **282**:755–62.
33. Basoglu M, Mineka S, Parker M et al, Psychological preparedness for trauma as a protective factor in survivors of torture, *Psychol Med* (1997) **27**:1421–33.
34. Kilpatrick DG, Saunders BE, Veronen LJ et al, Criminal victimization: lifetime prevalence, reporting to police, and psychological impact, *Crime & Delinquency* (1987) **33**:479–89.
35. Winfield I, George LK, Swartz M, Blazer DG, Sexual assault and psychiatric disorders among a community sample of women, *Am J Psychiatry* (1990) **147**:335–41.
36. Green BL, Lindy JD, Grace MC et al, Buffalo Creek survivors in the second decade: stability of stress symptoms, *Am J Orthopsychiatry* (1990) **60**:43–54.
37. Green BL, Grace MC, Lindy JD et al, Buffalo Creek survivors in the second decade: comparison with unexposed and nonlitigant groups, *J Appl Soc Psychol* (1990) **20**:1033–50.
38. Smith EM, North CS, McCool RE, Shea JM, Acute postdisaster psychiatric disorders: identification of persons at risk, *Am J Psychiatry* (1990) **147**:202–6.
39. Shore JH, Vollmer WM, Tatum EL, Community patterns of posttraumatic stress disorders, *J Nerv Ment Dis* (1989) **177**:681–5.
40. McFarlane AC, The aetiology of post-traumatic morbidity: predisposing, precipitating and perpetuating factors, *Br J Psych* (1989) **154**:221–8.
41. Bromet EJ, Parkinson DK, Schulberg HC et al, Mental health of residents near the Three Mile Island reactor: a comparative study of selected groups, *J Prev Psych* (1982) **1**:225–76.
42. Cwikel J, Abdelgani A, Goldsmith JR et al, Two-year follow-up study of stress-related disorders among immigrants to Israel from the Chernobyl area, *Environ Health Perspect* (1997) **105**:1545–50.
43. Havenaar JM, Rumyantzeva GM, Van den Brink W et al, Long-term mental health effects of the Chernobyl disaster: an epidemiological survey of two former Soviet regions, *Am J Psychiatry* (1997) **154**:1605–7.
44. Fukuda S, Morimoto K, Mure K, Maruyama S, Posttraumatic stress and change in lifestyle among the Hanshin-Awaji earthquake victims, *Prev Med* (1999) **29**:147–51.
45. Garrison CZ, Bryant ES, Addy CL et al, Post-traumatic stress disorder in adolescents after Hurricane Andrew, *J Am Acad Child Adolesc Psychiatry* (1995) **34**:1193–201.
46. La Greca AM, Silverman WK, Wasserstein SB, Children's predisaster functioning as a predictor of posttraumatic stress following Hurricane Andrew, *J Consult Clin Psychol* (1998) **66**:883–92.
47. Green BL, Grace MC, Lindy JD et al, Levels of functional impairment following a civilian disaster: the Beverly Hills supper club fire, *J Consult Clin Psychol* (1983) **51**:573–80.
48. Brooks N, McKinlay W, Mental health consequences of the Lockerbie disaster, *J Trauma Stress* (1992) **5**:527–43.
49. Fitzpatrick KM, Boldizar JP, The prevalence and consequences of exposure to violence among African-American youth, *J Am Acad Child Adolesc Psychiatry* (1993) **32**:424–30.
50. Michels R, Marzuk PM, Progress in psychiatry, *N Engl J Med* (1993) **329**:628–38.
51. McFarlane AC, Papay P, Multiple diagnoses in posttraumatic stress disorder in the victims of a natural disaster, *J Nerv Ment Dis* (1992) **180**:498–504.

52. Breslau N, Davis GC, Peterson EL, Schultz LR, Psychiatric sequelae of posttraumatic stress disorder in women, *Arch Gen Psychiatry* (1997) 54:81–7.
53. Chilcoat HD, Breslau N, Posttraumatic stress disorder and drug disorders: testing causal pathways, *Arch Gen Psychiatry* (1998) 55:913–17.
54. Andreski P, Chilcoat HD, Breslau N, Posttraumatic stress disorder and somatization symptoms: a prospective study, *Psychiatry Res* (1998) 79:131–8.
55. Boscarino JA, Chang J, Electrocardiogram abnormalities among men with stress-related psychiatric disorders: implications for coronary heart disease and clinical research, *Ann Behav Med* (1999) 21:227–34.
56. Long N, Chamberlain K, Vincent C, The health and mental health of New Zealand Vietnam war veterans with postraumatic stress disorder, *N Z Med J* (1992) **105**:417–19.
57. Shalev A, Bleich A, Ursano RJ, Posttraumatic stress disorder: somatic comorbidity and effort tolerance, *Psychosomatics* (1990) **31**:197–203.
58. Beckham J, Kirby AC, Feldman ME et al, Prevalence and correlates of heavy smoking in Vietnam veterans with chronic posttraumatic stress disorder, *Addict Behav* (1997) 22:637–47.
59. Koss MP, Koss PG, Woodruff WJ, Deleterious effects of criminal victimization on women's health and medical utilization, *Arch Intern Med* (1991) 151:342–7.
60. Walker EA, Unutzer J, Rutter C et al, Costs of health care use by women HMO members with history of childhood abuse and neglect, *Arch Gen Psychiatry* (1999) 56:609–13.
61. Shore JH, Tatum E, Vollmer WM, Psychiatric reactions to disaster: the Mt. St. Helen's experience, *Am J Psychiatry* (1986) **143**:590–5.
62. McFarlane AC, The longitudinal course of post traumatic morbidity, *J Nerv Ment Dis* (1988) 176:30–9.
63. King DW, King LA, Foy DW et al, Posttraumatic stress disorder in a national sample of female and male Vietnam veterans: risk factors, war-zone stressors, and resilience-recovery variables, *J Abnorm Psychol* (1999) **108**:164–70.
64. King LA, King DW, Fairbank JA, Resilience-recovery factors in post-traumatic stress disorder among female and male Vietnam veterans: hardiness, postwar social support, and additional stressful life events, *J Pers Soc Psychol: Personality Processes and Individual Differences* (1998) 74:420–34.
65. Fontana A, Rosenheck R, Posttraumatic stress disorder among Vietnam theater veterans: a causal model of etiology in a community sample, *J Nerv Ment Dis* (1994) **182**:677–84.
66. Gurvits TV, Lasko NB, Schachter SC et al, Neurological status of Vietnam veterans with chronic posttraumatic stress disorder, *J Neuropsychiatry Clin Neurosci* (1993) **150**:183–8.
67. Engel CC, Engel AL, Campbell SJ et al, Posttraumatic stress disorder symptoms and precombat sexual and physical abuse in Desert Storm veterans, *J Nerv Ment Dis* (1993) **181**:683–8.
68. Fontana A, Schwartz LS, Rosenheck R, Posttrauamtic stress disorder among female Vietnam veterans: a causal model of etiology, *Am J Public Health* (1997) **87**:169–75.
69. Gurvits TV, Gilbertson MW, Lasko NB et al, Neurological soft signs in chronic posttraumatic stress disorder, *Arch Gen Psychiatry* (2000) 57:181–6.
70. Solomon Z, Benbenishty R, Mikulincer M, The contribution of wartime, pre-war, and post-war factors to self-efficacy: a longitudinal study of combat stress reaction, *J Traumatic Stress* (1991) 4:345–61.
71. Solomon Z, Mikulincer M, Benbenishty R, Locus of control and combat-related post-traumatic stress disorder: the intervening role of battle intensity, threat appraisal, and coping, *Br J Clin Psychol* (1989) **28**:131–44.
72. Vincent C, Long N, Chamberlain K, Relation of military service variables to posttrauamtic stress disorder in New Zealand war veterans, *Mil Med* (1994) **159**:322–6.
73. Atkeson BM, Calhoun KS, Resnick PA, Ellis EM, Victims of rape: repeated assessment of depressive symptoms, *J Consult Clin Psychol* (1982) **50**:96–102.

3

Diagnostic dilemmas in assessing post-traumatic stress disorder

Berthold PR Gersons

Introduction

The introduction of the DSM-III,[1] ICD-10[2] and DSM-IV[3] has helped psychiatrists to become more precise in assessing psychiatric disorders. In DSM-III post-traumatic stress disorder (PTSD) has been introduced for the first time in psychiatry as a coherent profile of signs and symptoms related to the experience of a traumatic incident. Large epidemiological studies have contributed to the validity of this disorder.[4,5] In the assessment of PTSD two flaws can however interfere with the correct establishing of the diagnosis of PTSD. The first flaw is that people do not talk easily about their traumatic experiences and doctors do not like to hear the terrible details. So much of the accuracy of the psychiatric interview concerning trauma depends on the skill to establish a trustful relationship with the patient and the acceptance of the need to listen to horrifying details. Also the patient is often unaware of any relationship between the symptoms of PTSD and the experience of the trauma. As we know in psychiatry the accuracy of the information which we get in the interview strongly depends on our willingness to listen. A non-judgemental attitude in the interview is a necessary prerequisite. The second flaw in assessing PTSD is the overwhelming affect that accompanies the report of someone who experienced trauma. For the listener, therefore, it sometimes seems self evident that traumatic experiences must result in some kind of disorder, especially PTSD. Asking about symptoms after listening to the details of a traumatic incident can look like an unneeded burden. Here the epidemiology of PTSD[4,5] has helped us enormously to understand the limited relationship between the experience of trauma and the development of PTSD. A minority of trauma victims develop PTSD.

Before starting treatment it is essential first to assess the diagnosis of PTSD. After treatment assessment is again necessary to evaluate the effectiveness of the intervention. Here we also see a dilemma. For patients it is often already very satisfactory to have experienced the intense emotions related to the trauma in the trusted setting with the therapist. The patient rarely judges the result of the treatment by evaluating the disappearance of symptoms. For the therapist the cathartic experience by the patient is often taken as proof of a well-established working-through of the traumatic experience. Also therapists do not always evaluate the treatment in a more objective fashion. Studies of debriefing after traumatic experiences, for instance, have shown a high satisfaction by the debriefed ones and by the debriefers themselves,[6–9] despite those who were debriefed showing higher symptom profiles in the follow-up compared to the non-debriefed (see Chapter 8). Important for the assessment of PTSD, therefore, is the precise assessment of symptoms. It also helps the patient to understand that he or she is not only suffering from traumatic experiences but also from symptoms resulting from the experience as well.

The assessment skills for PTSD consist of the skills to assess trauma in all its gruesome details and to assess symptoms which may be the result of the incident(s). In this chapter we will first pay attention to the assessment of trauma and its dilemmas. After this we will continue with the symptoms of PTSD. There are specific structured interviews and self-report instruments developed for the assessment of PTSD. These will be mentioned but not presented in detail. There are also other techniques to help to establish the diagnosis of PTSD using psychophysiological measures, neuroimaging and neurohormonal measures. These techniques will not be discussed here. Then we will discuss the issue of the trauma spectrum disorders and comorbidity in PTSD.

Dilemmas in the assessment of trauma

In DSM-IV[1†] diagnostic criteria for PTSD trauma are described as follows:

The person has been exposed to a traumatic event in which both of the following were present:

(1) the person experienced, witnessed, or was confronted with an event or events that involved actual or threatened death or serious injury, or a threat to the physical integrity of self or others
(2) the person's response involved intense fear, helplessness, or horror.

From the definition follows the distinction between the actual traumatic event and the person's reaction.

Traumatic event

The definition does not describe exactly what a traumatic event means. There are characteristics concerning the actual role of the person involved in the event:

- The person must be exposed to an event.
- The person must survive the event.
- The event can be an experience of the person him- or herself.
- The event can be an experience of others in which the person is a witness.

The conditions which result from the definition, for instance, suggest the following examples. A person who has been a victim of an automobile accident and who lost consciousness for the incident itself did not consciously experience the traumatic incident.

†Because DSM-IV favours a more precise description of symptoms compared to ICD-10 we will quote from the DSM-IV definition of PTSD.

However, when the person later on, for instance in the hospital, hears her husband died in the incident and as was the case in our hospital also experiences her leg is broken, she has to cope with two traumatic events following the incident. This is important to understand because the re-experience symptoms of the event can only evolve when someone consciously went through the incident. Another example was a police officer who could not work because of illness on a specific day. In her place another officer was killed in the police car. She developed symptoms quite similar to PTSD and she tried to reconstruct the event. She felt guilty because she thought she should have been the one to be killed and not her fellow police officer. This assessment of the actual involvement in the incident is important in treatment when this implies imaginal exposure. It is another question if such exposure can be helpful in such situations, but the nature of re-experiencing is essentially different. For the assessment it is important to analyse very precisely the actual involvement in the traumatic situation with the patient.

In the DSM-IV definition of trauma the examples mentioned are:

- actual death;
- threatened death;
- serious injury;
- threat to the physical integrity of self;
- threat to the physical integrity of others.

These events can become traumatic for the person who experienced, witnessed or was confronted with the event. From our police studies[10,11] we therefore made the distinction between *threatening* and *depressive* experiences. The threatening ones are those incidents in which one is the victim. The depressive experiences are those events in which one witnesses the traumatic incident. This distinction is important because it makes the traumatic experience very different. In a threatening experience one's fight–flight stress responses are activated to reach safety. This is important for instance for survivors of fires, robberies and rapes. But in the same instances those who were not threatened become overwhelmed by the helplessness of seeing others get hurt or die. Here also the fight–flight responses can become activated but more to flee from the horrible experience and from the intense feeling of helplessness. An 18-year-old girl witnessed a robbery in daylight. Her office manager asked her to accompany her to put a cassette with the money of the day into the deposit box of the bank. The box was located outside the bank. When they approached the bank one of the two boys put a gun on the head of the office manager. She gave the cassette to boy and the boys disappeared in the crowd. The girl was not threatened at all by the boys who actually did not take notice of her. But she witnessed the threat and later on started to get re-experiences of this scene. She was not at all used to such events. Ursano et al[12] for instance wrote about the risk factor for emergency workers, in that they seem to be more at risk of developing PTSD when the corpses resemble their family or children. The confrontation with death and destruction is in itself a frequent experience for rescue workers but when they associate the victims with those closest to them the traumatic experience can result in PTSD. Here we are reminded of an aspect of the definition of the stressor criterion mentioned in the DSM-IIIR description of PTSD: . . . an event outside the range of usual human experience and that would be markedly distressing to almost anyone . . . This criterion has been abandoned in DSM-IV because the stressors as we know from epidemiology were much more common human experiences than thought before. However, it is still important because one usual experience can make the difference.

By focusing in the definition on (threatening) death or on injury, too much attention is sometimes only paid to the result of some act. In fact, in the re-experiencing, the result of the act not only returns to mind, like a dead body, also do the details of the actual happenings themselves. A man survived an air crash in which the plane crashed on the runway because of a storm. This was accompanied by an enormous noise, the plane turned round and the walls of the cabin started to crumble which resulted in one of the stewardesses falling over him. The air crash in itself is of course a traumatic event. But the traumatic experiences, which can come back as symptoms in PTSD, are these specific aspects of the threatening happening. In this case, for instance, the trembling of the plane, the noise of the crash, the falling down of the stewardess and the view of a crumbling cabin became the traumatic details.

Violent behaviour of someone else can become the reminder of the incident. Here also specific moments are often re-experienced. This is also meant by the adjective 'serious' to injury. Here the threat is the most important aspect of the event. An important aspect of an incident is often that it is unexpected. A person driving came along an accident. He saw a tractor with a white stick behind it. A moment later he found out it was someone's leg where the flesh had been stripped off. The adjunctive 'serious' in usual medical language is used for the critical condition of the victim. To make a critical incident into a traumatic experience the unexpected unwelcome details are usually essential. For instance, someone tried by resuscitation to keep an old man alive. However, under the pressure of his act the rescuer broke the ribs of the person. In the re-experiencing he relives the noise of the moment the ribs broke.

The person's reaction: intense fear, helplessness and horror

In contrast to DSM-III it is not only the experience of a traumatic event that is necessary for the diagnosis but also the response of intense fear, helplessness and horror. For instance, a threat to one's own physical integrity will specifically give these intense reactions. This is the case with rape, sexual abuse in childhood and with torture. Rape is always accompanied by threat and some kind of violence. Here also the reminders give a clue to the traumatic aspects of the experience, such as the use of a knife or the threat 'I will kill you if you tell anyone else'. Fear also plays an important role in the aftermath of the event. Shame is often not mentioned for all traumatic events but is usually very strongly felt in the three types of event. Here the assessment skills are important. Questioning about the trauma not only involves facts but also extreme emotions. The traumatized person often tries to suppress the intense emotional reminders. The victim also protects the interviewer from being confronted with the repulsive details and the extreme emotions. For instance, a woman who was raped by a group of youngsters had a lot of difficulties telling all the terrible details of the experience. There had been moments when one of the boys had put the gun into her vagina and other moments when he put it to her head. It is extremely difficult to tell these horrid details and they are also very difficult to listen to. These elements are most important in treatment, so for the patient it is important that the therapist will listen without hesitation to these details. So one has to ask questions like:

- Did you feel fear?
- What were the most frightening experiences?

- Did you feel helpless?
- At which moments did you feel most helpless?
- Did you feel horror?
- At which moments did you feel most horror?
- Do you feel ashamed to tell these things?

Abuse in childhood is also often connected with violence and neglect and here shame and helplessness play an important role in the traumatization of the person. A special issue in the assessment of sexual traumas is the need for the patient to trust the therapist. This is, of course, not self-evident. Judith Herman[13] calls our attention to a 'stabilization phase' in which the person can test the therapist about the safeness of the treatment situation. It must be realized that the assessment phase can be complicated by the need for safeness. The traumatized person not only suffers from the events but also from the disappearance of trust in other human beings. This is also the case with torture victims. The consulting room, which feels safe to other trauma victims, can all too greatly resemble the torture room in that it is disconnected from the outside world. Basoglu et al[14] has paid attention to the development of psychological preparedness for torture. This can be repeated in the therapist's consulting room.

Horror is another emotion which is often difficult to describe. An example of horror is the following: In 1992 in Amsterdam a plane crashed on a neighbourhood.[15] This caused a fire as high as the apartment buildings that were struck by the plane. 'Eyewitnesses' not only experienced this unbelievable scene but also heard the shouting and crying of burning people, some of them jumping off the balconies. Such extreme emotions are characteristic for traumatic experiences. Fear is often recollected as 'I felt the adrenaline flow through my body'. One remembers fear as a somatic experience of increased heartbeat, trembling of the legs, being rooted to the ground and unable to speak, having cold hands, etc.

For the therapist there are risks in connection with listening to the events and especially being confronted with the extreme emotions. This is called 'secondary traumatization' or 'vicarious traumatization'.[16] It is well known in psychiatry that it is essential for a good interview that an empathic, understanding relationship with the patient is developed. The patient will only tell his or her story and detail symptoms when he or she can trust the therapist. The attitude, therefore, must be a listening and accepting one as such attitudes stimulate the patient to continue to tell. But with trauma histories this is much more complicated. The patient is afraid the interviewer will not take the story and the complaints seriously, or is afraid because of the gruesome details. For instance, after listening to the story of burning people jumping from the balconies the therapist can start dreaming about it. Treatment of a survivor of a plane crash can make the therapist fearful of flying. Secondary traumatization refers to a sort of 'infectious' effect of listening to trauma stories. One feels saddened and helpless, and traumatic details can cause the interviewer to develop nightmares of such incidents. Thus PTSD can endanger the mental health of the interviewer. It is therefore advised to limit the number of trauma patients one has to interview or to treat. Also supervision is very highly recommended when working with trauma patients.

Symptom assessment

Even in the assessment of the traumatic event a lot of elements of symptoms are encompassed. The symptom profile of PTSD has been divided into three sections:

- re-experiencing symptoms;
- avoidance symptoms;
- hyperarousal symptoms.

In the interview a person often realizes that the re-experience symptoms are related to the traumatic event so they are more easily reported. The other two groups of symptoms are less well known to the sufferer and therefore less connected to the experience of the event. A clear problem in DSM-IV when asking about the different symptoms is the lack of frequency or intensity measures. In the structured interviews for PTSD this is mostly better defined.

Re-experience symptoms

These are:

> B. The traumatic event is persistently reexperienced in one (or more) of the following ways:
>
> (1) recurrent and intrusive distressing recollections of the event, including images, thoughts, or perceptions;
> (2) recurrent distressing dreams of the event;
> (3) acting or feeling as if the traumatic event were recurring (includes a sense of reliving the experience, illusions, hallucinations, and dissociative flashback episodes, including those that occur on awakening or when intoxicated);
> (4) intense psychological distress at exposure to internal or external cues that symbolize or resemble an aspect of the traumatic event;
> (5) physiological reactivity on exposure to internal or external cues that symbolize or resemble an aspect of the traumatic event.

In the re-experience symptoms there are some important characteristics:

- the person involved does not have control over the occurrence of the symptoms;
- the re-experience is a perceptional one which resembles actual experience;
- the perceptional quality of the remembrance is essentially different from telling a story.

By 'persistent' is meant that nearly every week such a symptom occurs. Quite typical is the recurrent nature of the symptoms. Mostly, specific episodes of the traumatic scene come back again and again. At moments of rest like before sleep when someone is most relaxed the person can be taken by surprise in reliving and seeing the terrible happening. They also come back in dreams. For instance, the partner may report that the bedclothes were wet and disordered or the person was talking and gesticulating during sleep. The reactions to cues that symbolize or resemble an aspect of the traumatic event are characteristic. Someone who survived an air crash ducks every time a plane crosses the sky. After a rape by a coloured person a woman feels frightened every time she sees a coloured person, even though she knows there is no real danger. Every element of the traumatic incident – sound, colour, scene, etc. – can act as the trigger of the conditioned fear response, which is accompanied by some kind of reminder or reliving. The physiological reactivity means that the confrontation with cues results in increased heartbeat, transpiration, feeling cold, trembling and so on.

Avoidance symptoms

These are:

> C. Persistent avoidance of stimuli associated with the trauma and numbing of general responsiveness (not present before the trauma), as indicated by three (or more) of the following:
>
> (1) efforts to avoid thoughts, feelings, or conversations associated with the trauma;
> (2) efforts to avoid activities, places, or people that arouse recollections of the trauma;
> (3) inability to recall an important aspect of the trauma;
> (4) markedly diminished interest or participation in significant activities;
> (5) feeling detachment or estrangement from others;
> (6) restricted range of affect (e.g., unable to have love feelings);
> (7) sense of a foreshortened future (e.g., does not expect to have career, marriage, children, or a normal life span).

Here two kinds of reaction are described: actual avoidance or numbing of general responsiveness. These symptoms strongly relate to the general stress response of fight and flight. The numbing also seems related to a third kind of response, which is known from animals: acting as if one were dead. In the interview one has to ask quite actively about avoidance behaviour. Often the person is so used to the avoidance that it is not perceived as an active strategy. In fact many of the normal activities before the traumatic events may not be taking place any more. Certain neighbourhoods will no longer be visited any more. Those who suffered war and camps avoid the scenes of endless streams of refugees on television. So in assessing avoidance symptoms one has to understand that the traumatic cue brings back the perceptual memories of the trauma. Also the intense pain, grief and helplessness are felt again; it feels like 'an open wound', a wound which will never completely close. Also fear is intense again and behind it extreme feelings of aggression are often hiding. The avoidance can also involve (like in C1) social withdrawal. Here the question: 'Do others perceive you as being changed after the incident?' helps. The answer is often: 'Yes, I was always actively involved but now I do not like to go out.' An example of how complicated this can be is the following. An officer who shot a person was complimented after returning to the police station. He was seen as a hero. However he felt terrible because he did not want to kill anybody. He felt guilty notwithstanding the rightness of the act in the terrible situation. He realized his colleagues had no idea about how dreadful he felt. They could not understand his withdrawal and in a certain way they did not like to see their hero withdrawn.

For the assessment of the inability to recall an important aspect of the trauma one has to investigate the traumatic incident very carefully. The traumatized person is not always aware of this symptom. A woman survived a killing in daylight while sitting with friends outside a café. She could only remember seeing a group of men coming near and then she remembered being in hospital crying. She was not hurt herself, but the actual traumatic moment was lost because of dissociation. Another well-known aspect of the remembering of traumatic incidents is the fact that the person feels very convinced of the details of the happening. For instance, I treated three people who survived the same crash. Their stories of the actual happening were very different with regard to details, and they felt threatened after being faced with the probability that their memory was not totally accurate. In the face of danger one must rely on only a few cues, which activates the stress response. From the work of Le Doux[17] we know our brains work to perceive these threatening cues which activate our fight–flight behaviour. Certain details are not taken into consideration or are lost. This is also meant by what is called 'tunnel vision'. The perception is restricted to endangering elements.

The symptoms listed under C4–7 overlap strongly with symptoms of depression. The interest in initiating activities or participation in something can be lost. The normal world from before has lost its safeness and can also seem less important. Here we see that the appreciation of the world, of what is important, can have changed tremendously. A United Nations military officer went to Bosnia to identify the corpses of killed inhabitants. In 1 month he saw remains of three hundred bodies in devastating surroundings of burned and destroyed houses. Before in his homeland he was an active participant in local activities in the area where he was living with his family. After this month he felt everything was unimportant. He also felt detached from his partner and even his children, which is a terrible feeling. In treatment it became clear that behind this was the feeling that he was unable as a father to safeguard their lives and he internally rehearsed the loss. Also this symptom of detachment is difficult to express because the person involved feels very guilty about it. The restricted range of affect also becomes clear from the fact the 'shine' of normal experience has been lost. The sense of a foreshortened future relates to the loss of control over one's life and over the lives one feels responsible for.

Hyperarousal symptoms

These are:

> D. Persistent symptoms of increased arousal (not present before the trauma), as indicated by two (or more) of the following:
>
> (1) difficulty falling or staying asleep;
> (2) irritability or outburst of anger;
> (3) difficulty concentrating;
> (4) hypervigilance;
> (5) exaggerated startle response.

These symptoms are more easily assessed. The sleeping problem can relate to the fear of the traumatic incident happening again. After the air crash in Amsterdam we saw people who could only sleep with the light on as well as the television set. Here the stimuli came in place of the increased need to scan the environment for endangering cues. Also awaking after 2 hours is common, as it seems dangerous not to be awake. To have no control over one's reactions becomes clear in the symptom of irritability or outbursts of anger. A shopkeeper was robbed under the threat of a gun just before closing time. He developed PTSD. One of the symptoms was his hypervigilance. He was afraid the robbery would happen again, and had much difficulty in being patient with his clients. His normal humour had faded away, so people no longer liked to visit his cheese shop. At home he showed irritability towards his wife and children. He changed, as partners often tell us happens. Children suffer because of the irritability of their parents. One can easily understand this irritability; the traumatized person seems to be constantly distinguishing dangerous stimuli from 'unimportant' stimuli. This is, in fact, the description of hypervigilance. One sees this in their behaviour also.

The person will take the chair in which the back is against the wall, so no one can get behind. A person who had been attacked very violently constantly slowed down when cycling because he feared the people cycling behind him. Also normal stimuli like the closing of a door can startle the person extremely. Difficulty in concentrating also relates to this 'scanning behaviour'. When danger is involved there is no difficulty; on the contrary, the person can be very active and remembers all kinds of details. But after reading two pages of a book he or she will forget the contents and have to start all over again. When going to a shop to buy food there is the risk of forgetting: the person needs to write a list at home before going to the shop.

The hyperarousal symptoms are quite disruptive. Normal relations and everyday activities become disordered. We see the person involved cope with it in less adaptive ways by avoidance and withdrawal.

Dissociative symptoms

Apart from the symptoms B3 'dissociative flashback episodes' and C3 'inability to recall an important aspect of the trauma' dissociative symptoms are not very well specified in the DSM-IV description of PTSD. Spiegel and others[18] have argued that PTSD should be seen as a disorder of memory. From this viewpoint more symptoms than the two mentioned above can be seen as distortion of normal memory functions like encoding, storage and retrieval of traumatic memories. Bremner and Marmar[19] have argued that dissociation should be seen as the main mechanism in the development of PTSD. An example is the lack of emotion experienced in remembering traumatic events. Without such accompanying emotions the incident, according to the definition, is not a traumatic one. Here we have the problem that such emotions can have been split off by dissociation, so the person remembers the incident but cannot remember the intense emotions. A specific accompanying symptom is often depersonalization or derealization, which are dissociative symptoms. It is well known that the traumatic incident can be forgotten especially from sexual child abuse. This is part of a major debate because some accuse therapists of 'implanting' such memories (as in false memory syndrome). One has to be very careful not to suggest such experiences, but one cannot ignore them. Especially when there is amnesia for long periods in childhood the possibility of childhood trauma must be seriously considered.

Marmar et al[20] has described a set of specific dissociative features of the traumatic experience which are quite common. These symptoms are called 'peritraumatic dissociation'. These symptoms are part of the traumatic experience of a person and they come back in the remembering of the event. For instance, a traumatic situation feels like 'endless' in time, while it is mostly a short moment. Also the incident can be experienced as 'a slow motion' scene in which sound can change or even be absent. Peritraumatic dissociation describes the changes in perception, especially in the time–space relation. A police officer who was sitting in his car shot through the windscreen at a man who took a woman hostage. The windscreen fell apart in a thousand particles. He, however, experienced it as a very slow falling down of the particles as if they were drops. It sounded like 'Christmas bells'. The traumatic value of an incident can therefore change the perception. The changes can have regard to time, sound or place but the experience can also be perceived as unreal or as though it were not really happening.

Structured instruments

Structured interviews and self-report instruments have the advantage of requiring fewer clinical skills. They also make the validity of assessment between groups better. Many instruments have been developed for epidemiological purposes and for research on PTSD. The oldest one, is the Impact of Events Scale (IES) of Horowitz et al.[21] It is often used because it gives a fine presentation of the re-experiencing and avoidance characteristics. However, it was developed long before the formulation of PTSD in DSM-III and IV, and hyperarousal symptoms are not part of this scale. IES is therefore not helpful for diagnosing PTSD, but the revised version is better for that purpose (IES-R). The Structured Clinical Interview for DSM-IV[22] is also available with a PTSD part. In research the Clinician Administered PTSD Scale for DSM-IV (CAPS-DX) is often used.[23] For epidemiological research with trained lay interviewers (not clinicians) the Composite International Diagnostic Interview[24] is available for PTSD assessment. Recently, Breslau et al[25] reported on a seven-item symptom list to discover PTSD in the community. Self-report instruments have been used in research and are sometimes recommended for use in clinical practice. These are the Davidson Trauma Scale (DTS),[26] the Self-rating Scale for PTSD (SRS-PTSD),[27] the Self-rating Inventory for Posttraumatic Stress Disorder (SID)[28] and the Posttraumatic Diagnostic Scale (PDS).[29] Most of the self-report instruments have been developed for special trauma populations, such as Vietnam veterans (CAPS), police and disaster victims,[28] and for rape victims.[29] There are no reports available about the usefulness in clinical practice, or comparative studies of the different instruments.

Trauma spectrum and comorbidity

In the ICD-10 classification[2] it is noted that PTSD is often accompanied by anxiety, depression or even obsessive-compulsive disorder. The consequence is that when a patient comes for assessment one should not only focus on PTSD as a result of the traumatic experience. Comorbidity of PTSD with other disorders, including the dissociative ones, is quite common. Therefore, some have argued for a so-called trauma spectrum of disorders.[30–32] Also PTSD can become complicated by addiction. *Acute stress disorder* (ASD) was recognized in DSM-IV.[3] There is also much interest in subthreshold manifestations of PTSD symptoms described as *partial PTSD*.[33] Herman[34] and van der Kolk et al[35] have pleaded for adding *complex PTSD* to DSM-IV. Much attention has been given to a partial relationship between the borderline personality disorder and early trauma. Complex PTSD has been developed to describe the long-term effect of PTSD on the personality.

In future research it will be necessary to pay more attention to trauma spectrum disorders. In the meantime clinicians should not stop short at assessment of PTSD alone.

Conclusion

In the assessment of the diagnosis of PTSD many dilemmas have been mentioned. Psychiatrists are mostly familiar with the difficulty of assessing psychotic symptoms, for example. Such skills are part of the professional expertise because for other doctors such assessment would prove extremely difficult. Disorders like PTSD which are related to traumatic events can on first acquaintance seem easier to assess. The classification in DSM and ICD has helped psychiatry tremendously by improving the reliability of the diagnosis of the different disorders. However, behind the short descriptions, definitions and sentences is concealed much clinical expertise and research which have made it possible to be much more precise in the assessment of PTSD. A special aspect of the skills for assessing PTSD is the impact of the horrible stories forming the basis for the diagnosis. It is important to understand that the patient often does not want to share the terrible experiences with the therapist, sometimes out of a desire to protect the therapist from the unpleasant details and with extreme emotions. For the clinician it is therefore necessary to realize what knowledge and skills are required to enable an assessment of PTSD. The risk of secondary traumatization has to be taken very seriously. Those who argue for seeing PTSD as a dissociative disorder help us to understand the symptoms from the view of a memory disorder. The use of structured instruments and self-rating inventories can be helpful, but as yet it is not known to what extent.

References

1. American Psychiatric Association, *Diagnostic and Statistical Manual of Mental Disorders*, 3rd edn (APA: Washington, DC, 1980).
2. World Health Organization, *The ICD-10 Classification of Mental and Behavioural Disorders; Clinical Descriptions and the Diagnostic Guidelines* (WHO: Geneva, 1992).
3. American Psychiatric Association, *Diagnostic and Statistical Manual of Mental Disorders*, 4th edn (APA: Washington, DC, 1994).
4. Kessler RC, Sonnega A, Bromet E, Nelson CB, Posttraumatic stress disorder in the national comorbidity survey, *Arch Gen Psychiatry* (1995) 52:1058–60.
5. Breslau N, Kessler RC, Chilcoat HD et al, Trauma and posttraumatic stress disorder in the community; the 1996 Detroit area survey of trauma, *Arch Gen Psychiatry* (1998) 55:626–32.
6. Kenardy JA, Webster RA, Lewin TJ et al, Stress debriefing and patterns of recovery following a natural disaster, *J Trauma Stress* (1996) 9:37–50.
7. Bisson JI, Jenkins PL, Psychological debriefing for victims of acute burn trauma, *Br J Psychiatry* (1997) 171:583.
8. Bisson JI, Jenkins PL, Alexander J, Bannister C, Randomized controlled trial of psychological debriefing for victims of acute burn trauma, *Br J Psychiatry* (1997) 171:78–81.
9. Carlier IVE, Van Uchelen JJ, Lamberts RD, Gersons BPR, Disaster-related posttraumatic stress in police officers; a field study of the impact of debriefing, *Stress Medicine* (1998) 14:143–8.
10. Carlier IVE, Gersons BPR, Partial PTSD; the issue of psychological scars and the occurrence of the PTSD symptoms, *J Nerv Ment Dis* (1995) 183:107–9.
11. Carlier IVE, Lamberts RD, Gersons BPR, Risk factors for posttraumatic stress symptomatology in police officers, *J Nerv Ment Dis* (1994) 185:4989–506.
12. Ursano RJ, Fullerton CS, Vance K, Kao TC, Posttraumatic stress disorder and identification in disaster workers, *Am J Psychiatry* (1999) 156:353–9.
13. Herman J, *Trauma and Recovery; the Aftermath of Violence – from Domestic Abuse to Political Terror* (Basic Books: 1992).
14. Basoglu M, Mineka S, Paker M et al, Psychological preparedness for trauma as a protective factor in survivors of torture, *Psychol Med* (1997) 27:1421–33.
15. Carlier IVE, Gersons BPR, Stress reaction in disaster victims following the Bijlmermeer plane crash, *J Trauma Stress* (1997) 10:329–35.
16. Figley CR, Compassion fatigue as secondary stress disorder: an overview. In: Figley CR, ed, *Compassion Fatigue: Secondary Traumatic Stress Disorder in Treating the Traumatized* (Brunner/Mazel: New York, 1995) 1–20.

17. LeDoux J, *The Emotional Brain. The Mysterious Underpinnings of Emotional Life* (Simon & Schuster: New York, 1996).
18. Butler LD, Spiegel D, Trauma and memory, Washington, Review of Psychiatry vol. 16, II-13–53.
19. Bremner JD, Marmar, CR, *Trauma, Memory, and Dissociation* (American Psychiatric Press: Washington, DC, 1998).
20. Marmar CR, Weiss DS, Schlengen WE et al, Peritraumatic dissociation and posttraumatic stress in male Vietnam theater veterans, *Am J Psychiatry* (1994) **151**:902–7.
21. Horowitz MJ, Wilner N, Alvarez W, Impact of event scale: a measure of subjective stress, *Psychosom Med* (1979) 41:209–18.
22. Spitzer RL, Williams JBW, Gibbon M, Structured Clinical Interview for DSM-III-R, Version NP-V. Biometrics Research Department, New York State Psychiatric Institute.
23. Blake D, Weathers F, Nagy D, A clinician administered PTSD scale for assessing current and lifetime PTSD: the CAPS-I, *Behav Ther* (1990) **18**:187–8.
24. Kessler RC, Andrews G, Mroczek D et al, The World Health Organization Composite International Diagnostic Interview Short-Form (CIDI-SF), *Int J Methods in Psychiatry Res* (1998) 7:171–85.
25. Breslau N, Peterson EL, Kessler RC, Schultz LR, Short screening scale for DSM-IV posttraumatic stress disorder, *Am J Psychiatry* (1999) **156**:908–11.
26. Davidson JR, Book SW, Colket JT et al, Assessment of a new self-rating scale for posttraumatic stress disorder, *Psychol Med* (1997) **27**:153–60.
27. Carlier IVE, Lamberts RD, Van Uchelen JJ, Gersons BPR, Clinical utility of a brief diagnostic test for posttraumatic stress disorder, *Psychosom Med* (1998) **60**:42–7.
28. Hovens JE, Van der Ploeg HM, Bramsen I et al, The development of the Self-Rating Inventory for Posttraumatic Stress Disorder, *Acta Psychiatr Scand* (1994) **90**:172–83.
29. Foa EB, Hearst-Ikeda D, Perry KJ, Evaluation of a brief cognitive-behavioral program for the prevention of chronic PTSD in recent assault victims, *J Consult Clin Psychol* (1995) **63**:948–55.
30. Bremner JD, Editorial: acute and chronic responses to psychological trauma: where do we go from here? *Am J Psychiatry* (1999) **156**:349–51.
31. Horowitz MJ, *Stress-Response Syndromes*, 2nd edn (Jason Aronson: Northvale, NJ, 1986).
32. Van der Kolk BA, McFarlane AC, Weiseath L, eds, *Traumatic Stress: the Effects of Overwhelming Experience on Mind, Body, and Society* (Guilford: New York, 1996).
33. Carlier IVE, Gersons BPR, Partial posttraumatic stress disorder (PTSD): the issue of psychological scars and the occurrence of PTSD symptoms, *J Nerv Men Dis* (1995) **183**:107–9.
34. Herman JL, Sequelae of prolonged and repeated trauma: evidence for a complex posttraumatic syndrome (DESNOS). In: Davidson JRT, Foa EB, eds, *Posttraumatic Stress Disorder: DSM-IV and Beyond* (American Psychiatric Press: Washington, DC, 1993).
35. Van der Kolk BA, McFarlane AC, Weiseath L, eds, *Traumatic Stress: the Effects of Overwhelming Experience on Mind, Body, and Society* (Guilford: New York, 1996).

4

Human brain-imaging and post-traumatic stress disorder

Andrea L Malizia and David Nutt

The study of post-traumatic stress disorder (PTSD) using imaging techniques offers a number of unique opportunities to investigate human brain function and its pathology. First, the disorder is by definition precipitated by an unusually intense stressor which is out of keeping with normal day-to-day experiences and which results in long-term brain changes. Since this powerful aetiological factor can be modelled by analogy in experimental animals with some of the standard behavioural pharmacology tests, this disorder provides a unique opportunity to examine neurochemical similarities and differences of response to stress between experimental animals and man. Secondly, three populations of sufferers can be delineated: patients who experience the trauma early on in life as in childhood sexual abuse, patients who experience the trauma in adult life but who have a previous axis I or axis II disorder and, finally, patients who experience trauma in adult life and who have no personal or family history of significant psychopathology. The separation of these groups of patients is important in that it may provide experimental data about the influence of premorbid factors on the neurochemistry and functional anatomy of pathological reactions to stress. Thirdly, PTSD is an anxiety disorder which is characterized by core anxiety symptoms and signs as well as distinctive additional features such as intrusive memories, flashbacks, dissociative experiences and anaesthesia. Hence the comparison of PTSD with other anxiety syndromes may help to define the core networks involved in pathological anxiety.

Human imaging has progressed considerably in the past decade and can be used to address some of the questions related to human brain anatomy, physiology, neurochemistry and pharmacology in vivo. This chapter reviews the studies that have made use of either magnetic resonance or emission tomography to investigate brain structure or function in PTSD. Clinical electrophysiology will not be reviewed here.

What are the effects of PTSD on brain anatomy?

PTSD is a condition which by definition occurs after an unusually severe stressful event. Acute stress is known to result in a physiological response which is mediated in part by ascending monoaminergic systems (noradrenaline, dopamine and serotonin) in the short term and by the hypothalamic–pituitary–adrenal (HPA) axis in the longer term whereby stress results in increased glucocorticoid (GC) concentration in plasma and brain. Recently, much attention has been devoted to the noxious effects of increased GC on neurons,[1] particularly in the hippocampus where it is thought that persistently high GC concentrations induce reversible atrophy of the dendritic spines (see Chapter 5). This process is followed by neurotoxicity where, over the course of months, high GC concentrations kill hippocampal neurons. These observations lead to the conclusion that prolonged periods of stress, leading to increased GC concentration, result in hippocampal atrophy in man, a theory supported by findings in depression (which is accompanied by HPA axis abnormalities in many patients), where atrophy is correlated with total period of illness.[2]

In PTSD severe stress is experienced repeatedly over a period of months, first because of the incident itself and then through the re-experience of the traumatic events which causes considerable distress. It should therefore follow that a reduction in hippocampal volume should be observed in patients with this condition and that the greatest damage should be seen in patients with the longest history of PTSD. Four magnetic resonance imaging (MRI) studies of PTSD patients have been performed and the results are shown in Table 4.1. These four studies have used volumetric MRI with manual segmentation of the hippocampus. Each study had a different criterion for definition of the hippocampus, since some investigators prefer to measure a clearly defined portion (for example, middle) rather than increasing noise by including areas with poor boundary definition.

On the whole, all studies report a decrease in hippocampal volume which is small except for Gurvits et al.[3] However, a firm conclusion from these studies is made difficult by the usual problem of the unlikely reporting in the literature of small negative studies. In addition, as in all PTSD studies, interpretation is made more difficult by considerable clinical methodological problems such as psychiatric comorbidity and substance and alcohol abuse. Some of these magnetic resonance investigations attempted to minimize these problems by careful matching and the use of multiple linear regression, but the direct effect of these factors cannot be categorically excluded. Finally, imaging confounds such as cohort sequence in scanning (that is, patients' group and controls' group being scanned at different times) can cause artefact which would result in the reported differences. This can be due to scanner drift, producing a significant bias in the grey values of the image. This potential problem is only reported in one paper[3] but should be explicitly excluded.

Despite the above limitations, the consistent reported picture is of reduced hippocampal volume in patients with PTSD which may be associated with clinically important variables such as severity of exposure, severity of dissociation or Wechsler memory score (see Table 4.1).

The observation of mild hippocampal atrophy is supported by the only published magnetic resonance spectroscopy (MRS) study.[4] This study shows significantly reduced NAA/Cr (*N*-acetylaspartate/creatinine) proton

Table 4.1 Studies of hippocampal and cortical volume in post-traumatic stress disorder (PTSD)

Author and method	PTSD patient group	Controls	Left hippocampus	Right hippocampus	Other
Bremner et al 1995[5] Volumetric MRI	Veterans (n=26) males	Healthy volunteers (n=22) Males Matched on many parameters	4% smaller (NS)	8% smaller (p=0.03)	Right hippocampal volume correlates to Wechsler Verbal Memory Score.
Bremner et al 1997[6] Volumetric MRI	Child abuse (n=17) 12 males	Healthy volunteers (n=17) Males Matched on many parameters	12% smaller (p=0.008)	5% smaller (NS)	Larger left temporal lobe and trend for larger amygdala in PTSD.
Gurvits et al 1996[3] Volumetric MRI	Veterans (n=7) males	Non-PTSD veterans (n=7) Healthy vols (n=8) Matched on many parameters Males	28% smaller (p<0.001)	30% smaller (p<0.001)	Subarachnoid space increased in all veterans. Total hippocampal volume decrease correlates to combat exposure.
Stein et al 1997[7] Volumetric MRI	Child sexual abuse (n=21) females	Healthy vols (n=21) Female Matched for age and education	5% smaller (p<0.05)	3% smaller (NS)	Left hippocampus volume decrease correlates to severity of dissociation.

MRI, magnetic resonance imaging; NS, not significant.

MRS ratios (an index of neuronal damage) in the right medial temporal lobe, and significant reduction in Cho/Cr (choline/creatinine) ratios (possibly an index of white matter damage) in the left medial temporal lobe in 21 veterans with PTSD compared with eight control veterans.

What is the significance and mechanism of hippocampal damage in PTSD?

The significance of a decrease in hippocampal volume is difficult to interpret as it may be a predisposing factor to developing PTSD rather than a consequence of the trauma. If mild hippocampal atrophy is a predisposing factor, then it may be possible to devise screening procedures to prevent vulnerable individuals from coming into contact with severe stressors as part of their jobs. The finding would be of great significance for biological psychiatry as it would link predisposition to psychological vulnerability to trauma.

If, however, the hippocampal changes are secondary to the trauma, it would be important to determine the mediating factor. This is unlikely to be a plain increase in GC as PTSD patients have been demonstrated to have normal or low cortisol levels in the blood and a hyperresponsive pituitary.[8] A case can be made that GC receptor sensitivity precipitates neuronal death (see Chapter 5) and in this case hippocampal neurons in PTSD would have hypersensitive GC receptors. It is difficult, however, to reconcile this concept with the human depression findings without invoking the contribution of other possible mediating factors (for example, noradrenaline release[9]).

This area merits further close scrutiny, and a study of structural brain scans in trauma victims in the immediate aftermath of the accident should help resolve the question.

Lateralization of hippocampal damage and PTSD

The evidence so far suggests that if lateralization is indeed present, then patients with adult-onset PTSD have smaller right hippocampi and patients with childhood-onset PTSD have smaller left hippocampi. It is likely that lateralization is an artefact of the small sample sizes. However, if these data were to be robustly replicated, the implication would be that patients with PTSD from childhood experiences or PTSD from adult trauma have smaller hippocampi in brain side by condition interaction where adult PTSD relates to right atrophy and childhood PTSD to left atrophy. The mechanism for this effect would have to be related either to predisposition before the traumatic event or to differences in brain connectivity between the adults and children.

Which areas of the brain are involved in symptom experience in PTSD?

The emergence of brain imaging techniques has allowed the investigation of the anatomical substrate for the experience of PTSD symptoms. These studies usually involve the subtraction of relative regional blood flow between a resting or control condition and an activation condition congruent with the trauma. In many of the PTSD studies appropriate controls were also included in order to ascertain whether the changes in brain metabolism were specific to PTSD patients or a general response to highly arousing stimuli.

The psychiatry imaging group at Massachusetts General Hospital in Boston has performed the most comprehensive set of studies (Table 4.2) using $C^{15}O_2$ positron emission tomography. With this technique the inhaled CO_2 changes into positron emitter labelled water in the lung and is then distributed via the circulation in the body. The partition of water between circulation and brain tissue is very close to 1 and therefore the recorded brain counts represent a map of relative blood flow in the brain during the experimental condition of interest. Only a limited number of scans can be performed with this technique because of the radioactive

Table 4.2 $C^{15}O_2$ PET post-traumatic stress disorder (PTSD) activation studies – the Boston series

Study	Patients	Controls	Comparison	Anterior temporal	Orbito-frontal	Insula	Cingulate	Hippocampus/ amygdala	Other frontal	Other
Rauch 1996[10]	Mixed (*n*=8) 6 females 2 males	None	Autobiographical scripts Trauma minus neutral	Increase right	Increase right	Increase right	Non= significant increase right	Non-significant increase right	Decrease left inferior	Increases Med temp ctx R visual ctx R sensorimotor ctx B
Shin 1997[11]	Veterans (*n*=7) males	Veterans (*n*=7) males	Perception War scenes minus neutral				PTSD Ant decr Ctrl mid & post increase		PTSD L inf decr Ctrl L inf decr	Ctrl increases Visual Middle frontal Postcentral Superior temporal
			Imagery War scenes minus neutral				PTSD Ant incr			PTSD decrease Inf parie, sup temp Ctrl increase visual, precuneus
			Perception War scenes minus negative				PTSD & Ctrl Post incr	Ctrl Amygdala decreases Parahippocampus increases	PTSD L inf decr	PTSD Precuneus increase Middle temp, supramarginal decreases Ctrl Increase visual
			Imagery War scenes minus negative				Ctrl Anterior increases		PTSD L inf decrease Ctrl Middle & inf increase	PTSD Middle inf temp increases Visual, precuneus decreases
Shin 1999[12]	Childhood sexual abuse (*n*=16) Females	Childhood sexual abuse (*n*=16) Females	Autobiographical scripts Trauma minus neutral	Both groups increase PTSD>Ctrl	Both groups increase PTSD>Ctrl	Ctrl Anterior increase	Ctrl Anterior increase	Larger decrease left parahippocampal gyrus PTSD vs ctrl	PTSD Decrease left inferior	Both groups decrease visual cortices

exposure to the subject, therefore the statistical power is limited.

In all the Boston studies patients were right-handed and had been off medication for at least 2 weeks. A total of 31 patients were studied, one study being completely on childhood sexual abuse victims and one on war veterans. In all the studies the exposure to the trauma-related stimuli (either autobiographical memories or imagery/perception of trauma scenes) produced an increase in emotional cognitions and physiological signs of increased arousal; these changes were far greater in magnitude in PTSD patients than controls.

Two studies employed autobiographical memories to induce emotion. In these studies the resting condition is listening to a script of neutral personal memories while the activated condition consists of listening to a script of memories of the traumatic event. Both studies showed a similar pattern of increased blood flow in the anterior cingulate, orbitofrontal cortex, anterior insula and anterior temporal pole while decreases in blood flow were observed in the left inferior frontal cortex. The anterior cingulate and anterior insula, however, were non-specifically activated by the experience of strongly emotionally laden memories irrespective of PTSD, as the volunteers re-experiencing traumatic events (but who had not developed PTSD) also activated these areas. Comparing PTSD patients with controls, orbitofrontal and anterior temporal activations were greater in PTSD patients but also present in victims who had not developed the disorder, while the left inferior frontal decreases were present only in the PTSD patients.

One of the Boston studies compared the activations produced by perception with imagery of war scenes of either negative or neutral stimuli in war veterans with and without PTSD. The pattern of regional blood flow change differed according to the paradigm employed and the only common pattern which emerged was of cingulate increases (albeit in different loci) and of left inferior frontal decreases.

Four other activation studies contribute to the current knowledge (Table 4.3). One employed a similar strategy to the Boston group by investigating victims of childhood sexual abuse with and without PTSD using autobiographical scripts of trauma minus neutral scripts.[13] This study showed a completely different pattern of regional blood flow change compared with the Boston group. In seemingly common areas the changes differ either by exact location (for example increases in the posterior rather than anterior insula) or by valence (decreases rather than increases in anterior cingulate).

One study documented a failure of parietal activation with an attentional task in PTSD patients when compared with controls.[14] The other two are from the same group. One study set out to test the hypothesis of an increase in medial prefrontal blood flow in PTSD victims when compared with healthy controls or veterans when listening to combat sounds compared with white noise[15] and indeed found such an increase. The other[16] found an increase in anterior cingulate blood flow with exposure to combat sounds irrespective of diagnosis as well as increases in left amygdala and a decrease in retrosplenial cortex particular to patients with PTSD.

The same group also described the changes in brain metabolism in one patient observed during a flashback which occurred by chance during an HMPAO SPECT study.[11] In this paradigm the images obtained by scanning represent the sum of the regional brain blood flow occurring in the first few minutes after injection of the ligand when, having listened to a tape of combat sounds, the subject experienced feeling 'back in Vietnam' and extreme distress. The scan demonstrated an alteration

Table 4.3 Other post-traumatic stress disorder activation studies

Study	Patients	Controls	Comparison	Insula	Cingulate	Hippocampus/ amygdala	Other frontal	Other
Bremner et al 1999[13] $H_2{}^{15}O$ PET	Child sexual abuse (n = 11) Females	Child sexual abuse (n = 11) Females	Autobiographical scripts Trauma minus neutral	Posterior increases PTSD> ctrl	Abuse memories: decreases subcallosal PTSD>ctrl Increases posterior	PTSD>ctrl Decreases R hippocampus	Increases PTSD>ctrl Sup and middle	Increases PTSD>ctrl motor cortex Decreases PTSD>ctrl inferior temporal supramarginal fusiform
Liberzon et al 1999[16] HMPAO-SPECT	War veterans (n = 12) Males	War veterans (n = 11) and healthy volunteers (n = 14)	Combat sounds minus white noise		All groups Increases anterior	PTSD Increases left amygdala		PTSD Decreases retrosplenial cortex
Zubieta et al 1999[15] HMPAO-SPECT	War veterans (n = 14) Males	War veterans (n = 11) and healthy volunteers (n = 14)	Combat sounds minus white noise				Increase medial prefrontal PTSD vs ctrl and veterans	
Semple et al 1996[14] $H_2{}^{15}O$ PET	Mixed + substance abuse (n = 8) Males	Healthy volunteers (n = 8) Males	Continuous performance task minus rest					Failure to activate parietal cortex with attentional task

in perfusion ratio between the thalamus and the cortex so that during the flashback the ratio of thalamic/cortical–basal ganglia metabolism was increased by 15%. This change in corticothalamic ratio could not be explained by changes due to hyperventilation and the authors interpreted it as representing a dissociative change in state of consciousness.

How do brain activations in PTSD compare with each other and with studies in other anxiety conditions?

It may seem from the above that no consistent picture emerges from the imaging studies thus far conducted in PTSD. In particular the total dissonance of two studies which at face value are very similar[12,13] is a cause for concern. Because of the differences in the laboratories, of the detail of the paradigms employed and of the relatively small numbers it is perhaps not surprising that differences are more striking than the similarities. This should not be seen as a failure or as something which is peculiar to human research, as was recently demonstrated by the differences in behavioural observations of genetically identical mice put in ostensibly identical equipment in different laboratories.[18] However, the message is clear: large studies employing comparable techniques in different laboratories are needed in order to generate robust analyses of a generalizable nature. Some testable hypotheses already emerge from the current work:

- Is decreased activity in the left inferior frontal lobe when exposed to emotionally arousing material a marker of PTSD? And, if so, what does this tell us about the neurobiology and psychology of the disorder? To make it clearer – does this represent a difficulty in engaging cortical systems related to language expression?
- The orbitofrontal cortex, anterior cingulate, anterior temporal pole and anterior insula are also activated in other anxiety disorders.[10,19] Does the activation of this represent a nodal circuit at the interface between the cognitive experience of anxiety and the physiological changes which occur with arousal? If so, how does this circuit relate to the other pathological experiences in PTSD?
- Are the decreases in activity in medial temporal lobe structures observed in some of the experiments related to atrophy?
- What are the differences and similarities in activation pattern when the same subject is exposed to different paradigms which produce an increase in cognitive malaise and a modulation of autonomic response?
- Is the finding of altered thalamocortical metabolic ratios reproducible in a large sample of subjects?

A further fundamental question emerges from these studies: what sort of information emerges from 'ecologically valid' studies which aim to observe the whole of the activated network? Would the understanding of the circuits be better served by the study of specific changes in activations generated by well-understood paradigms (such as the emotional Stroop for instance)? In our opinion both kinds of approach are useful. The global activation studies serve the purpose of highlighting the areas implicated in the expression of the clinically relevant psychopathology. The alterations in function of these areas are, however, better understood by the use of well-validated paradigms which test specific neuropsychological functions. Finally, both have to be studied in order to understand the effect of pharmacological manipulations.

Imaging neurochemical changes in PTSD

Alterations of noradrenergic and serotonergic function have been observed in patients with PTSD, possible cholecystokinin B (CCK-B) involvement has been postulated from animal experiments, while, contrary to panic disorder, no observation has been made of benzodiazepine–gamma amino butynic acid–A ($GABA_A$) dysregulation in this disorder. Imaging studies of receptor binding in PTSD are absent, partly because of the absence of relevant ligands.

An alternative strategy to radioligand emission tomography is the observation of changes in regional brain metabolism or blood flow following pharmacological challenge. Only one such study has been reported in the literature to date.[20] This investigation by the Yale group examined the differences in regional metabolic rate after the administration of yohimbine to patients with PTSD and healthy volunteers. The study employed ^{18}FDG PET as the measure of metabolism. FDG is an analogue of deoxyglucose. It accumulates almost irreversibly in tissue after going through the first step of glycolytic metabolism. As such, analysis of ^{18}FDG scans provides a measure of integrated regional metabolic activity over a period of tens of minutes after the injection into the circulation. Yohimbine is an alpha-2 noradrenergic antagonist. As such, it has both presynaptic effects which result in an increase in phasic release of noradrenaline from the presynaptic terminal and a postsynaptic effect in antagonizing the effects of noradrenaline on postsynaptic neuronal activity. The effects of noradrenaline are inhibitory on postsynaptic neurons; however, the metabolic effects depend on the extent of noradrenergic activation. Low levels of noradrenergic release are postulated to increase regional metabolism through an increase in local synaptic work which is responsible for a large proportion of the local metabolic requirements. At higher levels of noradrenergic activity, however, a net decrease in local metabolism is observed. This occurs, presumably, because the reduction in the number of active local interneurons becomes predominant in comparison to the increased synaptic transmission at noradrenergic synapses. Although noradrenergic modulation affects vascular responsivity, this can be corrected for in ^{18}FDG PET and is therefore not a confounding factor.

This study demonstrated that yohimbine generates a global small increase in grey matter metabolism in healthy volunteers, while patients with PTSD respond with a moderate global decrease in grey matter metabolism. These effects were maximal in the orbitofrontal cortex and significant in the prefrontal, parietal and temporal cortices and were accompanied by significant behavioural activation in PTSD patients. The authors interpreted this observation as evidence of increased sensitivity to the noradrenergic releasing properties of yohimbine in PTSD, in line with their previous pharmacological observations in this patient group and consistent with the observation that the alpha-2 agonists clonidine and guanfacine can be of therapeutic value.

Conclusions

PTSD, like other anxiety-related conditions, has been relatively little studied with imaging tools. Yet these are the most powerful way of relating human brain function and chemistry to psychopathology.[21] To date the findings have to be, at best, regarded as pilot data. These are, however, useful in having generated hypotheses which will be testable in larger cohorts. In particular the issues of hippocampal atrophy and decreased blood flow in Broca's area with symptom provocation and alterations in the ratio of thalamic/cortical activity merit further attention. In many respects PTSD is worthy of a major effort in biological psychiatry, as the condition is close to many animal models which have already produced abundant evidence of neurochemical and physiological alterations following repeated stress. The mapping of these to human empirical evidence should be able to produce strong clinical science.

References

1. Sapolsky RM, Why stress is bad for your brain, *Science* (1995) 273:749–50.
2. Sheline YI, Sanghavi M, Mintun MA, Gado MH, Depression duration but not age predicts hippocampal volume loss in medically healthy women with recurrent major depression, *J Neurosci* (1999) 19:5034–43.
3. Gurvits TV, Shenton ME, Hokama H et al, Magnetic resonance imaging study of hippocampal volume in chronic, combat-related posttraumatic stress disorder, *Biol Psychiatry* (1996) 40:1091–9.
4. Freeman TW, Cardwell D, Karson CN, Komoroski RA, In vivo proton magnetic resonance spectroscopy of the medial temporal lobes of subjects with combat-related posttraumatic stress disorder, *Magn Reson Med* (1998) 40:66–71.
5. Bremner JD, Randall P, Scott TM et al, MRI-based measurement of hippocampal volume in patients with combat-related posttraumatic stress disorder, *Am J Psychiatry* (1995) 152:973–81.
6. Bremner JD, Randall P, Vermetten E et al, Magnetic resonance imaging-based measurement of hippocampal volume in posttraumatic stress disorder related to childhood physical and sexual abuse – a preliminary report, *Biol Psychiatry* (1997) 41:23–32.
7. Stein MB, Koverola C, Hanna C et al, Hippocampal volume in women victimized by childhood sexual abuse, *Psychol Med* (1997) 27:951–9.
8. Yehuda R, Levengood RA, Schmeidler J et al, Increased pituitary activation following metyrapone administration in post traumatic stress disorder, *Psychoneuroendocrinology* (1996) 21:1–16.
9. Petty F, Chae Y, Kramer G et al, Learned helplessness sensitizes hippocampal norepinephrine to mild restress, *Biol Psychiatry* (1994) 35:903–8.
10. Rauch SL, van der Kolk BA, Fisler RE et al, A symptom provocation study of posttraumatic stress disorder using positron emission tomography and script-driven imagery, *Arch Gen Psychiatry* (1996) 53:380–7.
11. Shin LM, Kosslyn SM, McNally RJ et al, Visual imagery and perception in posttraumatic stress disorder. A positron emission tomographic investigation, *Arch Gen Psychiatry* (1997) 54:233–41.
12. Shin LM, McNally RJ, Kosslyn SM et al, Regional cerebral blood flow during script-driven imagery in childhood sexual abuse-related PTSD: a PET investigation, *Am J Psychiatry* (1999) 156:575–84.
13. Bremner JD, Narayan M, Staib LH, Southwick SM et al, Neural correlates of memories of childhood sexual abuse in women with and without postraumatic stress disorder. *Am J Psychiatry* (1999) 156:1787–95.
14. Semple WE, Goyer PF, McCormick R et al, Attention and regional cerebral blood flow in posttraumatic stress disorder patients with substance abuse histories, *Psychiatry Res* (1996) 67:17–28.
15. Zubieta JK, Chinitz JA, Lombardi U et al, Medial frontal cortex involvement in PTSD symptoms: a SPECT study, *J Psychiatr Res* (1999) 33:259–64.
16. Liberzon I, Taylor SF, Amdur R et al, Brain activation in PTSD in response to trauma-related stimuli, *Biol Psychiatry* (1999) 45:817–26.
17. Liberzon I, Taylor SF, Fig LM, Koeppe RA, Alteration of corticothalamic perfusion ratios

during a PTSD flashback, *Depression & Anxiety* (1997) 4:146–50.

18. Crabbe JC, Wahlsten D, Dudek BC, Genetics of mouse behavior: interactions with laboratory environment, *Science* (1999) 284:1670–2.
19. Malizia AL, What do imaging studies tell us about anxiety disorders? *J Psychopharmacol* (1999) 13:372–8.
20. Bremner JD, Innis RB, Ng CK et al, Positron emission tomography measurement of cerebral metabolic correlates of yohimbine administration in combat-related posttraumatic stress disorder, *Arch Gen Psychiatry* (1997) 54:246–54.
21. Rauch SL, Savage CR, Alpert NM et al, The functional neuroanatomy of anxiety: a study of three disorders using positron emission tomography and symptom provocation, *Biol Psychiatry* (1997) 42:446–52.

5

Neuroendocrinology

Rachel Yehuda

Introduction

Post-traumatic stress disorder (PTSD) is associated with a unique and somewhat paradoxical neuroendocrine profile in that corticotrophin releasing factor (CRF) levels appear to be increased in this disorder even though ambient cortisol levels are low.[1] In this sense, the hypothalamic–pituitary–adrenal (HPA) axis alterations in PTSD are different from those observed in studies of acute and chronic stress and major depressive disorder, because the latter conditions are associated with both increased CRF and cortisol levels.[2] There is converging evidence to support the idea that the HPA axis is particularly sensitive to negative feedback inhibition in PTSD. The increased sensitivity to negative feedback inhibition is reflected by a hypersuppression of cortisol in response to dexamethasone administration,[3–8] an increased concentration and sensitivity of lymphocyte glucocorticoid receptors,[3,5,9,10] and an augmented adrenocorticotropic hormone (ACTH) response to metyrapone administration.[11] The enhanced negative feedback of cortisol is also accompanied by a more dynamic circadian release of cortisol under basal conditions.[12] This review will summarize the evidence for the enhanced negative feedback model in PTSD and discuss some of the implications of this alteration.

The neuroendocrine response to stress

Exposure to stress results in the initiation of concurrent and instantaneous biological responses that assess the salience of a stressor and help the organism organize a behavioral response. One of the most immediate neuroendocrine responses to stress involves the coordinated sympathetic discharge that causes increases in heart rate and blood pressure.[13] Walter Cannon initially described this as the 'fight or flight' reaction.[14] It is now clear that the sympathetic changes described by Cannon allow a greater perfusion of blood glucose to muscles and vital organs and result in increased energy to skeletal muscles, which allow the organism better to fight or flee adverse situations.[13]

The HPA response to stress involves a more complex set of chemical reactions, and requires a slightly longer time frame. Brain neuropeptides stimulate the paraventricular nucleus of the hypothalamus to stimulate the release of corticotrophin factor (CRF; or corticotropin hormone, CRH), vasopressin and other regulatory neuropeptides.[15] The release of CRF stimulates, among other things, the pituitary release of adrenocorticotrophin hormone (ACTH), and this hormone, in turn, stimulates the release of cortisol from the adrenal glands. This is the basic HPA axis stress-response cascade (reviewed by Chrousos and Gold[16]).

All things being equal, stress – particularly acute stress – results in a dose-dependent increase in both catecholamines and cortisol. The greater the severity of the stressor, the higher the levels of both hormones. However, the actions of these two systems appear to be synergistic. Whereas catecholamines facilitate the availability of energy to the body's vital organs, cortisol's role in stress is to help contain, or shut down, sympathetic activation and other neuronal defensive reactions that have been initiated by stress.[17] In one sense, then, cortisol functions as an 'anti-stress' hormone. As these stress-activated biological reactions shut down, cortisol levels also suppress the HPA axis via the negative feedback inhibition of cortisol on the pituitary, hypothalamus, hippocampus, and amygdala.[18–19] Indeed, these sites contain a large concentration of glucocorticoid receptors,[19–20] and are important targets of action of cortisol.[21] Once the acute stressor has been removed, and the amygdala no longer detects the external threat, it helps activate negative feedback inhibition of the HPA axis in tandem with the hippocampus,[21] leading to the restoration of basal hormone levels.

The hippocampus is the brain region that has most frequently been implicated in mediating the negative feedback effects of glucocorticoids.[21] This organ's role in negative feedback inhibition is supported by numerous animal studies which have demonstrated that lesioning portions of the hippocampus results in delayed feedback control, whereas administration of cortisol directly onto the hippocampus results in an enhancement of negative feedback inhibition.[22,23] Hippocampal glucocorticoid receptors are thought to be critical not only in the regulation of negative feedback inhibition, but also in the modulation of circadian rhythms of cortisol.[21] Glucocorticoid receptors in this brain region additionally control the expression of genes responsible for cognitive integration, and circumscribed memory functions under both basal and stress-induced conditions.[21] Indeed, changes in hippocampal morphology have been noted in PTSD,[24] and may be related to changes in both cortisol negative feedback inhibition and circumscribed memory functions.[25]

The above discussion highlights the fact that the direct action of glucocorticoids at several target tissues in the peripheral nervous system and limbic system ultimately controls the biobehavioral responses to acute stressors and the process that terminates this response. Chronic stress can also result in sustained increases in cortisol. However, depending on the nature of the stressor, the HPA axis may also become tonically inhibited due to a chronic adaptation of the organism to the stressor. This response would result in normal or lower than normal cortisol levels.[26] Selye referred to this tonic inhibition of the HPA axis following chronic stress as 'adrenal exhaustion'.[27] Under these conditions the entire HPA axis appears to be suppressed, with no evidence of suprahypothalamic activation of the HPA axis (for example, increased CRF levels). Thus, in classic stress theory, stressors that result in the activation of CRF release from paraventricular neurons in the hypothalamus also result in elevated cortisol levels, whereas lower levels of cortisol are thought to result directly from a cessation of activation by CRF.

Neuroendocrine alterations in PTSD

Brain CRF concentrations appear to be elevated in PTSD, as indicated by increased concentrations of this peptide in the cerebrospinal fluid (CSF).[28,29] There is also specific evidence of increased hypothalamic CRF release, as determined by the ACTH response to metyrapone administration[11] (see later). However, ambient cortisol levels are not higher in PTSD as they are in major depression[2,12,30,31] – a disorder that is also characterized by CRF hypersecretion.[32] In fact in several studies cortisol concentrations have been found to be lower in PTSD subjects than normal comparison groups, other psychiatric patients, or similarly exposed non-PTSD groups.[10,30,33,34] The studies published to date by our group have produced rather consistent results, with means of cortisol ranging from around 33 μg/day to 40 μg/day in PTSD groups regardless of age, gender, or type of trauma.[10,33,34] The range we have observed in PTSD is comparable to that initially published by Mason and colleagues,[30] who used a similar laboratory methodology for the analysis of cortisol and gave subjects similar directions regarding the importance of performing the collection on days when true 'baseline' (unstimulated and unstressed) conditions could be met.

Some studies of 24-hour urinary cortisol excretion have not replicated the finding that cortisol levels are lower in PTSD compared to other subject groups. We have described elsewhere the methodological errors or collection procedures that might distort urinary cortisol values.[26] It is relatively easy to suspect a hormone value as being spurious because normal values for urinary cortisol excretion over a 24-hour period are well documented in endocrinology textbooks, and are known to be between 20 and 90 μg/day. As indicated in Table 5.1, cortisol levels for both PTSD and normal subjects in some studies have been reported to be either outside this normal range, or at the very high end of it.[35–37]

We have been able to confirm our observations of low urinary cortisol with a 24-hour plasma cortisol study in which blood samples were obtained every 30 minutes around the clock. The data quite compellingly demonstrated lower cortisol levels in the evening in PTSD subjects, whereas morning levels were comparable to normals.[12] Other changes in circadian rhythm were also noted. PTSD subjects showed a greater dynamic range of cortisol over the diurnal cycle compared to normals, as estimated by the amplitude-to-mesor ('signal-to-noise') ratio of cortisol over the diurnal cycle, and demonstrated evidence of a stronger circadian rhythm as evidenced by an increased goodness-of-fit of the 24-hour single oscillator cosinor model to the raw cortisol data.

Studies examining single-point cortisol levels in plasma and salivary samples have also found evidence of low cortisol. In general, single-point estimates do not provide an optimal methodology for testing the hypothesis of low cortisol, owing to the enormous amount of moment-to-moment variability in

Table 5.1 Summary of urinary cortisol levels across all post-traumatic stress disorder (PTSD) studies published to date

Study	PTSD	Normal control Psychiatric control[a]	Trauma control
Mason et al 1986[30]	33.3	51.0[a]	–
Yehuda et al 1990[33]	40.9	62.8	–
Yehuda et al 1993[10]	38.6	69.0[a]	–
Yehuda et al 1995[34]	32.6	51.9	62.7
Pitman and Orr 1990[35]	107.3	–	80.5
Lemieux and Coe 1994[36]	111.8	87.8	83.1
Maes et al 1998[37]	840.0	118.0	–
		591.0[a]	

[a]: In Mason et al 1986[30] psychiatric subjects included major depressive disorder (*n*=8), mania (*n*=8), schizophrenia (*n*=7), paranoid schizophrenia (*n*=12). In Yehuda et al 1993[10] psychiatric subjects included major depressive disorder (*n*=10), mania (*n*=7), psychotic disorder (*n*=9) and panic disorder (*n*=6). For the Maes et al 1998 study,[37] all psychiatric subjects had major depressive disorder (*n*=10). For Mason et al 1986,[30] Yehuda et al 1990,[33] Yehuda et al 1993,[10] and Yehuda et al 1995,[34] mean cortisol levels in PTSD subjects were significantly lower than those in other groups. In the Lemieux and Coe 1994[36] and Maes et al 1998[37] studies, PTSD subjects had significantly higher subjects than normal and trauma-exposed groups. In the Pitman and Orr 1990 study,[35] there were no significant differences in cortisol levels between PTSD and trauma-exposed subjects.

Data represent mean cortisol levels (expressed as µg/day) for PTSD and control groups in the seven published studies to date.

cortisol release as well as individual differences in the stress of venipuncture. Studies employing large sample numbers, however, provide more power to detect subtle group differences and may overcome sources of between-subject error. In a large study of 2490 veterans, Boscarino reported significantly lower cortisol levels in combat veterans with the heaviest combat exposure, including the subset of 293 veterans with PTSD.[38] Goenjian et al[6] demonstrated that basal salivary cortisol levels were lower in children who had been close to the epicenter of the Armenian earthquake 5 years earlier, and who still had substantial PTSD symptoms, compared to children who had been further away from the epicenter and who, as a group, had fewer symptoms; Heim et al[7] found lower basal salivary cortisol in women with chronic pelvic pain who had a high prevalence of sexual trauma and PTSD, compared to women without sexual trauma or PTSD. Jenssen et al also reported lower basal plasma cortisol levels in combat veterans before and after sodium lactate infusion.[39]

Other studies have demonstrated low plasma cortisol in trauma survivors who appear to have been symptomatic at the time of assessment, but were not specifically evaluated for PTSD. Low plasma cortisol levels were also observed in a sample of 29 detainees who were studied shortly after being liberated from a prisoner of war camp in Bosnia,[40] and in a group of 84 refugees who had fled from East to West Germany who were still symptomatic 6 weeks after their arrival in West Berlin.[41] In another study cortisol levels were analysed in 91 subjects, who included male detainees released from the Bosnian concentration camps, displaced persons evacuated from their Croatian town after occupation by the Serbians, and civilians living in Zagreb during the war, and were found to be significantly decreased in subjects 'expressing a severe psychological response'.[42]

Why are cortisol levels low in PTSD?

The presence of low cortisol levels in trauma survivors has been intriguing because these levels are counterintuitive to the idea that stress (and psychiatric symptoms) would be associated with high cortisol levels. One of the important questions that has arisen regarding the data concerns when in the course of adaptation to trauma are low basal cortisol levels first observable. In the above-mentioned studies, cortisol levels were obtained generally several months, years, or even decades following exposure to the stressor. This has led some investigators to hypothesize that the low basal cortisol levels in PTSD reflect a chronic adaptation of the HPA axis. Implicit in this hypothesis is the possibility that if cortisol levels were to have been obtained while the individual was undergoing the traumatic event, or at least in the immediate aftermath of it, then cortisol levels would have been found to be elevated – particularly in individuals who would subsequently develop long-term psychiatric problems and/or PTSD. In fact, this idea that cortisol levels must have been extremely high at the time of the trauma in individuals who develop PTSD has been stated numerous times in the literature as if it were an obvious, foregone conclusion.[25]

In this regard, it is interesting to consider the provocative observations by Bourne et al, who measured urinary cortisol metabolites in Vietnam soldiers while they were stationed in Vietnam, during a threat of imminent enemy attack.[43] Contrary to stress theory that might have predicted that cortisol levels would be quite high in individuals undergoing this stressful situation, the investigators actually found lower levels of the cortisol metabolite 17-hydroxycorticosteroid compared to normal. This study raised the possibility that cortisol levels can be low in response to an extremely traumatic experience.

Studies examining trauma survivors while they are experiencing an extremely stressful situation are rare due to the impracticality, and in most cases, unfeasibility, of obtaining such observations in experimental research settings. Indeed, it was almost 30 years after these observations that investigators attempted to measure the hormonal response to a traumatic event while it was occurring, or at least, in its immediate aftermath. Recently, however, two studies have examined the cortisol response to trauma within hours after the trauma occurred. These studies are quite different in scope and design from Bourne et al's investigation because they have attempted directly to relate the acute cortisol response to a traumatic event with the subsequent development of PTSD.

In one study, McFarlane et al measured the cortisol response to motor vehicle accidents in persons appearing to the emergency room in the immediate aftermath (usually within 1–2 hours) of this trauma.[44] Six months later subjects were evaluated for the presence or absence of psychiatric disorder. In subjects who had developed PTSD, the cortisol response in the immediate aftermath of the motor vehicle accident was significantly lower than the cortisol response of those who subsequently developed major depression. The data are presented in Figure 5.1. The mean cortisol levels following motor vehicle accidents in those who did not subsequently develop psychiatric disorder were in between that of those who developed PTSD or major depression.[44,45] This study suggests that PTSD-like HPA axis alterations are present in the immediate aftermath of a traumatic event.

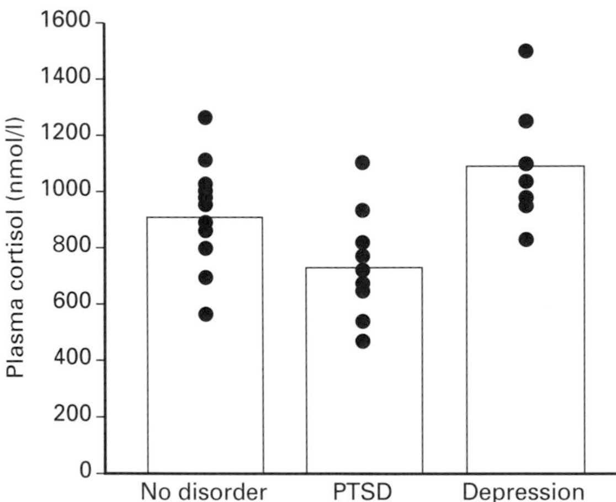

Figure 5.1. Cortisol levels in trauma survivors in the immediate aftermath of a motor vehicle accident. Data from 38 subjects are shown and are redrawn from Yehuda et al 1998.[45] Results of a two-way ANOVA (group × gender) revealed a main effect of diagnosis (F=4.59; df=2,35; p=0.02), but no main effect of gender or group × gender interactions. Covariates were: minutes post-accident, time of day, severity of trauma, past post-traumatic stress disorder (PTSD). No covariate was significant.

Resnick et al demonstrated that women with a prior history of rape or assault had lower cortisol levels immediately after rape than women without such histories.[46] Cortisol levels did not predict the subsequent development of PTSD in these women (possibly owing to the small sample size). Thus, cortisol levels in the immediate aftermath of a traumatic event may be predicted by factors that precede trauma exposure, or by previous exposure.

The two prospective longitudinal studies above demonstrate that the acute cortisol responses to trauma in individuals who develop PTSD, or who show characteristic risk factors for PTSD such as prior exposure to trauma, may be different from those of individuals who do not develop PTSD in response to a similar trauma, or do not have prior trauma histories.

One question raised by these studies is whether or not individuals may have had low cortisol levels even *before* the traumatic event, or had some abnormality that accounts for their aberrant response to the traumatic event they sustained. In this regard, we have previously demonstrated that cortisol levels are low in the high-risk group of adult children of Holocaust survivors.[47] Adult children of Holocaust survivors are three times more likely to develop PTSD compared to demographically matched comparison subjects.[48] Risk of PTSD is greater in offspring whose parents had chronic PTSD compared with those whose parents did not develop or sustain PTSD.[49] Although low cortisol was present in offspring with their own PTSD, it was also associated with the specific risk factor of parental PTSD in the offspring, and was present in high-risk offspring (those with parental PTSD) who had not been exposed to traumatic events and therefore had not developed PTSD. These types of studies need to be performed on a wider scale with multiple high-risk groups before this issue is resolved. Ultimately, the best resolution of this question will necessitate prospective studies that assess cortisol levels in persons before and after they experience traumatic events, or the study of other groups at risk for PTSD (for example, owing to increased familial risk for the development of PTSD).

Implications of low cortisol in the immediate aftermath of a trauma

If cortisol levels were low in the immediate aftermath of a traumatic event, this might have important biological consequences for trauma survivors. The model we have previously set forth is that the failure of cortisol to completely contain the SNS response results in the initial problem of a failure of normal memory consolidation.[50] Indeed, there is substantial evidence that catecholamines, particularly epinephrine, enhance memory consolidation in laboratory rats.[51] This effect appears to be at least in part modulated by adrenal steroids, since removing the adrenal glands of animals makes them more sensitive to the effects of epinephrine on memory consolidation.[52] Furthermore, when such animals are given replacement doses of glucocorticoids, they become less sensitive towards the memory-enhancing effects of epinephrine.[53]

Pitman has hypothesized that PTSD results from an exaggerated response of neuropeptides and catecholamines at the time of the trauma.[54] He has suggested that the increased levels of these stress hormones initiate a process in which memories of the traumatic event might be 'overconsolidated' or inappropriately remembered due to an exaggerated level of distress. This is indeed possible because the primary mechanism through which catecholamines facilitate memory formation is by maintaining organisms in a heightened state of arousal.[51] Certainly, the failure of cortisol to shut down other neuropeptides would facilitate this effect, and also explain why non-PTSD patients do not 'overconsolidate' their traumatic memories. Importantly, the proposed mechanism allows not only for the increased formation of distressing memories, but also explains why reminders of the traumatic event are accompanied by distress in individuals with PTSD. Indeed, there is some evidence from prospective studies that individual differences in the SNS response to trauma are related to the subsequent development of PTSD. Shalev et al collected heart rate data from trauma survivors who appeared at the emergency room in the immediate aftermath of a traumatic event, but who did not have significant physical injury.[55] Mean heart rate levels at the time of the trauma were significantly higher in the 23.4% (of 86) subjects who developed PTSD as determined at a 4-month follow-up. The mean heart rate in the PTSD group remained higher at the 1-week follow-up, however, by 1 month and 4 months, there were no group differences. Importantly, subjects who did not develop PTSD also had elevated heart rate (83.2 beats per minute) at the emergency room, because they were expressing a stress response. The groups did not differ in initial blood pressure, and the results remained significant when adjusted for age, event severity, intensity of the subjective response, and peritraumatic dissociation.

It is interesting to consider in tandem the observations that low cortisol and elevated heart rate were separately associated with the development of PTSD, particularly in light of the role of SNS–HPA interactions in stress.[56] Under normal stress-activated conditions, cortisol levels would ultimately inhibit the adrenergic system. However, it may be that some trauma survivors have higher heart rates in the immediate aftermath of a traumatic event because there has been a failure of cortisol to contain this specific response. In support of this idea is the observation that cortisol and MHPG levels – measured from the same blood sample in the aforementioned rape survivors – appeared to be related to different aspects of the traumatic experiences.[57] While cortisol levels were related to prior history, MHPG levels in these rape victims were associated with the severity of the trauma. Moreover, in the women who did not subsequently develop PTSD there was a significant correlation between cortisol and MHPG levels, which is consistent with the normal stress response, whereas in the women who did subsequently develop PTSD, this relationship was lacking. Thus, the HPA and sympathetic nervous system responses to trauma may literally be 'dis-associated' in those who subsequently develop PTSD. These preliminary data suggest a possible mechanism for why only some individuals would develop a PTSD-like response, whereas others may recover. They also offer a testable hypothesis regarding the role of risk factors in determining whether or not there will be a normative stress response.

One could further theorize that the increased dose of distress every time there are traumatic reminders might activate stress responsive systems, and primarily CRF. Thus, CRF would be expected to be hyper-released due to the intense anxiety brought about by memories that have been inappropriately paired with distress, which are then accompanied by higher levels of catecholamines. We have previously suggested that CRF hypersecretion activates the pituitary to release ACTH. However, because there is an increased sensitivity of glucocorticoid receptors (which account for why cortisol levels might be low in the first place), the HPA axis becomes progressively more sensitive to cortisol (and stress) as it continues to be exposed to CRF.

The HPA paradox in PTSD

That there might be evidence of suprapituitary activation by CRF in the face of low or even normal ambient cortisol levels would be an unusual combination of circumstances. The increased CRF levels imply that the brain is attempting to stimulate an HPA axis response. Thus, if CRF levels are increased, the HPA axis can hardly be called underactive. The paradox here is that, for whatever reason, the activation of hypothalamic CRF does not culminate in an increased cortisol response in PTSD.

Our research has attempted to resolve this seeming inconsistency by identifying and testing a model that explains how cortisol levels would be low in the face of suprapituitary activation by CRF. Because data in our laboratory have demonstrated an increased number of glucocorticoid receptors and increased sensitivity of the glucocorticoid receptors as evidenced by the low-dose dexamethasone suppression test (DST) (reviewed below), we were led to hypothesize that the neuroendocrine alteration in PTSD is one of an enhanced negative feedback inhibition of cortisol.[1]

The model of enhanced negative feedback offers an explanation for how cortisol levels can be low under conditions of CRF activation (that is, stress). In this model (Figure 5.2), chronic CRF release[34] leads to an altered responsiveness of the pituitary. However, because the number and sensitivity of glucocorticoid receptors are increased, negative feedback inhibition is strengthened resulting

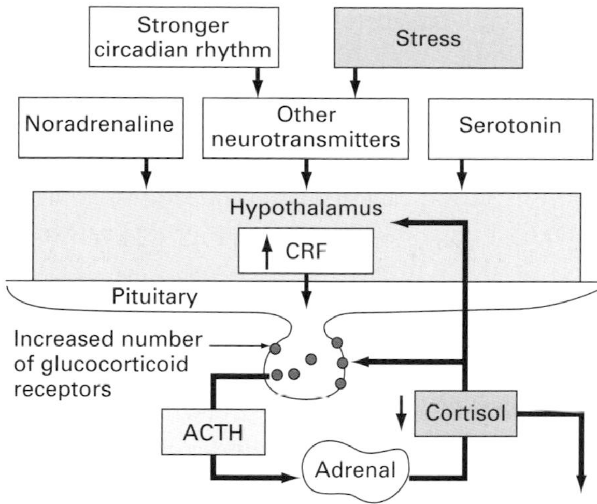

Figure 5.2. Schematic diagram of hypothalamic–pituitary–adrenal alterations in post-traumatic stress disorder (PTSD).

Our group has found several alterations in (nonelderly) PTSD including: (a) stronger circadian rhythm as reflected by an enhanced 'signal-to-noise' or amplitude-to-mean ratio and by a significantly higher goodness of fit of the raw data to a cosinor model of the raw cortisol data;[12] (b) increased suprapituitary activation, possibly reflecting increased hypothalamic CRF release, as evidenced by the ACTH response to metyrapone;[11] (c) increased number and sensitivity of lymphocyte glucocorticoid receptors, as reflected both by an increased number of receptors, and an enhanced down-regulation of those receptors following dexamethasone administration;[3,4,9,10] (d) a decreased level of cortisol;[10,33,34] and (e) an enhanced cortisol response to dexamethasone (that is, enhanced negative feedback inhibition).[3–10]

in an attenuation of tonic cortisol levels. The enhanced negative feedback response contrasts with the well-known cascade in depression, in which chronic CRF release results in an erosion of negative feedback inhibition and resultant hypercortisolism, and glucocorticoid receptor down-regulation.[2] The model implies that low cortisol is not the salient feature of the neuroendocrinology of PTSD. Rather, low cortisol is a downstream manifestation of a more primary alteration, which is an enhanced negative feedback inhibition resulting from an increased glucocorticoid receptor sensitivity.

Glucocorticoid receptor responsiveness in PTSD

As previously mentioned, the physiological and behavioral effects of cortisol depend on the ability of this hormone to bind to glucocorticoid receptors. These receptors are located in the cytosol of cells. Once bound, the steroid–receptor complex translocates into the cell nucleus. This process initiates the transcription of mRNA and the synthesis of proteins that alter the structure and function of cells.[58] Our group has demonstrated that urinary cortisol concentrations and lymphocyte glucocorticoid receptor numbers are not always inversely correlated,[10] which supports the notion that there can be critical individual differences in the number and functional activity of the receptors. In turn, individual differences in glucocorticoid receptor sensitivity would potentially also explain why everyone does not respond to stress in the same manner.

Cortisol exerts its actions by binding to one of two types of receptors: (a) the mineralocorticoid receptor (MR, type 1), or (b) the glucocorticoid receptors (GR, or type 2). The affinity of mineralocorticoid receptors for cortisol is approximately 10 times higher than that of glucocorticoid receptors, therefore, mineralocorticoid receptors are occupied by cortisol under basal conditions, while glucocorticoid receptors become increasingly occupied after stress, and at the circadian peak. Glucocorticoid receptors are thought to be involved in negative feedback following stress-activated increases in cortisol.

Our studies, and those of others, have been limited to measuring type II glucocorticoid receptor sensitivity on human lymphocytes. However, animal studies have demonstrated similarities in glucocorticoid receptor sensitivity in the hippocampus and lymphocytes.[59] With the increased development of radioligands for use in positron emission tomography studies, it will soon be possible to visualize and quantify the number and sensitivity of glucocorticoid receptors in the brain. For now, measurement of receptor number (and sensitivity) in lymphocytes represents the current state of the art in the assessment of glucocorticoid receptors.

In major depression, the number and sensitivity of lymphocyte type II glucocorticoid receptors is lower than normal.[10,60,61] Therefore, although high cortisol levels are present in major depression, the decreased sensitivity of the receptor may actually result in an attenuation of the normal biobehavioral effects of steroids. This phenomenon has been referred to as 'glucocorticoid resistance'.[62] The occurrence of a glucocorticoid resistance explains why depressed patients with very high cortisol levels do not show evidence of endocrinological disorders such as Cushing's syndrome (a disease characterized by excessively high release of cortisol).

In contrast to the decreased number of glucocorticoid receptors observed in major depression and stress, the number of lymphocyte glucocorticoid receptors appears to be increased in PTSD compared to normals, trauma survivors without PTSD, and other psychiatric groups.[3,9,10] Stein et al have recently shown that glucocorticoid receptor numbers are also increased in number in adult survivors of childhood sexual abuse compared to a nonabused nonpsychiatric group of women ($p = 0.07$).[5]

Not only are there a greater number of glucocorticoid receptors in PTSD, the receptors also appear to be more sensitive. This was determined by examining glucocorticoid receptor levels on lymphocytes before and after dexamethasone administration. Dexamethasone administration resulted in a significant decrease or down-regulation of the lymphocyte glucocorticoid receptor number in combat veterans with PTSD but not in trauma survivors without PTSD or normal controls, suggesting that the glucocorticoid receptors of PTSD subjects show a greater response to the administration of the synthetic steroid.[3]

One of the well-known manifestations of the diminished glucocorticoid sensitivity in major depression is the reduced cortisol negative feedback inhibition of the HPA axis, which can be measured using the dexamethasone suppression test (DST).[63] Dexamethasone is a synthetic steroid that mimics the effects of cortisol and affects negative feedback inhibition at the level of the pituitary. The strength of the negative feedback inhibition can therefore be determined by measuring the magnitude of the cortisol inhibition following the administration of this steroid. The higher the cortisol levels (that is, the less inhibition) following dexamethasone, the weaker the negative feedback inhibition.

The initial DST studies in PTSD used the 1.0 μg dose of dexamethasone.[64–68] However, the studies tended not to find evidence for a nonsuppression of cortisol following dexamethasone in nondepressed PTSD patients, and most also failed to demonstrate nonsuppression in depressed PTSD patients (except for the findings of Kudler et al,[67] who did note nonsuppression in about half of their subjects with PTSD). Halbreich et al[65] noted that the low mean cortisol observed (0.90 + 0.53 μg/dl) was well below the cutoff for nonsuppression and suggested the possibility of a hypersuppression in PTSD.

Halbreich et al's suggestion of hypersuppression of the HPA axis led us to administer lower doses of dexamethasone (0.50 and 0.25 µg) in order to cause a partial suppression of cortisol in the comparison group and to determine whether PTSD subjects would show significantly lower post-dexamethasone cortisol levels. Using lower doses of dexamethasone, we observed augmented suppression in combat veterans with PTSD compared to nonexposed subjects.[3] The increased responsiveness to dexamethasone was also present in combat veterans with PTSD who met the diagnostic criteria for concurrent major depression,[4] and importantly, was not present in trauma survivors without PTSD.[3] The finding of an enhanced cortisol suppression to 0.50 µg dexamethasone in veterans has now been independently replicated in adult survivors of childhood sexual abuses,[5] adult sexual abuse,[7] children exposed to natural disasters,[6] and Desert Storm returnees[8] (see Figure 5.3).

Further evidence for the enhanced negative feedback theory has been provided by the results of the metyrapone stimulation test.

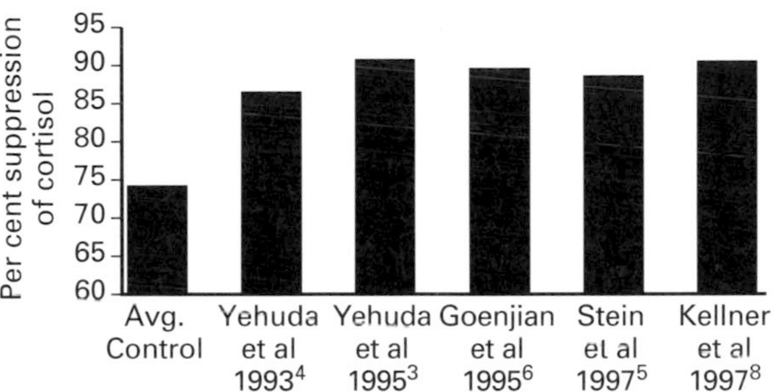

Figure 5.3. Cortisol suppression following a low dose (0.50 mg) of dexamethasone.

Data represent the percentage suppression of cortisol in the PTSD group for the published studies indicated. The Average Control group represents the mean percentage suppression across all studies that utilized a nontraumatized, nonpsychiatric comparison group.[3–5]

Metyrapone is a drug that blocks the conversion of 11-deoxycortisol (the immediate precursor of cortisol) into cortisol and therefore provides a pharmacological mechanism that allows removal of negative feedback inhibition for several hours.[69] Metyrapone administration resulted in an augmented ACTH response in combat veterans with PTSD compared to nontraumatized men, who showed ACTH increases in the normal endocrinologic range.[11] The increased ACTH response to metyrapone demonstrates that when the pituitary is unconstrained by negative feedback inhibition, there is clearly evidence of suprapituitary activation (increased CRF). It therefore follows that under basal conditions, the increased negative feedback inhibition at the level of the pituitary results in lower ambient cortisol levels.

Implications of enhanced negative feedback inhibition for other biological alterations in PTSD

If the brain glucocorticoid receptors are more sensitive in PTSD this might explain some of the recent findings of smaller hippocampal volumes in this disorder. The hippocampus is an area that is rich in glucocorticoid receptors. The current explanation promulgated in the literature is that smaller hippocampal volumes occur as a result of increased cortisol levels, released in response to the traumatic event, that cause neurotoxicity and ultimately reduced volume.[70] However, as stated above, cortisol levels are neither low in the immediate aftermath of a trauma, nor during the chronic PTSD illness. However, if PTSD were characterized not only by increased sensitivity of lymphocyte glucocorticoid receptors but also of hippocampal glucocorticoid receptors, this could increase the vulnerability of the hippocampus to atrophy even if cortisol levels were not increased. Indeed, it is the activation of receptors that leads to the cascade that results in the events (that is, primarily activation of glutamate receptors) that contribute to the neuronal degeneration following stress. That glucocorticoid responsiveness is a more relevant contributor to hippocampal alterations than cortisol per se also explains why not all trauma survivors develop smaller hippocampal volumes following trauma exposure.

Conclusions

Neuroendocrine alterations in PTSD, particularly those relating to the HPA axis, do not resemble those that have been described in classic studies of stress or major depression. If one considers these findings in the context of the fact that PTSD is not a universal stress response (as described in Chapter 2 of this volume), these data can be more readily understood. Indeed, PTSD represents a situation where there has been a failure of restitution of the body to its pre-stress baseline. The biological findings appear to mirror this phenomenon. It appears that there may be biological risk factors that determine the responses that are most likely to result in a PTSD syndrome. These biological risk factors may be related to the prior stress history of the person experiencing a traumatic event. As our understanding of the biology of PTSD grows, we will be able to understand the developmental biological progression of PTSD as well as its implications for the pathophysiology and treatment of the disorder.

References

1. Yehuda R, Hypothalamic–pituitary–adrenal in PTSD. In: Yehuda R, McFarlane AC, eds, Psychobiology of Posttraumatic Stress Disorder. Annals of the New York Academy of Sciences. 821:437–41, 1997.
2. Holsboer F, Neuroendocrinology of mood disorders. In: Bloom FE, Kupfer DJ, eds, *Psychopharmacology: The Fourth Generation of Progress* (Raven: 1995).
3. Yehuda R, Boisoneau D, Lowy MT et al, Dose–response changes in plasma cortisol and lymphocyte glucocorticoid receptors following dexamethasone administration in combat veterans with and without PTSD, *Arch Gen Psychiatry* (1995) **52**:583–93.
4. Yehuda R, Southwick SM, Charney DS et al, Enhanced suppression of cortisol following dexamethasone in combat veterans with PTSD and major depression, *Am J Psychiatry* (1993) **150**:83–6.
5. Stein MB, Yehuda R, Koverola C et al, Enhanced dexamethasone suppression of plasma cortisol in adult women traumatized by childhood sexual abuse. *Biol Psychiatry* (1997) **42**:680–6.
6. Goenjian AK, Yehuda R, Pynoos RS et al, Basal cortisol and dexamethasone suppression of cortisol among adolescents after the 1988 earthquake in Armenia, *Am J Psychiatry* (1995) **153**:929–34.
7. Heim C, Ehlert U, Hanker JP et al, Abuse-related posttraumatic stress disorder and alterations of the hypothalamic–pituitary–adrenal axis in women with chronic pelvic pain, *Psychosom Med* **60**:309–18.
8. Kellner M, Baker DG, Yehuda R, Salivary cortisol in Operation Desert Storm returnees, *Biol Psychiatry* (1997) **41**:849–50.
9. Yehuda R, Lowy MT, Southwick SM et al, Increased lymphocyte glucocorticoid receptor number in PTSD, *Am J Psychiatry* (1991) **149**:499–504.
10. Yehuda R, Boisoneau D, Mason J et al, Relationship between lymphocyte glucocorticoid receptor number and urinary-free cortisol excretion in mood, anxiety, and psychotic disorder, *Biol Psychiatry* (1993) **34**:18–25.
11. Yehuda R, Levengood R, Schmeidler J et al, Increased pituitary activation following metyrapone

administration in PTSD, *Psychoneuroendocrinology* (1996) **21**:1–16.

12. Yehuda R, Teicher MH, Levengood R et al, Circadian rhythm of cortisol regulation in PTSD, *Biol Psychiatry* (1996) **40**:79–88.
13. Mountcastle ZB, *Medical Physiology,* 13th edn, (CV Mosby: St Louis, 1973).
14. Cannon WB, Emergency function of adrenal medulla in pain and major emotions, *Am J Physiol* (1914) **3**:356–72.
15. Rivier CL, Plotsky CM, Mediation by corticotropin releasing factor (CRF) of adenohypophysis hormone secretion, *Ann Rev Physiol* (1986) **48**:475–94.
16. Chrousos GP, Gold PW, The concepts of stress and stress system disorders: overview of physical and behavioral homeostasis. *JAMA* **267**:1244–52.
17. Munck A, Guyre PM, Holbrook NJ, Physiological functions of glucocorticoids in stress and their relation to pharmacological actions, *Endocr Rev* (1984) **93**:9779–83.
18. deKloet ER, Reul JMHM, Feedback action and tonic influence of glucocorticoids on brain function: a concept arising from heterogeneity of brain receptor systems, *Psychoneuroendocrinology* (1987) **12**:83–105.
19. Jacobson L, Sapolsky RM, The roles of the hippocampus in feedback regulation of the hypothalamic–pituitary–adrenocortical axis, *Endocr Rev* (1991) **12**:118–34.
20. Reul JMHM, de Kloet ER, Two receptor systems for corticosterone in rat brain: microdistribution and differential occupation, *Endocrinology* (1985) **117**:2502–11.
21. McEwen BS, deKloet ER, Rostene W, Adrenal steroid receptors and actions in the nervous system, *Physiol Rev* (1987) **66**:1121–88.
22. Sapolsky RM, Krey LC, McEwen BS, Glucocorticoid sensitive hippocampal neurons are involved in terminating the adrenocortical stress response, *Proc Natl Acad Sci* (1984) **81**:6174–7.
23. Plotsky PM, Otto S, Sapolsky RM, Inhibition of immunoreactive corticotropin-releasing factor secretion into the hypophyseal-portal circulation by delayed glucocorticoid feedback, *Endocrinology* (1987) **119**:1126–30.
24. Bremner JD, Randall P, Scott TM et al, MRI-based measurement of hippocampal volumes in patients with combat-related posttraumatic stress disorder, *Am J Psychiatry* (1995) **152**:7.
25. Golier J, Yehuda R, Southwick SM, Memory in adult trauma survivors. In: Appelbaum PS, Uyehara LA, Elin MR, eds, *Trauma and Memory: Clinical and Legal Controversies* (1998.
26. Yehuda R, Giller EL, Southwick SM et al, Hypothalamic–pituitary–adrenal dysfunction in post-traumatic stress disorder, *Biol Psychiatry* (1991) **30**:1031–48.
27. Selye H, *Selye's Guide to Stress Research* (Van Nostrand Reinhold: 1980).
28. Bremner JD, Licino J, Darnell A et al, Elevated CSF corticotropin-releasing factor concentrations in posttraumatic stress disorders, *Am J Psychiatry* (1997) **154**:624–9.
29. Baker DG, West SA, Nicholson WE et al, Serial CSF corticotropin-releasing hormone levels and adrenocortical activity in combat veterans with posttraumatic stress disorder, *Am J Psychiatry* (1999) **156**:985–8.
30. Mason JW, Giller EL, Kosten TR et al, Urinary-free cortisol levels in posttraumatic stress disorder patients, *J Nerv Ment Dis* (1986) **174**:145–59.
31. Sacher EJ, Hellman L, Roffwarg HP, Disrupted 24-hour patterns of cortisol secretion in psychotic depression, *Arch Gen Psychiatry* (1973) **28**:19–24.
32. Nemeroff CB, Widerlov E, Bissette G et al, Elevated concentrations of CSF corticotropin releasing factor-like immunoreactivity in depressed patients, *Science* (1984) **226**:1342–4.
33. Yehuda R, Southwick SM, Nussbaum G et al, Low urinary cortisol excretion in patients with PTSD, *J Nerv Men Dis* (1990) **178**:366–309.
34. Yehuda R, Kahana B, Binder-Brynes K et al, Low urinary cortisol excretion in Holocaust survivors with PTSD, *Am J Psychiatry* (1995) **152**:982–6.
35. Pitman R, Orr S, Twenty-four hour urinary cortisol and catecholamine excretion in combat-related PTSD, *Biol Psychiatry* (1990) **27**:245–7.
36. Lemieux AM, Coe Cl, Abuse-related posttraumatic stress disorder: evidence for chronic neuroendocrine activation in women, *Psychosom Med* (1994) **57**:105–15.
37. Maas M, Lin A, Bonaccorso S et al, Increased 24-hr urinary cortisol excretion in patients with posttraumatic stress disorder and patients with major depression, but not in patients with fibromyalgia, *Acta Psychiatr Scand* (1998) **98**:328–35.
38. Boscarino JA, PTSD, exposure to combat, and lower plasma cortisol among Vietnam veterans: findings and clinical implications, *J Consult Clin Psychology* (1996) **64**:191–201.
39. Jenssen CF, Keller TW, Peskind ER et al, Behavioral and plasma cortisol responses to sodium

lactate infusion in posttraumatic stress disorder, *Am J Psychiatry* (1997)**154**: 266–8.

40. Dekaris D, Sabioncello A, Mazuran R et al, Multiple changes of immunologic parameters in prisoners of war, *JAMA* (1993) **270**:595–9.
41. Bauer M, Priebe S, Graf KJ et al, Psychological and endocrine abnormalities in refugees from East Germany: Part II. Serum levels of cortisol, prolactin, luteinizing hormone, follicle stimulating hormone and testosterone, *Psychiatry Res* (1984) **51**:75–85.
42. Kocijan-Hercigonja D, Sabioncello A, Rijavec M et al, Psychological condition hormone levels in war trauma *J Psychiatr Res* (1996) **30**:391–9.
43. Bourne PB, Rose RM, Mason JW, 17-OHCS levels in combat: special forces 'A' team under threat of attack, *Arch Gen Psychiatry* (1968) **19**:135–40.
44. McFarlane AC, Atchison M, Yehuda R, The acute stress response following motor vehicle accidents and its relation to PTSD. In: Yehuda R, McFarlane AC, eds, Psychobiology of Posttraumatic Stress Disorder. Annals of the New York Academy of Sciences. **821**:437–41. 1997.
45. Yehuda R, McFarlane AC, Shalev AY, Predicting the development of posttraumatic stress disorder from the acute response to a traumatic event, *Biol Psychiatry* (1998) **44**:1305–13.
46. Resnick HS, Yehuda R, Pitman RK et al, Effect of previous trauma on acute plasma cortisol level following rape, *Am J Psychiatry* (1995) **152**:1675–7.
47. Yehuda R, Parental PTSD as a risk factor for PTSD. In: Yehuda R, ed, *Risk Factors for Posttraumatic Stress Disorder*, Progress in Psychiatry Series (American Psychiatric Association: Washington, DC, 1999).
48. Yehuda R, Schmeidler J, Wainberg M et al, Increased vulnerability to posttraumatic stress disorder in adult offspring of Holocaust survivors, *Am J Psychiatry* (1998) **155**:1163–72.
49. Yehuda R, Schmeidler J, Giller EL, Siever LJ, Relationship between PTSD characteristics of Holocaust survivors and their adult offspring, *Am J Psychiatry* (1998) **155**:841–3.
50. Yehuda R, Harvey P, Relevance of neuroendocrine alterations in PTSD to cognitive impairments of trauma survivors. In: Read D, Lindsay S, eds, *Recollections of Trauma: Scientific Research and Clinical Practice*, published proceedings from the 1995 NATO Conference on Trauma and Memory, in Port Bourgenay, France (Plenum Press: 1997).
51. De Wied D, Croiset G, Stress modulation of learning and memory processes. In: Jasmin G, Proschek L, eds, *Stress Revisited 2: Systemic Effects of Stress. Methods Achieve Exp Pathol* (Karger: Basel, 1991) 167–99.
52. De Wied D, Neurohypophyseal hormone influences on learning and memory processes. In: Lynch G, McGaugh JL, Weinberger NM, eds, *Neurobiology of Learning and Memory* (Guilford: New York, 1984) 289.
53. Borrell J, De Kloet ER, Vertseeg DHG, Bohus B, Inhibitory avoidance deficit following short-term adrenalectomy in the rat: the role of adrenal catecholamines, *Behavioral Neurobiology* (1983) **39**:241.
54. Pitman RK, Posttraumatic stress disorder, hormones, and memory, *Biol Psychiatry* (1989) **26**:645–52.
55. Shalev AY, Sahar T, Freedman S et al, A prospective study of heart rate responses following trauma and the subsequent development of PTSD, *Arch Gen Psychiatry* (1998) **55**:553–9.
56. Yehuda R, Southwick SM, Perry BD et al, Interactions of the hypothalamic–pituitary–adrenal and catecholaminergic system in posttraumatic stress disorder. In: Giller, EL, ed, *Biological Assessment and Treatment of PTSD*, Progress in Psychiatry Series (American Psychiatric Association: Washington, DC, 1990) 115–34.
57. Yehuda R, Resnick HS, Schmiedler H et al, Predictors of cortisol and MHPG responses in the acute aftermath of rape, *Biol Psychiatry* (1998) **43**:855–9.
58. Svec F, Minireview, Glucocorticoid receptor regulation, *Life Sci* (1985) **35**:2359–66.
59. Lowy MT, Quantification of type I and II adrenal steroid receptors in neuronal, lymphoid, and pituitary tissues, *Brain Res* (1989) **503**:191–7.
60. Whalley LJ, Borthwick N, Copolov D, Glucocorticoid receptors and depression, *BMJ* (1986) **292**:859–61.
61. Gormley GJ, Lowy MT, Reder AT et al, Glucocorticoid receptors in depression: relationship to the dexamethasone suppression test, *Am J Psychiatry* (1985) **142**:1278–84.
62. Lowy MT, Gormley GJ, Reder AT, Immune function, glucocorticoid receptor regulation and depression. In: Miller AH, ed, *In Depressive Disorders and Immunity* (American Psychiatric Association: Washington, DC, 1989).
63. Stokes PE, Pick GR, Stoll PM et al, Pituitary–adrenal functioning in depressed patients: resistance to dexamethasone suppression, *J Psychiatr Res* (1975) **12**:271–81.

64. Dinan TG, Barry S, Yatham LN et al, A pilot study of a neuroendocrine test battery in posttraumatic stress disorder, *Biol Psychiatry* (1990) 28:665–72.
65. Halbreich U, Olympia J, Carson S et al, Hypothalamic–pituitary–adrenal activity in endogenously depressed post-traumatic stress disorder patients, *Psychoneuroendocrinology* (1989) 14:365–70.
66. Kosten TR, Wahby V, Giller E et al, The dexamethasone suppression test and thyrotropin-releasing hormone stimulation test in PTSD, *Biol Psychiatry* (1990) 28:657.
67. Kudler H, Davidson J, Meador K et al, The DST and post-traumatic stress disorder, *Am J Psychiatry* (1987) 144:1068–71.
68. Olivera AA, Fero D, Affective disorders, DST, and treatment in PTSD patients: clinical observations, *J Trauma Stress* (1990) 3:407–14.
69. Lisansky J, Peake G, Strassman RJ et al, Augmented pituitary corticotropin response to a threshold dosage of human corticotropin-releasing hormone in depressives pretreated with metyrapone, *Arch Gen Psychiatry* (1989) 46:641–9.
70. Sapolsky R, *Stress, the Aging Brain and the Mechanisms of Neuron Death* (MIT Press: Cambridge, MA, 1992).

6

Brain mechanisms and neurotransmitters

Nick J Coupland

A substantial body of preclinical research into the effects of aversive stress can inform our understanding of post-traumatic stress disorder (PTSD), although it is unrealistic to expect preclinical findings to provide a model for all aspects of the disorder. Traumatic stress is associated with a wide variety of psychopathology, including dissociation, depression, anxiety disorders, somatization, impaired relationships, substance abuse, self-harm, and revictimization in addition to the cardinal symptoms that currently define PTSD. The development of PTSD is influenced both by aspects of the traumatic events, such as their proximity, type, duration, outcome and the involvement of significant others, and by aspects of the traumatized person, including their age, sex, family history, developmental experiences and past psychiatric history. There are limits to animal studies for understanding this human complexity, but they do have an important role in identifying components of responses to aversive stress that can be further investigated in humans as clinical research tools become available. Studies of mild aversive stressors in humans have confirmed the operation of some of the mechanisms shown in animals, such as aversive conditioning.[1,2] The advantage of studies of mild stress is that they can investigate the acquisition phase of conditioned responses, which is not possible for PTSD itself. However, it should not be assumed that the mechanisms of PTSD can simply be extrapolated from such studies. Severe stress may engage additional processes and PTSD may involve an abnormal pattern of engagement of responses to severe stress (see Chapter 5). At this early stage of research, neurobiological investigations of PTSD have mainly used cross-sectional designs with two types of control group: healthy subjects and subjects exposed to similar trauma without subsequently developing PTSD. The latter controls are used to determine whether abnormalities are associated with trauma exposure or with the clinical disorder, but this approach still cannot determine if abnormalities represent changes in state or vulnerability traits. In order to address this, longitudinal studies of the evolution of PTSD in the aftermath of trauma are now being employed and studies in high-risk groups could also be feasible.[3,4] The lack of post-treatment biological studies in PTSD is perhaps an indicator of the early state of research in the field.

The defense system

Studies of the reactions of PTSD patients to trauma reminders show that a variety of responses may be elicited, including the negative affects of anxiety, fear, anger, disgust, shame, and sadness, neuroendocrine and cardiorespiratory activation, and sensory, cognitive, and motor responses, such as dissociation, altered pain sensitivity, flashbacks, intrusive memories, enhanced startle reflexes, the urge to escape, and vocalization of distress.[5,6] In animals the physiological and behavioral components of response can readily be measured, but memories and affects have to be inferred from behavior, rather than from verbal reports. Fear is the affect that can most readily be inferred, because of the well-defined pattern of responses that follows threat. A number of structures that are conserved across mammalian species respond to aversive threat and so function as a defense system that mediates fear, although they also subserve other adaptive roles (see Figure 6.1). The defense system both reacts acutely to danger and triggers long-term adaptations that may prepare the animal to cope with its recurrence. Acute reactions include visceral and simple motor responses,

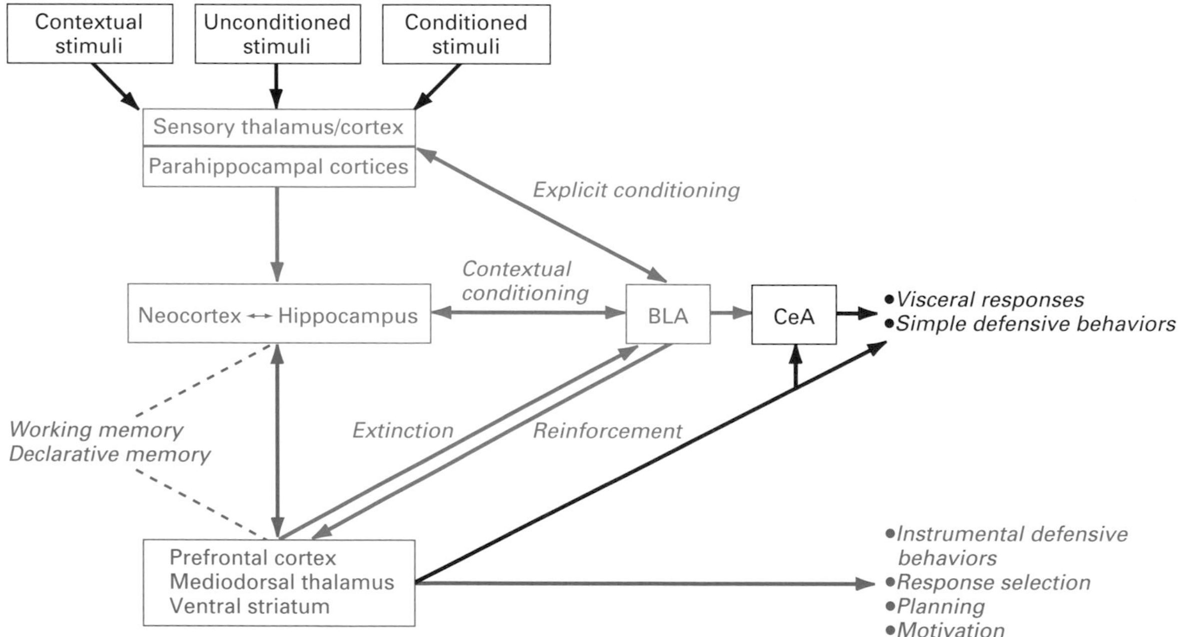

Figure 6.1. Simplified diagram of defense system. The basolateral complex of the amygdala (BLA) is highlighted as the major influence in forming aversive associations (blue). Outputs through the central nucleus of the amygdala (CeA) initiate visceral and simple motor responses (red). Outputs through ventral striatum, prefrontal cortex, and thalamus mediate more complex controlled behaviors that are informed by conscious memory (green), but can release visceral and simple motor outputs when appropriate.

Table 6.1 Fear responses activated by the central nucleus of the amygdala

Region	Response
Lateral periaqueductal gray	Escape Fighting Vocalization Nonopioid analgesia
Ventrolateral periaqueductal gray	Freezing Opioid analgesia
Parabrachial nucleus	Respiration
Hypothalamus	Escape Fighting Increased heart rate and blood pressure ACTH response
Caudal pontine reticular nucleus	Potentiated startle response
Locus coeruleus	Noradrenaline response
Ventral tegmental area	Dopamine response
Basal forebrain	Acetylcholine response
Raphe nuclei	Serotonin response

ACTH, adrenocorticotropic hormone.

mediated by a variety of structures that receive outputs from the central nucleus of the amygdala (CeA: see Table 6.1). Adaptations include the modification of these simple outputs and the development of more complex behavioral and cognitive responses, mediated by networks involving the hippocampus, mediodorsal thalamus, prefrontal cortex, and ventral striatum. In addition, the engagement of the defense system activates the diffuse monoaminergic and cholinergic systems, which modulate the processing of aversive stimuli and execution of responses.

Fear conditioning and negative reinforcement

Fear stimuli can be divided into two broad classes: unlearned and learned. Unlearned stimuli, which for rodents include raised, open or bright areas, novelty, pain, or the sight or odor of predators, evoke fear responses on the animal's first exposure. In contrast, in learned fear, stimuli that do not initially evoke fear do so after the animal has come to associate them with fear-inducing stimuli. One type of learning that has been studied intensively is *fear conditioning*, in which a neutral stimulus such as a tone or light flash (the *conditioned stimulus*) is repeatedly paired in time with an aversive stimulus such as a foot shock (the *unconditioned stimulus*), until the conditioned stimulus elicits the pattern of response (the *conditioned response*) that was initially elicited only by the unconditioned stimulus. The expression of conditioned visceral and simple motor responses depends on the CeA, which can activate multiple output relays (Table 6.1).[7,8] This role of the amygdala has been most clearly elucidated through studies of the acoustic startle and freezing responses. Acoustic startle is a strong motor reflex of the face, neck, and shoulders in response to a sudden loud noise, that is mediated via projections from the cochlear nerve roots to the caudal pontine reticular nucleus (CPRN) and from there to spinal motorneurons. Aversive stimuli potentiate acoustic startle via projections from the CeA and the closely related bed nucleus of the stria terminalis (BNST), that pass to the CPRN both directly and through relays such as the periaqueductal gray (PAG).[9] The unconditioned response to moderate foot shock normally includes an activity burst of running and jumping mediated via the dorsolateral PAG, followed by freezing, in which the animal adopts a rigid motionless posture that is mediated by the ventrolateral PAG. After repeated tone–shock pairings animals show conditioned freezing to the presentation of a tone.[7] Destruction or inactivation of the CeA after fear conditioning blocks conditioned startle and freezing potentiation by disrupting the CeA outputs to the CPRN and the ventrolateral PAG. The acquisition of conditioned fear requires that the conditioned stimulus become linked with unconditioned stimulus, so that it can then activate the outputs of the CeA. Several lines of evidence show that this convergence takes place in the lateral/basolateral complex of the amygdala (BLA), which receives a variety of sensory inputs. Sensory information about the conditioned stimulus is relayed through the thalamic nuclei and perirhinal cortex to the BLA. Sensory information about the unconditioned stimulus also reaches the BLA, in the case of foot shock via the thalamus and the somatosensory and insular cortex. The convergence in time of pain and sensory signals strengthens synaptic connections between their pathways within the BLA, such that either signal can then activate projections to the CeA. Increasing evidence suggests that this process involves long-term potentiation (LTP) within the BLA.[10] Inactivation of the BLA or its sensory inputs impairs the acquisition and expression of conditioned fear to auditory and visual cues. The sensory modalities of taste and smell access the amygdala via its medial nucleus.

Additional circuits are needed to support more complex stimulus–response relationships, including links between unconditioned and conditioned stimuli that are separated in time, learning about environments that may be associated with threat, modifying stimulus–response relationships when contingencies change, and planning and executing more complex responses than those generated by the CeA. These circuits particularly involve the connections of the BLA with the hippocampal and parahippocampal cortex, orbital, insular, medial prefrontal and anterior cingulate cortex, mediodorsal thalamus, and ventral striatum, influencing motor output through connections to the dorsal striatum and pallidum. The prefrontal regions also have predominantly inhibitory outputs to the CeA and projections directly to many of the same targets as the CeA, a pattern that is consistent with the modulation both of conditioned responses and of the same output systems, but based on more controlled and less reflexive stimulus processing.[11,12]

Standard fear conditioning is a form of *delay conditioning*, in which the unconditioned stimulus is presented during or immediately at the offset of the conditioned stimulus. The timing parameters of delay conditioning may be required for the stimuli to become associated within the BLA, as described above, because LTP requires the convergence of depolarizing inputs within a window of about 200 ms. However, fear can also be conditioned by *trace conditioning*, in which the conditioned and unconditioned stimuli occur in a regular relationship, but are separated by an interval. Lesions of the hippocampus impair trace conditioning in animals and in humans, despite having no effect on delay conditioning. Clinical studies have shown that trace conditioning activates the hippocampus and that its strength is associated with awareness of the stimulus pairing, whereas delay conditioning can occur in the complete absence of conscious knowledge.[13,14] The relationship of hippocampal functioning to conscious or declarative knowledge is considered later. The possible mechanism of trace conditioning can be related to emerging ideas about how the hippocampus forms rapid continuous representations of sequences of complex stimuli.

Although a detailed discussion is beyond the scope of this chapter, several recent articles have reviewed evidence that the hippocampus stores information about spatial and temporal relationships as sequences of perceptions.[15,16] These are encoded and stored in the short term as networks of preferentially connected hippocampal neurons called *context fields*, that over a longer time frame can influence storage in parahippocampal and/or neocortical networks. Individual neurons in such networks fire in relation to specific components of a sequence of events. For example, when an animal is exploring an environment in which it is given varying olfactory cues at specific locations, some neurons fire in response to locations, some to olfactory stimuli, some to complex polymodal stimuli, and some in relation to responses emitted by the animal. Parts of the same sequence will more readily coactivate the other components than unrelated neurons, allowing the retrieval of information separated in time. Representations may be strengthened by repetition, for example by exploration of an environment, and possibly by neurotransmitter influences on sensory inputs to and connectivity within the hippocampus. The set of connections that maps locations and experiences for a specific environment has been called a *memory space*.[15] It is hypothesized that a component stimulus can evoke memories by preferentially activating the other parts of the network to which it is most strongly linked. Over longer time periods representations become more strongly established in other cortical areas, such that the hippocampus is not required to evoke recall. Thus the hippocampus can link events in trace conditioning over longer time periods than can LTP within the BLA.

The hippocampus is also involved when environmental stimuli that are not explicitly paired to aversive unconditioned stimuli become fear conditioned. When animals are placed back into an apparatus in which they have been fear conditioned, they show fear even in the absence of the conditioned stimulus. In this case they have become *contextually conditioned* to environmental features of the training apparatus. Contextual conditioning can be acquired rapidly, even with a single shock, but it may not occur if there was only very brief exposure to the apparatus before the shock, a finding called the *immediate shock effect*. Unpaired *preexposure* to the apparatus during a separate session strengthens subsequent contextual conditioning in the face of an immediate shock.[17] Lesions of the hippocampus block contextually conditioned freezing, without necessarily modifying delay conditioning to an explicitly paired cue.[7] It can be hypothesized that this is because the representation of the context depends on the development of a context field within the hippocampus. There is a temporal gradient to the effects of hippocampal lesions on contextual conditioning, such that it is not impaired after a longer period following training, which may be because by this stage a representation has become better established in the parahippocampal cortex or neocortex.[18] One important finding using preexposure has been that when distinct features of the context are preexposed individually, this does not strengthen subsequent contextual conditioning. On the other hand, preexposure to a few of the elements in the same spatial relationship as in the testing context does enhance contextual conditioning.[19] This suggests that representations that link the elements during preexposure provide more potent cues for contextual conditioning. The immediate shock effect suggests that aversive stimuli may interfere with the subsequent development of a contextual representation, but not with one that has already been established by preexposure. It should be noted that not all experiments have confirmed the involvement of the hippocampus in contextual conditioning and that questions concerning the timing of lesions, their location within the hippocampus and adjacent structures, and the effects of lesions on motor activity remain to be answered.[20]

The expression of fear conditioning through the CeA appears to be particularly relevant to the intense physical reactions of PTSD patients to threat cues, such as tachycardia, hyperventilation, feeling paralysed with fear, or the escape response of falling to the ground when a car backfires. In psychophysiological studies of veterans with PTSD, recordings of gunfire or images of combat have activated fear responses consistent with the preclinical expression of fear conditioning. Patients have shown larger heart rate, blood pressure, neuroendocrine, skin conductance and muscle tension responses than trauma-exposed controls without PTSD.[5,21] The likelihood that these responses were conditioned has been supported by evidence that the patients were not more reactive to more general aversive stressors, although exaggerated acoustic startle responses have been shown during the threat of shock.[22,23] There appear to be substantial intersubject differences in the degree to which particular components of response are activated, such that these are not correlated within a group of patients. This should caution against drawing conclusions that conditioned fear is not present if only a limited range of responses has been tested.[24] Despite the preclinical evidence for amygdala activation, this has been inconsistent in neuroimaging studies of trauma cue exposure.[25] Recent studies have shown that the amygdala is activated in humans during aversive delay and trace conditioning paradigms, but only transiently.[1,2,13] Failure to show amygdala activation in PTSD may be because of limitations of temporal or spatial resolution, or because deactivations of inhibitory outputs and activations of excitatory outputs are both involved. It may be noted that other negative emotions relevant to PTSD, such as disgust, can also be conditioned in animals and have been coactivated with fear in patients by trauma cues.[6] Amygdala activations and psychophysiological responses to trauma may therefore not be related solely to the component of fear.

Preclinical studies of partial contextual cues or how aversive cues may be linked within context fields might help to understand how fear generalizes. In a clinical example, a patient had driven home and walked up to his daughter's bedroom, where he found her hanged body in a white dressing gown. He reported that afterwards parts of the drive to his house and seeing hanging decorations or white towels would trigger intense distress and flashbacks. Towels only distressed him if they were hanging over a shower rail and not on the towel rail or the side of the bath. This is reminiscent of the differential potency for contextual conditioning of partial contexts and individual contextual elements during preexposure. Activation of linked elements from a context field might be more likely to activate other parts of the field than single elements. His responses on driving home also fits with the idea that contexts may involve sequences of behavior. The preclinical finding that immediate shock interferes with contextual conditioning suggests that traumatic stress might disrupt the ability to form sequential representations, which may be relevant to the fragmentation of trauma recall that is discussed further in the sections on memory and neurotransmission.

In contrast to studies of fear conditioning, there has been relatively little work on the structures that mediate the influence of aversive stimuli on complex behaviors. In humans lesions of the orbitomedial cortex and amygdala have been shown to impair the ability to use aversively salient information to guide decision-making.[26,27] Recent preclinical studies have begun to investigate negatively reinforced tasks that use instrumental avoidance. Negative reinforcement involves changes in behaviors that are followed by aversive consequences and instrumental avoidance involves the controlled utilization of a behavior to avoid an aversively conditioned stimulus. The first study compared the effects of BLA and CeA lesions on a task where the animal had to learn to press a lever to avoid a stimulus aversively conditioned with footshock. Lesions of the BLA, but not of the CeA, impaired performance of this behavior.[28] In a second study more selective lesions were made in the BLA, showing that although lateral nucleus lesions impaired both responses, explicitly conditioned freezing was selectively impaired by CeA lesions, whereas controlled escape in response to the conditioned stimulus was selectively impaired by destruction of the basal amygdaloid nucleus.[29] This suggests that the amygdala may gain access to circuits mediating instrumental behavior through the basal nucleus, rather than the CeA. Substantially more work has been done on appetitive conditioning of instrumental responses, showing that they are mediated by networks involving the ventral striatum, mediodorsal thalamus, anterior cingulate, and prefrontal cortex, with the strength or vigor of responding influenced by dopaminergic projections from the ventral tegmental area. If the BLA influences this network through projections that are distinct from those to the CeA, this might explain how some patients with PTSD show cognitive and behavioral symptoms without physiological reactivity.[5]

The orbitomedial cortex is important in overriding prior associations when contingencies change, for example when the pairing of a cue with a reward is switched.[30,31] *Extinction* is the gradual loss of fear conditioning when the conditioned stimulus is repeated without further pairing with the aversive unconditioned stimulus. In extinction the aversive association in the BLA seems to be inhibited rather than removed, because whereas explicit cue conditioning requires repeated training, fear can be rapidly reinstated even long after extinction by a single stimulus–shock pairing, or by the presentation of the conditioned stimulus in a different context, suggesting that a dormant association has been reactivated.[32] Orbitomedial lesions can impair the extinction of fear conditioning and also facilitate its acquisition, suggesting a tonic inhibitory influence over the amygdala.[33,34] The latter may have adaptive value in suppressing CeA-based responses to enable more complex stimulus analysis and behavior to supervene when the threat is not immediate. Neuroimaging studies of fear conditioning in healthy volunteers have shown activation of the orbitomedial cortex, although this has not been associated definitively with extinction at this time.[35]

In patients with PTSD, neuroimaging studies have shown differences in the activity of the medial prefrontal cortex including reduced blood flow during symptom provocation, compared with trauma-exposed controls.[36,37] This could reflect an impaired ability to inhibit the amygdala and thereby to extinguish or otherwise modulate conditioned responses to trauma (see also Chapter 4). Given that orbitomedial lesions may enhance fear acquisition, such an impairment could also increase severity of acute stress responses and provide one explanation of how they predict subsequent PTSD. Major depression has recently been associated with altered blood flow and with the loss of glia and possibly neurons in the orbitomedial cortex.[38,39] It is possible that functional or neuroanatomical deficits in this region are implicated in the associations between PTSD and a current, past or family history of depression.[40]

Traumatic memory, amnesia and dissociation

Memories, flashbacks, and nightmares about the trauma are cardinal symptoms of PTSD. Trauma recall is often associated with intense arousal and is also notable for its vivid sensory qualities, intrusiveness, and lack of integration within a narrative of the events, often with at least partial amnesia for some aspects of the experience.[41] For example, when recounting his history, a technician vividly recalled every detail of the checks he had performed on a chemical reaction vessel, his realization that a faulty gasket was going to burst, and his conviction that he would be killed. However, his escape from the building complex remained a complete blank and his next memories were of his throat and chest burning, a terror of suffocation, fleeting impressions of colleagues being present, and then a clearer awareness of being admitted to hospital. A transition in memory appeared in his case to occur at the point of trauma, but in other cases, particularly involving prolonged or repeated trauma, substantial memory deficits may occur for all aspects of the events. In addition to the striking features of traumatic memories, PTSD can also involve deficits in the ability to learn new information, manifested clinically as absent-mindedness or as memory gaps for periods of time and evident in formal psychological tests of memory.[25,42]

Explicit, conscious retention of facts and events is called *declarative memory*. *Procedural* or *implicit memory* involves other types of retention, such as conditioning, improvements in skills with practice and priming (where prior exposure to a complete cue, such as a word, facilitates the subsequent recognition of that cue from an incomplete fragment, such as a word stem). *Working memory* is a short-term buffer that allows new or retrieved information to be held 'on line' during cognitive or motor operations. Preclinical and neuroimaging studies show the involvement in working memory of a network that includes the dorsolateral prefrontal cortex, thalamus, hippocampus, posterior cortical regions and cerebellum.[43] Information in working memory is rapidly lost unless continually updated or *encoded* into longer-term memory stores. *Retrieval* is the reactivation of memories from storage. The establishment of long-term memories appears to take place in stages of *consolidation*. It is postulated that as information is fed forward into the hippocampus, neurons are activated to produce a continuous representation of inputs. Several factors may modulate encoding by influencing how strongly connections between neurons become stabilized as new or updated context fields. Encoding is influenced by factors including actual repetition of events, cognitive operations on the contents of working memory (such as mental rehearsal as an internal repetition of events), comprehension of information (perhaps because this updates a complex context field, as opposed to establishing a new one), and emotional arousal and attention, which engage neurotransmitters that modulate neuronal connectivity. Signals are fed back from the hippocampus to the neocortex or parahippocampal cortices to develop networks that form the basis of long-term memory representations.[44] The unique role of the hippocampus in this process is not its ability to form associations, but that it can do so rapidly, with the capacity for salient representations to become stabilized for incorporation into long-term stores. The neurophysiological basis of interconnecting networks involves switching between two patterns of synaptic activity, feedforward of sensory inputs into the hippocampus that activate firing sequences, and intrinsic activity within the hippocampus that facilitates the development of interconnections between the active neurons via LTP. In the hippocampus this switching appears to depend on oscillatory firing activity at the rate of 3.5–7 Hz (the hippocampal theta rhythm), which rhythmically alters the activity of $GABA_B$ receptors that suppress intrinsic neuronal activity relative to sensory inputs.[16,45] The duration of a burst of theta activity in the human hippocampus has recently been shown to be related to the size of a working memory load.[46] The timing and strength of stages of consolidation appear to be related to neurotransmitter influences within and across stages of the sleep–wake cycle. As an example, feedforward of signals into the hippocampus is also enhanced over feedback into the parahippocampal cortices and neocortex by acetylcholine. The decrease in acetylcholine release between waking and slow-wave sleep would favor a shift from short-term storage of inputs to their consolidation into longer-term stores.[44] Other rhythms also appear to be involved in associative processes, for example gamma oscillations in the 30–70 Hz range may play a role in the binding together of sensory inputs into global perceptions in the neocortex, perhaps involving switching between subcorticocortical and corticocortical connections.[45]

Traumatic and nontraumatic memories could differ at multiple stages of these processes, but it is not possible to be certain from retrospective clinical studies whether differences arise from altered attention, working memory, encoding, consolidation, stability of long-term storage, or retrieval. The extent to which attention can be involved is suggested by descriptions of the attentional shifts that can take place during trauma, from external events to internal sensations, the planning of actions and fantasies about possible outcomes or interventions.[47] In the case of the technician, the impaired clarity of his recall of escape compared with that of his prior checking may have involved such a shift of attention. In addition traumatic stress might interfere with the ability to encode memories, as suggested preclinically by the immediate shock effect on contextual conditioning. This would be consistent with preservation of memory for events leading up to the trauma, for which representations may already have been encoded, as in preexposure studies.

Preclinical studies have suggested how memories of events preceding a stressor can be enhanced. These studies tested the effects of fear-related arousal on memory consolidation, using avoidance as a behavioral measure of declarative memory.[48] Two extensively researched paradigms involve single-trial inhibitory avoidance learning, in which a rodent is given a shock when it moves from a brightly lit to a dark compartment, or when it steps from an elevated to a lower platform. When placed back on the light or elevated section of the apparatus, the animal has to inhibit responses to these aversive settings to avoid the more severely aversive area. A review of many studies of these tasks suggests that the hippocampus, parahippocampal cortices, and neocortex are essential for memory consolidation, but that after long periods only the neocortex is required for retrieval.[49] This parallels contextual fear conditioning and human lesion studies, where hippocampal damage leads to a temporal gradient of memory loss.[18,50] Although the amygdala is not crucial for the consolidation or retention of inhibitory avoidance, consolidation is enhanced by emotional arousal and this effect requires an intact BLA. Temporary inactivation of the BLA during the consolidation period impairs avoidance, whereas BLA inactivation just before retention testing does not.[48] Elicitation of emotional arousal via the amygdala may therefore selectively enhance the longer-term encoding of sequences containing aversive events from the continuous stream of information reaching the hippocampus. Healthy volunteer studies of memory consolidation show parallels with the animal data, in that neuroimaging measures of amygdala activity at the time of viewing emotive films have been found to correlate with later declarative memory of the films' content, and amygdala but not hippocampal deficits are associated with a loss of the arousal effect.[51,52]

It can be postulated that the intensity of traumatic memories may occur through amygdala activation. The mechanisms by which some trauma memories may be impaired are more open to speculation. Deficits in encoding might result from suppression of sensory inputs to the hippocampus. For example, stress has been shown to produce biphasic effects on sensory inputs, with an early enhancement, but followed by a more slowly developing attenuation.[53] Stress might also interfere with the formation of context fields within the hippocampus, perhaps explaining how vivid traumatic memories can occur in isolation from a narrative sequence of events. In this situation fear might become predominantly linked to isolated perceptions, or even to unconscious associations, through the parahippocampal cortices and amygdala-based delay conditioning.[54] In one study, a patient with hippocampal damage showed fear conditioning of skin conductance to a tone paired with shock, despite having no declarative memory of the training sessions.[55] Other studies have used conditioned stimuli that were so brief that subjects lacked conscious awareness of them, yet they still developed aversively conditioned responses associated with amygdala activation.[56]

Symptoms of peritraumatic dissociation include marked derealization or depersonalization, changes in the quality of perceptions and sense of time, and memory gaps, indicating an impaired ability to form integrated polymodal representations of the internal and external environment.[42] This can be hypothesized to involve disruption of the capacity of the hippocampus to form a continuous and polymodal sensory record, although changes in the inputs from sensory thalamus, the binding of stimuli into perceptions in association cortex, or the feedback of hippocampal representations into cortex may also be involved. There is indirect evidence that may be consistent with ongoing changes in these processes in established PTSD, in the form of abnormalities in event-related potentials (ERPs).[57–60] ERPs are partly generated by the time-locking of rhythmic oscillations to stimuli, such that altered ERPs in PTSD may indicate abnormalities of the binding or cognitive processing of sensory inputs.[61] Peritraumatic dissociation is an important predictor, not only of the development of PTSD, but also of repeated dissociative states.[62,63] It is presumably triggered by neurotransmitter changes that occur with severe stress, or in a sensitized defense system (see next section). The trauma of child abuse appears particularly to be associated with later dissociation and in some cases substantial amnesia, which might result because anticipatory fear induces dissociation early within repeated abuse episodes. There is evidence that dissociation in women with sexual abuse histories is associated with smaller hippocampal volumes.[64] A not uncommon opinion of dissociation is that it is a self-protective strategy, but an alternative view is that the breakdown of functions that underlies dissociation and amnesia is in fact a herald of more serious long-term consequences.

Sensitization and hyperarousal

Multiple traumas lead to a higher prevalence of PTSD than single events and early life trauma also predicts the development of PTSD after further adult events. The onset of PTSD may also occur long after the events, a finding that is not readily explicable in terms of simple conditioning (see Chapters 1 and 2). *Sensitization* may help to explain some of these findings. In preclinical studies, sensitization is an increase in response to repeated stimuli, for example, an increase in unconditioned fear with repeated foot shock. Although it refers to response magnitude rather than the development of conditional associations, it can be difficult to divorce from contextual conditioning experimentally. Moderately aversive stressors lead to *context-dependent* sensitization, which is only elicited back in the same training environment. In natural settings this would be adaptive, preparing the animal for defense in situations where threat could be predicted to recur. More strongly aversive stressors may become *context-independent*. *Cross-sensitization* can also occur between different aversive stressors, or between aversive stressors and drug intoxication or withdrawal.[65] These processes that magnify and generalize stress responses across settings may contribute to PTSD, which by definition involves intense stressors. Delayed onsets may occur because of sensitization to repeated conditioned cues, or because responses are amplified by later cross-sensitization with nontraumatic stressors or drug use. Changes in specific transmitter systems are considered in later sections, but on a more general level the mechanisms may include both LTP and lasting changes in the genetic regulation of neurotransmitters, intracellular messengers, and cellular structure in pathways mediating defense. Such long-term changes have been most clearly exemplified in studies of the stress of early maternal deprivation in rats. When the animals reach adulthood and in the absence of further intervening stressors, they show marked changes in mRNA expression for multiple elements of the defense system that are associated with increased physiological and behavioral responsiveness to stressors.[66,67]

The hyperarousal category of PTSD symptoms includes sleep disturbance, impaired concentration, increased vigilance, irritability, and an exaggerated startle response. This is a mixed group of symptoms, some suggesting continuous phenomena and others enhanced cue-responsiveness, and the term 'arousal' itself has multiple meanings. Arousal may be characterized in numerous ways: behaviorally by active or quiet reflective waking and by different sleep stages, autonomically by skin conductance or heart rate, electrophysiologically by electroencephalographic (EEG) rhythms, and neurochemically by the activity of diffuse transmitter systems. It generally implies alertness and a readiness for information processing or action and therefore interacts with attentional and motor performance, but is not equivalent to them.[68] Attentional performance can be inferior during states both of low or high arousal, giving rise to an inverted U-shaped relationship. EEG activation involves a transition from slow synchronized activity to fast desynchronized activity, which depends critically on cortical cholinergic inputs from the basal forebrain and serotonergic inputs from the midbrain raphe nuclei. Acetylcholine and serotonin block slow synchronized activity and induce fast rhythms directly, whereas other transmitters such as noradrenaline, dopamine, and histamine modulate the EEG indirectly via the cholinergic and serotonergic systems.[69]

One question that arises clinically is the extent to which hyperarousal is manifest as basal abnormalities in physiological indices, or is cue-related. It is hard to exclude anticipatory fear if abnormalities are found prior to trauma cue exposure, and unintended conditioned responses can also occur, for example if acoustic startle stimuli resemble gunfire. In general it appears that basal autonomic changes are not consistently present in chronic PTSD and the lack of increased responses to nontraumatic stress cues suggests that autonomic arousal is mainly conditional.[5,22] Despite the clear presence of sleep disorders in PTSD patients objective polysomnographic changes have not consistently been demonstrated. Increases in phasic movements, particularly during rapid eye movement (REM) sleep, and increased awakenings have been found in some studies.[70–75] Counterintuitively to the idea that hypervigilance for external threat disrupts their sleep, PTSD patients have been found to maintain slow-wave and REM sleep through higher levels of noise than controls.[76,77] The surprising lack of objective impairments in some studies may be related to the insensitivity of sleep staging to brief phasic events, or to an absence of threat cues, or to increased perceived safety when sleeping in the laboratory. A recent home-based study of nocturnal activity in prepubertal children has shown marked increases in movement and decreased sleep in those with documented abuse histories, compared with controls.[78] Home-based polysomnographic studies should also be pursued. The psychophysiological and sleep studies suggest that although hyperarousal symptoms are separated from the reexperiencing category in DSM-IV, they may not necessarily be 'basal' phenomena, but a consequence of the frequency of trauma reminders in daily life. A further clinical factor is that secondary stressors, resulting from the impact of PTSD on relationships, employment, and finances, may also increase some of these symptoms.

PTSD patients show information processing biases towards trauma cues, which may be an aspect of hypervigilance.[79,80] In Stroop paradigms subjects have to read out a set of words displayed in a neutral color and then name the print colors in which words in a second set are displayed. The second task takes longer, because reflexive processing of word meanings interferes with the processing of the color names. In emotional modifications of the Stroop task, additional interference takes place for words with particular salience for a patient group and PTSD patients show delayed color naming for trauma-related words. In other paradigms patients have also shown biases towards recalling trauma-related words, when prompted by ambiguous word stems.[81] Biasing of attention and selection for possible threat may contribute to the frequency and generalization of fear responses.

Neurotransmitters and cellular mechanisms

Differences in neurotransmission that result from or confer vulnerability to stress may occur at many levels, including neurotransmitter metabolism, release or uptake, receptor or second messenger function, gene regulation, neuronal and glial production, differentiation, and death, and patterns of neuroanatomical connection. I will focus mainly on neurotransmitters, because the previous chapter has highlighted some of the other issues in relation to the hypothalamic–pituitary–adrenal (HPA) axis.

Corticotropin-releasing hormone (CRH) and urocortin

Two related excitatory peptide neurotransmitters, CRH and urocortin, and two CRH receptor subtypes, CRH_1 and CRH_{2a}, have been identified in neurons. In addition to their role in the HPA axis, CRH and CRH_1 receptors are widely distributed throughout the neocortex and defense system.[82] CRH projections from the CeA and probably the BNST target the PAG, the parabrachial nuclei, the CPRN and the nuclei of the diffusely projecting monoamine and cholinergic systems.[83,84] Central injections of CRH increase unconditioned and conditioned fear and the acquisition of inhibitory avoidance.[82] Aversive stress can increase CRH mRNA expression and CRH release in the amygdala, independently as well as in association with effects on the HPA axis.[85] Nonselective CRH antagonists reduce fear when injected centrally or specifically into the CeA. Selective CRH_1 antagonists, or genetic manipulations that reduce CRH_1 receptors, can also attenuate the effects of unconditioned stressors and fear conditioning. The role of urocortin and CRH_{2a} receptors, for which it has a greater affinity than CRH, is less clear, partly because of species differences in their distribution. Central urocortin injections are anxiogenic, but since they can activate CRH_1 receptors, the physiological role of urocortin may depend how selectively it is compartmentalized with CRH_{2a} receptors, which may mediate stress-induced suppression of feeding and reproductive behavior.[82]

The maternal deprivation model of early life stress sensitizes multiple CRH parameters in adulthood, including increases in CRH and CRH receptor mRNA in the CeA and many of its targets in association with enhanced behavioral, noradrenergic, and neuroendocrine responses to aversive stressors.[66,67] Shorter-term sensitization induced by stress in adults can be blocked by CRH antagonists. Studies comparing sensitization of acoustic startle with startle potentiation by CRH have suggested that sensitization may also occur in the BNST.[86] Drug withdrawal increases CRH release at multiple sites in the defense system, which contribute to cross-sensitization with stress.[86a,87] An important difference between the CRH receptors in extrahypothalamic sites and the HPA axis is that the former are up-regulated and the latter down-regulated by glucocorticoids, which may permit the maintenance or enhancement of fear responses to an early recurrence of threat.[88] If extrahypothalamic and HPA axis CRH were both inhibited by glucocorticoids, then a stress-induced glucocorticoid surge could suppress defense when it is particularly likely to be needed.

In PTSD patients cerebrospinal fluid (CSF) and presumably extrahypothalamic levels of CRH are increased.[89,90] This abnormality is shared with patients with major depression, suggesting that increased CRH might mediate some of the overlap between these disorders. Sensitization of CRH systems would be a plausible mechanism for the increased risk of PTSD that is conferred by multiple trauma or early life stress, and CRH activity might also drive some of the alterations in other neurotransmitters described below. CRH antagonists have recently reached clinical testing and with the future development of labeled compounds for neuroimaging this should greatly increase our understanding of the role of this transmitter.

Glutamate

Glutamate is the main excitatory neurotransmitter, which acts via several types of receptor, including the *N*-methyl-*D*-aspartate (NMDA) and non-NMDA inotropic receptor subtypes, and the G-protein coupled metabotropic glutamate receptors. Glutamate is involved in fast, point-to-point neurotransmission, in long-term changes in synaptic connectivity by initiating long-term potentiation and depression (LTP and LTD), and in trophic and neurotoxic effects. NMDA-dependent LTP has been shown to take place in the BLA during tone–shock pairings and in the hippocampus during inhibitory avoidance learning, contributing to conditioning and declarative memory.[7,49] LTP of CeA efferents to the PAG and hypothalamus also contributes to the stress-induced sensitization of defense.[91] Non-NMDA receptor antagonists impair the retrieval of fear conditioning and inhibitory avoidance.[7,49] Unconditioned aversive stressors increase glutamate release in the prefrontal cortex and hippocampus, an effect that is at least partly glucocorticoid dependent.[92] Stress-related effects on glutamate release and receptor function could therefore be involved in several aspects of PTSD.

Glutamate dysfunction has also been hypothesized as a mechanism of dissociation, through interference with sensory transmission and association as a result of altered thalamocortical, corticocortical, or hippocampal connectivity.[42] Interference with hippocampal encoding might also act as a mechanism for dissociative amnesia. The main support for this hypothesis is indirect, in that the NMDA antagonists ketamine and phencyclidine induce marked dissociation in volunteers. Blockade of NMDA receptors can acutely increase glutamate release by reducing excitation of inhibitory γ-aminobutyric acid (GABA) neurons, which may increase fast transmission through non-NMDA receptors.[93] Lamotrigine, an anticonvulsant that may decrease glutamate release, has been shown to reduce ketamine-induced dissociative symptoms in healthy volunteers.[42] Stress-induced increases in glutamate could also interfere with neuronal and glial proliferation, or contribute to hippocampal neuronal toxicity.[94,95] If glutamate is linked both with dissociation and trophic effects, this could predict associations between dissociation and reduced hippocampal volumes, as have been reported following childhood sexual abuse. Recent studies showing that adult neurogenesis occurs in the neocortical association areas would predict additional neuroanatomical and functional abnormalities of these regions in PTSD, that might also contribute to dissociation.[96] Although these hypotheses remain very speculative, they are clinically relevant because a small controlled study has demonstrated clinical benefit from lamotrigine in antidepressant-resistant PTSD.[97] Agents that reduce glutamate transmission may have potential in established PTSD and as preventive agents in subjects with the risk factor of peritraumatic dissociation.

GABA

GABA (γ-aminobutyric acid) is the main inhibitory neurotransmitter of the brain and is widely distributed through the defense system in interneurons and long inhibitory projections. Benzodiazepines, alcohol, and neurosteroids modulate $GABA_A$ receptor activity via different binding sites.[98] Agents that enhance GABA actions, such as benzodiazepines used clinically and allopregnenalone, the main neurosteroid metabolite of progesterone, are classed as agonists and produce anxiolysis, sedation, amnesia, and inhibition of the HPA axis. Agents that reduce GABA activity are classified as inverse agonists and can trigger fear. Benzodiazepine antagonists displace agonists and inverse agonists, but with few effects of their own. One such agent is flumazenil, which is in clinical use to reverse benzodiazepine-induced sedation. GABA modulators are active when injected locally into the amygdala, medial hypothalamus and PAG, suggesting that there is tonic inhibition of these defense regions by GABA.[99] Changes in GABA can have multiple effects on memory, affecting working memory, encoding and consolidation through direct effects on hippocampal and cortical neurons and indirect effects via changes in monoaminergic and cholinergic activity.[48,49]

There is substantial $GABA_A$ receptor heterogeneity due to the variety of subunits from which receptors can be assembled.[98] Stress and repeated drug use, particularly of alcohol, can impair GABAergic inhibition through reduced receptor numbers, changes in their subunit composition, reduced agonist or increased inverse agonist neurosteroid availability, or changes in receptor phosphorylation.[100] Early maternal deprivation in rats has also been shown to produce lasting reductions in the expression of mRNAs for $GABA_A$ receptor subunits and glutamic acid decarboxylase, the main synthetic enzyme for GABA.[66] This mechanism of long-term stress sensitization can be prevented by pharmacological enhancement of GABA activity at the time of stress and is subject to species differences in GABA function that might confer vulnerability or resilience to the long-term effects of stress.[101–103]

GABA appears to produce tonic inhibition of the defense system in humans, because pentylenetetrazole, which reduces GABA effects, used to be employed for convulsive therapy and produced marked anxiety and dissociation prior to seizure onset.[104] A benzodiazepine inverse agonist has also induced profound anxiety in volunteers.[105] However, there has been little systematic study of the GABA system in PTSD. The main finding to date has been that PTSD patients have reduced benzodiazepine binding in the rostral medial prefrontal cortex.[25] If this has pathophysiological effects then the reduction of cortical benzodiazepine sites that occurs with alcohol dependence might contribute to PTSD symptoms in comorbid patients.[106] Treatment of PTSD with benzodiazepines at doses that reduced anxiety did not ameliorate exaggerated acoustic startle, but this does not necessarily implicate an abnormality of GABA function.[107] Flumazenil can precipitate panic attacks in patients with panic or premenstrual dysphoric disorders, suggesting altered $GABA_A$ receptor responsivity, but this did not occur in PTSD despite its comorbidity with panic.[108,109] Patients with major depression show reduced cortical levels of GABA, which might also be a factor in PTSD, given the effects of early life stress on glutamic acid decarboxylase.[66]

Noradrenaline

The brain stem locus coeruleus (LC) projects to most of the defense system. LC neurons can fire in tonic or phasic modes. Tonic firing diminishes progressively with deepening sleep and is quiescent during REM sleep. During waking tonic LC firing increases with alertness and activity. Alpha-2 antagonist drugs and electrical stimulation increase tonic LC firing, leading to EEG and behavioral activation, disrupted sleep, and fear at high levels.[110] Tasks that require focused attention on discrete stimuli elicit phasic bursts of LC firing, which are required for good performance, but quickly habituate to repetitive stimuli that lack rewarding or aversive properties. Phasic firing is less likely during high or low levels of tonic firing, which are associated with drowsy inattention or restless visual scanning of the surroundings respectively. Forebrain activation by the LC is mediated via stimulation of the basal forebrain cholinergic system (see Figure 6.2), so that a role of the LC may be to recruit this system in response to novel or emotionally salient stimuli.[69] Noradrenergic lesions specifically impair focused attention in the presence of distracting stimuli.[68] Recent studies have suggested a possible mechanism for this effect.[110] Noradrenaline decreases spontaneous neuronal firing, but prolongs depolarization to inputs, enhancing signal detection in the cortex. LC firing may be regulated by electrical coupling between the dendrites of LC neurons.[111] Increased coupling may produce low tonic firing due to averaging of spontaneous neuronal activity, but strong phasic activity to inputs, because LC neurons would fire as a unit, leading to bursts of noradrenaline release that are time-locked to the stimuli. The timing of noradrenaline release to salient stimuli and relative lack of release during nonsalient stimuli would therefore act to focus attention on behavioral targets and not distractors. Low coupling during high levels of stress-induced tonic activity, perhaps driven by CRH (see next paragraph), would reduce phasic bursts. In this case noradrenaline release that is not time-locked to salient stimuli would enhance inputs indiscriminately, producing distractibility and hypervigilance.

In addition to its role in attention, noradrenaline has biphasic effects on memory, enhancing working memory and arousal-

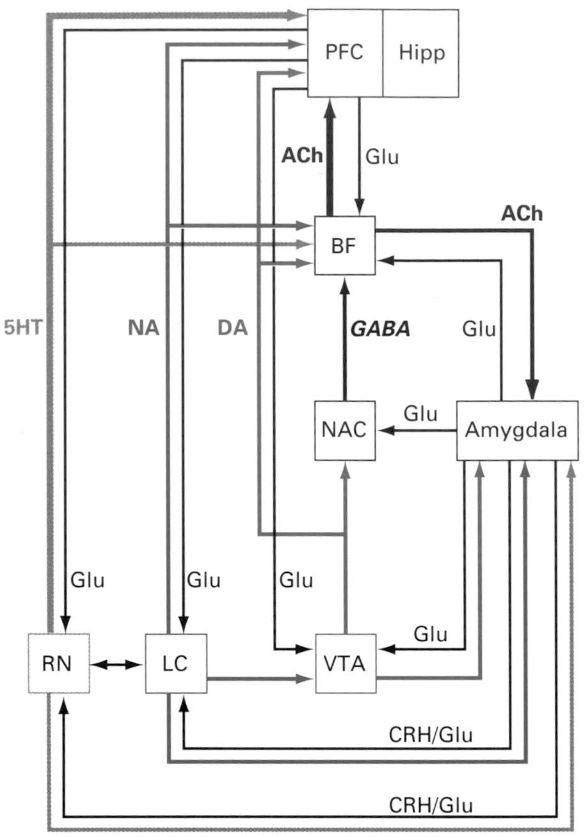

Figure 6.2. Simplified diagram of diffuse transmitter inputs to forebrain. Acetylcholine (red) and serotonin (purple) both produce direct forebrain EEG activation (thick lines), whereas noradrenaline (green) acts indirectly via basal forebrain cholinergic neurons and dopamine (blue) does so via inhibition of an inhibitory γ-aminobutyric acid input to the basal forebrain. Conditioned fear activates the acetylcholine, noradrenaline, and dopamine projections to the forebrain, which facilitate attention and memory processes, whereas serotonin can suppress them. Dopamine influences response selection and increases motivation in relation to emotionally salient stimuli, whereas serotonin is involved in response inhibition. Stress-induced sensitization of CRH activity influences monoamine function. Amygdala, amygdala and bed nucleus of the stria terminalis; PFC, prefrontal cortex; Hipp, hippocampus; NAC, nucleus accumbens; VTA, ventral tegmental area; BF, basal forebrain; LC, locus caeruleus; RN, raphe nuclei.

related consolidation of inhibitory avoidance at moderate levels, but impairing them at high concentrations.[48,112,113] Human studies have shown that centrally but not peripherally acting beta-antagonists reduced the enhancement of memory consolidation by emotional arousal.[114,115] The alpha-2 antagonist yohimbine increased consolidation at the dose used, but the additional prediction that higher, anxiety-inducing doses would impair it has not been tested.[113] A recent preclinical study of inhibitory avoidance has shown that the reactivation of memories during retention is associated with additional consolidation, which can be reduced by administration of a beta-antagonist. This suggests the possibility that repeated arousal associated with trauma recall may act to maintain hippocampal processing of trauma memories and contribute to their persistent intrusiveness.[116]

Several inputs regulate the LC. Brain stem nuclei which project to the autonomic relays controlling sympathetic and parasympathetic function also project to the core of the LC, perhaps coordinating central activation with peripheral autonomic function.[117] The medial prefrontal cortex, CeA, BNST, and paraventricular nucleus project to LC dendrites and the cortical and amygdaloid inputs presumably influence the LC on the basis of stimulus salience.[83,118] Some inputs are CRH neurons and others such as the projections from the medial prefrontal cortex are glutamatergic. The LC is activated by aversive stimuli and by CRH, which show both sensitization and cross-sensitization to each other. Stress-induced LC firing can be blocked by local injection of CRH antagonists.[119–121] In addition to CRH mechanisms, stress-sensitization of noradrenergic function can also occur through increased tyrosine hydroxylase, the rate-limiting enzyme for catecholamine synthesis and through down-regulation of presynaptic alpha-2 adrenoceptors that modulate LC firing and release from its terminals.[122]

The preclinical data suggest that PTSD may involve increased tonic firing of a stress-sensitized noradrenergic system. Early clinical studies measured peripheral noradrenaline and metabolites with inconsistent results, perhaps because these measures are very limited as indices of sympathetic activity or central noradrenergic function.[123,124] The latter has been studied using challenge tests with the noradrenaline reuptake inhibitor desipramine or with yohimbine. Growth hormone responses to desipramine did not differentiate PTSD patients and controls, but this response is a postsynaptic marker and desipramine acutely decreases LC firing, so that the paradigm does not address the question of increased presynaptic activity.[125] Yohimbine, which enhances LC firing in animals, produced a greater increase in acoustic startle in PTSD patients compared with combat controls and healthy volunteers, suggesting a heightened noradrenergic response.[126] In three separate studies yohimbine has also been shown to provoke panic attacks, flashbacks, dissociative symptoms, and cardiovascular activation in PTSD at doses that had little effect on controls.[127,128] Changes in brain metabolism in one of these studies were abnormal in PTSD patients, showing decreases in several regions, instead of the increases that occurred in controls .[129] In preclinical studies noradrenaline can increase brain metabolism and blood flow, but reduces them at high levels, so that this neuroimaging study provides the best evidence to date of noradrenergic hyperactivity in PTSD. The medial prefrontal cortex has a particularly high density of adrenoceptors and conditioned activation of high levels of noradrenaline release could be responsible for reductions in blood flow during trauma cue exposure. Noradrenergic hyperactivity would be a plausible mechanism for high levels of fear, hypervigilance and impaired concentration (focused attention) in PTSD. Episodes of dissociation and memory gaps in PTSD might involve impairing effects of intense noradrenergic stimulation on thalamic sensory relays, cortical sensory processing, working memory, and consolidation.

Several treatments that have some clinical benefit in PTSD modify central noradrenergic function. The alpha-2 agonists clonidine and guanfacine, tricyclic antidepressants, monoamine oxidase inhibitors, selective serotonin reuptake inhibitors, and benzodiazepines can all reduce LC firing. Given the recent identification of electrotonic coupling as a potential mechanism of LC control, it will be important to identify how this might be modified by stress and whether the variable effectiveness of these treatments may be related to their effects on coupling.

Dopamine

Dopamine projections from the substantia nigra to the dorsal striatum are involved in motor actions such as orientation and sequencing, and those from the ventral tegmental area (VTA) to the prefrontal cortex, amygdala, hippocampus, and ventral striatum/nucleus accumbens (see Figure 6.2) are involved in attention, working and declarative memory, conditioning, and behavioral motivation. Dopamine neurons can fire phasically or tonically and tonic firing may inhibit phasic bursts via autoreceptors. Phasic firing of the VTA can be elicited by inputs from the prefrontal cortex, hippocampus, amygdala, and accumbens.[130] It is triggered by cues that predict rewards, but habituates quickly to repetitive signals and expected rewards, appearing to act as an alerting signal to motivationally salient contingencies.[11,131,132] It is not clear if aversive stress can stimulate phasic firing as well as tonic activity, but it does increase dopamine release from the terminals of VTA neurons, particularly in the prefrontal cortex.[133] The effects of dopamine on output neurons include a suppression of spontaneous activity and prolongation of depolarization to inputs via D-1 receptors.[130] Similarly to noradrenaline this enhances working memory, but can impair it at high levels released during stress.[112] In the BLA, dopamine enhances inputs from sensory cortex and reduces inhibitory prefrontal inputs and might act to engage the BLA in processing external cues for their emotional salience.[134] Consistent with this possibility, inactivation of the VTA or blockade of D-1 receptors in the BLA impaired the retrieval of conditioned fear.[135] Given that aversive stressors activate projections from the amygdala to VTA, this may lead to a positive feedback loop that maintains the engagement of the amygdala during perceived threat.[136] In the hippocampus dopamine enhances the consolidation of inhibitory avoidance.[49] The nucleus accumbens is densely interconnected with the prefrontal cortex, amygdala, VTA, and basal forebrain cholinergic system. Dopamine has been postulated to have a dual role in the accumbens, acting in the shell region to increase attention to stimuli, perhaps via recruitment of the basal forebrain, and in the core to influence the engagement of behavioral responses.[11,137] This has been described as an enhancement of motivational salience, which influences the allocation of attentional and behavioral resources to obtain rewards (or avoid threat) and has been dissociated from hedonic responses that involve pleasure when a reward is actually consumed.[138] Repeated stress and psychostimulant administration can sensitize both the dopamine system and motivational salience for threat, producing cross-sensitization to each other.[65]

Several features of PTSD might plausibly involve changes in dopamine function. A stress-sensitized dopamine system may attune the amygdala to external sensory stimuli, increase their motivational salience via the accumbens, and enhance the allocation of attentional resources via the basal forebrain to produce hypervigilance. Enhanced retrieval of aversive associations in the BLA may also contribute to attentional biases to perceived threat. In schizophrenia positive symptoms are associated with a sensitized dopamine response to amphetamine, which may also underlie psychostimulant-induced psychosis.[139] It is therefore possible that stress-sensitization of dopamine responses may contribute to the paranoia that occurs in some PTSD patients.[140,141] Experienced clinicians often use antipsychotics in PTSD with paranoid symptoms, but this is based on anecdotal evidence. If stress predominantly leads to tonic dopamine activity, then secondary inhibition of phasic firing might interfere with the processing of reward cues and contribute to impaired motivation, emotional numbing, and possibly estrangement, if social interactions lose their rewarding properties. An intensified allocation of attention to threat would lead to preoccupation with the trauma, perhaps contributing to the compulsive quality that is sometimes apparent, together with competition for processing resources with other activities, which may lead to impaired concentration. Alterations in dopaminergic modulation of sensory inputs, or working and declarative memory, could contribute to impaired concentration, dissociation, and memory deficits. Cross-sensitization between drugs of abuse and traumatic stress may also contribute to the development or maintenance of PTSD. Currently these possibilities are in the realm of speculation, although the neuroimaging displacement techniques used in schizophrenia could also be applied to study amphetamine- and stress-induced changes in dopamine receptor occupancy in PTSD.

Acetylcholine

The cholinergic system consists of basal forebrain neurons that project to the neocortex, hippocampus, and amygdala and brain stem neurons in the pedunculopontine and laterodorsal tegmental nuclei that project to the basal forebrain, thalamus, and the pontine center controlling REM sleep.[137] The effects of acetylcholine at the cellular level are complex, with effects mediated by multiple muscarinic and nicotinic receptor subtypes, but it again appears to increase responses to inputs and enhance signal detection. At the functional level cholinergic nuclei are involved in attention, cortical activation, and the control of the sleep–wake cycle, producing fast desynchronous EEG activity and contributing to the generation of event-related potentials during both waking and REM sleep.[137,142] Similarly to the other diffuse transmitter systems, the attentional effects of acetylcholine probably depend on the timing of its release based on inputs to the basal forebrain. These include glutamatergic inputs from the prefrontal cortex, amygdala, and brain stem, and a GABAergic input from the nucleus accumbens (see Figure 6.2). It has been postulated that these inputs engage the basal forebrain in routine, habitual attentional processing, but that it can also be recruited by catecholamine inputs that are more specifically activated by novel and emotionally salient stimuli.[69,142]

Acetylcholine facilitates afferent input to the hippocampus and the development of context fields, which may contribute to the encoding and consolidation of memories.[44] Activation of acetylcholine by catecholamines plays a role in emotionally enhanced consolidation, because the positive effect of noradrenergic agonists on inhibitory avoidance learning can be blocked by muscarinic antagonists.[48] Acetylcholine also inhibits the feedback of signals from the hippocampus to the parahippocampal cortices and neocortex, which is thought to prevent retroactive interference with ongoing sensory processing by memories. High levels of acetylcholine during active waking or REM sleep would therefore lead to predominant information flow into the hippocampus. During quiet reflective waking or slow-wave sleep, lower levels of acetylcholine would switch the predominant flow to feedback, allowing an influence of hippocampal information on cortical representations. During REM sleep this hippocampal influence would be suppressed, but the lack of serotonin and noradrenaline activity is thought to increase corticocortical connectivity, enhancing the development of cortical associations and long-term memory representations.[44]

Aversive stressors lead acutely to cortical and hippocampal acetylcholine release; however, intense cholinergic activation produced by marked stress or the administration of anticholinesterases has biphasic effects on acetylcholine function.[143,144] Muscarinic receptor activation regulates the expression of several genes involved in cholinergic metabolism, decreasing the availability of acetylcholine. Acute enhancement is therefore followed by a more sustained depression of cholinergic function.[144] Direct evidence as to the functional consequences is lacking, but stress has been shown to have biphasic effects on the gating of sensory inputs to the hippocampus, with acute facilitation followed by a period of inhibition.[53] It would be of interest if this is cholinergically mediated, because it might be a mechanism for the admixture of enhanced and impaired memories in PTSD.

Ongoing changes in acetylcholine release in PTSD, due to conditioned fear or other types of trauma recall, can be hypothesized to contribute to hypervigilance, nightmares, and increased phasic movements during REM sleep. Increases or decreases in acetylcholine function have both been postulated to contribute to psychotic symptoms in schizophrenia and dementias. Decreases in acetylcholine could do so because of the loss of suppression of feedback from the hippocampus, which has been suggested to cause retroactive interference with sensory processing by hippocampal memory traces.[44,145] The mechanisms by which dopaminergically driven disinhibition of the basal forebrain might produce psychotic symptoms have been described in an earlier section.[146] Which, if any, of these mechanisms are operative may involve dynamic changes, with conditioned cholinergic activation followed by a counter-regulatory depression. In cases of PTSD following combat experience or Japanese terrorist attacks with sarin, it is also possible that anticholinesterase exposure might have contributed to the development of the disorder.[147] Although pyridostigmine bromide, which is used prophylactically by the military, does not normally cross the blood–brain barrier, it has been suggested that some individuals may be susceptible because of differences in metabolism.[148] Deficits in cholinergic function might also contribute to the recrudescence of PTSD that can occur with the onset of dementia.[149] An increasing number of ligands is becoming available for neuroimaging studies of the cholinergic system, which should lead to more direct clinical investigations of PTSD patients.

Serotonin

Serotonergic projections arise from the medial (MRN) and dorsal raphe nuclei (DRN) in the brain stem, which receive mixed inhibitory and excitatory inputs from the LC, PAG, lateral hypothalamus, and other limbic regions via the habenula, projecting to the prefrontal cortex, amygdala, hippocampus, thalamus, and basal ganglia.[150,151] Serotonergic neurons are quiescent during REM sleep, increase their firing from slow-wave sleep to waking, and can directly activate the cortical EEG.[69] It has been suggested that many of the effects of serotonin involve processes that are suppressed during locomotor activity, because their firing rate is otherwise stable.[152] For example, serotonin can suppress neocortical responses to sensory inputs and under some conditions it impairs aspects of attention, learning, and memory.[153] There is a CRH input to the DRN, which it appears has mixed excitatory and inhibitory effects, suggesting that stress-induced activation and sensitization of CRH function may alter serotonergic activity.[154] Stress may also regulate the serotonergic system at the receptor level, because $5HT_{1A}$, $5HT_6$, and $5HT_7$ receptors in the hippocampus are down-regulated by glucocorticoids, which also modulate the serotonergic inhibition of sensory inputs to the amygdala.[155,156] Acoustic startle is inhibited by serotonin and facilitated by tryptophan depletion and $5HT_{1A}$ agonists, which both decrease serotonin release.[157] Serotonin has inhibitory effects over the fight and flight region of the PAG, which is mediated via $5HT_{1A}$ receptors, but can also mediate excitation via $5HT_{2C}$ receptors.[158,159] Finally serotonin is involved in trophic functions, stimulating the proliferation of new hippocampal neurons and the activity of brain-derived neurotrophic factor.[160]

Low levels of serotonergic function are associated with impulsivity, irritability, aggression, and suicidality,[161,162] the former of which can also be induced acutely in susceptible subjects by tryptophan depletion.[163] In a recent study tryptophan depletion was also found to impair the ability to shift response set according to changes in emotional contingencies.[164] These findings may be linked through changes in response inhibition within the prefrontal cortex and fenfluramine-induced serotonin release has been found to increase cerebral metabolism in the orbitomedial and cingulate cortex.[68,165,166] It may be speculated that serotonergic deficits lead to impaired extinction of conditioned fear and increase the expression of inwardly or outwardly directed anger in PTSD.

Impulsivity, irritability, aggression, and suicidality are associated with PTSD, sometimes as part of comorbid borderline personality disorder, in which they are linked with a history of childhood trauma.[167,168] This relationship may be complex, as impulsive patterns of behavior could increase the risk of trauma exposure, as well as trauma altering serotonin function. Impulsive-aggressive and borderline subjects have shown reduced neuroendocrine responses to serotonergic agents, and reduced serotonin synthesis and metabolic responses to fenfluramine in the orbitomedial or cingulate cortex.[166,169,170] Although selective serotonin reuptake inhibitors are the most effective group of treatments for PTSD (see Chapter 9), there have been few pathophysiological studies of the serotonin system in the disorder. Combat veterans with PTSD were found to have decreased prolactin responses to fenfluramine that were associated with measures of aggression.[171] The serotonergic agent *m*-chlorophenyl piperidine (mCPP), which has mixed partial agonist and antagonist effects at different receptor subtypes, induced panic attacks and flashbacks in a subgroup of combat veterans with PTSD.[127] mCPP is anxiogenic in several disorders, so that it is unclear whether this represents a primary abnormality of serotonergic function.[172] Studies of serotonin transporters that used platelet assays have been inconsistent and central neuroimaging measures have not yet been reported.[173–176] Given that replicated serotonergic abnormalities have been found in major depression and with impulsive-aggressive personality traits and that variations in the genetic regulation of the serotonin system influence such traits, there is clearly scope for the application of such approaches to PTSD.[177]

Opioids

Unconditioned and conditioned stressors trigger the release of endogenous opioids in the amygdala and PAG, leading to stress-induced analgesia that can be blocked by opioid antagonists.[178,179] Opioids are also involved in hedonic responses and their interactions with the dopamine system are also important in the development of motivational salience.[138] Opioid dysfunction might therefore play a role in emotional numbing and loss of motivation in PTSD. Brain stem noradrenergic nuclei can be inhibited by opioids and simultaneous blockade of opioid and alpha-2 adrenoceptors precipitates panic attacks in healthy subjects.[180] Opiate withdrawal leads to rebound CRH and noradrenergic activation and abstinence symptoms can be exacerbated by yohimbine and ameliorated by alpha-2 adrenoceptor agonists.[87] Opiate dependence and withdrawal may therefore exacerbate PTSD symptomatology. At the level of the BLA, opioids influence the modulation of arousal by noradrenaline and its effects on memory consolidation.[48]

In combat veterans with PTSD naloxone-reversible analgesia has been triggered by viewing combat films, consistent with the preclinical finding of conditioned stress-induced opioid release.[181] Three studies of circulating opioid levels have been reported, finding normal levels of methionine enkephalin and both normal or decreased levels of β-endorphin in veterans with PTSD.[182–184] The last of these studies also found elevated CSF levels of β-endorphin. There are therefore insufficient well-replicated findings to confirm the suspected involvement of opioid dysfunction in the pathophysiology of PTSD.[185]

Other transmitters

Peptide neurotransmission occurs under conditions of high neuronal firing activity and is therefore particularly relevant to stress, with a variety of peptides being implicated in stress-related effects on fear, anxiety, and memory. Vasopressin fibers project from the medial amygdala and BNST to the hippocampus and lateral septum. Vasopressin is released during stress and mnemonic tasks, enhancing the encoding and consolidation of declarative memory, and it is also involved in aggressive behavior.[186,187] Odors are important in the functions of the medial amygdala vasopressin system in rodents, so that it is not clear that the same functions are served in humans, although effects on declarative memory have been found.[188] Odors can act as potent trauma cues for some PTSD patients. A pilot study has shown that patients with PTSD have enhanced sensitivity to the panic-inducing properties of cholecystokinin tetrapeptide.[189] Similarly to the effects of chronic stress in animals, PTSD patients show decreased basal and yohimbine-induced levels of neuropeptide Y, that are correlated with the degree of combat exposure.[124] Neurokinin receptors are involved in several elements of defense, including activation of the locus caeruleus, PAG-mediated flight behavior, and defensive aggression, and antagonists of these receptors are currently undergoing clinical trials in mood and anxiety disorders.[190–192] There is a burgeoning area of research into stress-sensitive regulators of neuronal plasticity, including intracellular messengers that regulate gene expression and trophic factors that affect cell growth and differentiation. For example, brain-derived neurotrophic factor, which has been shown to play a role in memory function, is down-regulated by stress in the hippocampus and up-regulated by antidepressant treatments.[193] Initial studies have also been performed on inflammatory cytokines, which have bidirectional links with HPA axis function and which could play a role in the associations between PTSD and physical morbidity.[194–196]

Conclusions

There is a substantial gap between preclinical understanding of responses to aversive stress and the confirmation that similar mechanisms play a role in PTSD. However, there are a number of areas in which there is a promising convergence of preclinical and clinical data. The best-established parallels currently are those relating conditioned fear to psychophysiological studies of responses to trauma cues, relating preclinical and clinical findings on the sensitization of central CRH and noradrenergic function and relating stress to deficits in hippocampal function and structure. Research in the field has accelerated in recent years and techniques are now available for many exciting studies, not least with the introduction of novel peptide antagonists to clinical therapeutic research.

Supported by the Alberta Heritage Foundation for Medical Research.

References

1. Buchel C, Morris J, Dolan RJ, Friston KJ, Brain systems mediating aversive conditioning: an event-related fMRI study, *Neuron* (1998) **20**:947–57.
2. LaBar KS, Gatenby JC, Gore JC et al, Human amygdala activation during conditioned fear acquisition and extinction: a mixed-trial fMRI study, *Neuron* (1998) **20**:937–45.
3. Shalev AY, Sahar T, Freedman S et al, A prospective study of heart rate response following trauma and the subsequent development of posttraumatic stress disorder, *Arch Gen Psychiatry* (1998) **55**:553–9.
4. Yehuda R, McFarlane AC, Shalev AY, Predicting the development of posttraumatic stress disorder from the acute response to a traumatic event, *Biol Psychiatry* (1998) **44**:1305–13.
5. Keane TM, Kolb LC, Kaloupek DG et al, Utility of psychophysiological measurement in the diagnosis of posttraumatic stress disorder: results from a Department of Veterans Affairs Cooperative Study, *J Consult Clin Psychology* (1998) **66**:914–23.
6. Rauch SL, van Der Volk BA, Fisler RE et al, A symptom provocation study of posttraumatic stress disorder using positron emission tomography and script-driven imagery, *Arch Gen Psychiatry* (1996) **53**:380–7.
7. Fendt M, Fanselow MS, The neuroanatomical and neurochemical basis of conditioned fear, *Neurosci Biobehav Rev* (1999) **23**:743–60.
8. LeDoux J, Fear and the brain: where have we been, and where are we going? *Biol Psychiatry* (1998) **44**:1229–38.
9. Koch M, The neurobiology of startle, *Prog Neurobiol* (1999) **59**:107–28.
10. Fanselow M, LeDoux J, Why we think plasticity underlying Pavlovian fear conditioning occurs in the basolateral amygdala, *Neuron* (1999) **23**:229–32.

11. Everitt B, Parkinson J, Olmstead M et al, Associative processes in addiction and reward. The role of amygdala–ventral striatal subsystems, *Ann N Y Acad Sci* (1999) **877**:412–38.
12. Price JL, Carmichael ST, Drevets WC, Networks related to the orbital and medial prefrontal cortex; a substrate for emotional behavior? *Prog Brain Res* (1996) **107**:523–36.
13. Buchel C, Dolan R, Armony J, Friston K, Amygdala-hippocampal involvement in human aversive trace conditioning revealed through event-related functional magnetic resonance imaging, *J Neurosci* (1999) **19**:10869–76.
14. Clark RE, Squire LR, Classical conditioning and brain systems: the role of awareness, *Science* (1998) **280**:77–81.
15. Eichenbaum H, Dudchenko P, Wood E et al, The hippocampus, memory and place cells: is it spatial memory or a memory space? *Neuron* (1999) **23**:209–26.
16. Wallenstein GV, Eichenbaum H, Hasselmo ME, The hippocampus as an associator of discontiguous events, *Trends Neurosci* (1998) **21**:317–23.
17. Kiernan MJ, Westbrook RF, Effects of exposure to a to-be-shocked environment upon the rat's freezing response: evidence for facilitation, latent inhibition, and perceptual learning, *Q J Exp Psychol B* (1993) **46**:271–88.
18. Anagnostaras SG, Maren S, Fanselow MS, Temporally graded retrograde amnesia of contextual fear after hippocampal damage in rats: within-subjects examination, *J Neurosci* (1999) **19**:1106–14.
19. Rudy J, O'Reilly R, Contextual fear conditioning, conjunctive representations, pattern completion, and the hippocampus, *Behav Neurosci* (1999) **113**:867–80.
20. Richmond M, Yee B, Pouzet B et al, Dissociating context and space within the hippocampus: effects of complete, dorsal, and ventral excitotoxic hippocampal lesions on conditioned freezing and spatial learning, *Behav Neurosci* (1999) **113**:1189–203.
21. Orr SP, Lasko NB, Metzger LJ et al, Psychophysiologic assessment of women with posttraumatic stress disorder resulting from childhood sexual abuse, *J Consult Clin Psychol* (1998) **66**:906–13.
22. Casada JH, Amdur R, Larsen R, Liberzon I, Psychophysiologic responsivity in posttraumatic stress disorder: generalized hyperresponsiveness versus trauma specificity, *Biol Psychiatry* (1998) **44**:1037–44.
23. Grillon C, Morgan CA 3rd, Davis M, Southwick SM, Effects of experimental context and explicit threat cues on acoustic startle in Vietnam veterans with posttraumatic stress disorder, *Biol Psychiatry* (1998) **44**:1027–36.
24. Liberzon I, Abelson JL, Flagel SB et al, Neuroendocrine and psychophysiologic responses in PTSD: a symptom provocation study, *Neuropsychopharmacology* (1999) **21**:40–50.
25. Bremner J, Alterations in brain structure and function associated with post-traumatic stress disorder, *Semin Clin Neuropsychiatry* (1999) **4**:249–55.
26. Bechara A, Damasio H, Damasio AR, Lee GP, Different contributions of the human amygdala and ventromedial prefrontal cortex to decision-making, *J Neurosci* (1999) **19**:5473–81.
27. Bechara A, Damasio H, Tranel D, Anderson SW, Dissociation of working memory from decision making within the human prefrontal cortex, *J Neurosci* (1998) **18**:428–37.
28. Killcross S, Robbins TW, Everitt BJ, Different types of fear-conditioned behaviour mediated by separate nuclei within amygdala, *Nature* (1997) **388**:377–80.
29. Amorapanth P, LeDoux J, Nader K, Different lateral amygdala outputs mediate reactions and actions elicited by a fear-arousing stimulus, *Nat Neurosci* (2000) **3**:74–9.
30. Dias R, Robbins TW, Roberts AC, Dissociation in prefrontal cortex of affective and attentional shifts, *Nature* (1996) **380**:69–72.
31. Nobre AC, Coull JT, Frith CD, Mesulam MM, Orbitofrontal cortex is activated during breaches of expectation in tasks of visual attention, *Nat Neurosci* (1999) **2**:11–2.
32. Falls WA, Davis M, Behavioral and physiological analysis of fear inhibition. In: Friedman MJ, Charney DS, Deutch AY, eds, *Neurobiological and Clinical Consequences of Stress: From Normal Adaptation to PTSD* (Lippincott-Raven: Philadelphia 1995) 177–202.
33. Morgan MA, LeDoux JE, Differential contribution of dorsal and ventral medial prefrontal cortex to the acquisition and extinction of conditioned fear in rats, *Behav Neurosci* (1995) **109**:681–8.

34. Morgan MA, Romanski LM, LeDoux JE, Extinction of emotional learning: contribution of medial prefrontal cortex, *Neurosci Lett* (1993) **163**:109–13.
35. Morris JS, Ohman A, Dolan RJ, A subcortical pathway to the right amygdala mediating 'unseen' fear, *Proc Natl Acad Sci USA* (1999) **96**:1680–5.
36. Bremner J, Narayan M, Staib L et al, Neural correlates of memories of childhood sexual abuse in women with and without posttraumatic stress disorder, *Am J Psychiatry* (1999) **156**:1787–95.
37. Bremner JD, Staib LH, Kaloupek D et al, Neural correlates of exposure to traumatic pictures and sound in Vietnam combat veterans with and without posttraumatic stress disorder: a positron emission tomography study, *Biol Psychiatry* (1999) **45**:806–16.
38. Drevets WC, Ongur D, Price JL, Neuroimaging abnormalities in the subgenual prefrontal cortex: implications for the pathophysiology of familial mood disorders, *Mol Psychiatry* (1998) **3**:190–1.
39. Rajkowska G, Miguel-Hidalgo J, Wei J et al, Morphometric evidence for neuronal and glial prefrontal cell pathology in major depression, *Biol Psychiatry* (1999) **45**:1085–98.
40. Davidson JR, Tupler LA, Wilson WH, Connor KM, A family study of chronic post-traumatic stress disorder following rape trauma, *J Psychiatric Res* (1998) **32**:301–9.
41. Van der Kolk BA, Fisler R, Dissociation and the fragmentary nature of traumatic memories: overview and exploratory study, *J Trauma Stress* (1995) **8**:505–25.
42. Chambers R, Bremner J, Moghaddam B et al, Glutamate and post-traumatic stress disorder: toward a psychobiology of dissociation, *Semin Clin Neuropsychiatry* (1999) 4:274–81.
43. Owen AM, The functional organization of working memory processes within human lateral frontal cortex: the contribution of functional neuroimaging, *Eur J Neurosci* (1997) **9**:1329–39.
44. Hasselmo M, Neuromodulation: acetylcholine and memory consolidation, *Trends Cog Neurosci* (1999) **3**:351–9.
45. Newman J, Grace A, Binding across time: the selective gating of frontal and hippocampal systems modulating working memory and attentional states, *Conscious Cogn* (1999) **8**:196–212.
46. Tesche C, Karhu J, Theta oscillations index human hippocampal activation during a working memory task, *Proc Natl Acad Sci USA* **97**:919–24.
47. Pynoos R, Steinberg A, Piacentini J, A developmental psychopathology model of childhood traumatic stress and intersection with anxiety disorders, *Biol Psychiatry* (1999) **46**:1542–54.
48. Cahill L, McGaugh JL, Mechanisms of emotional arousal and lasting declarative memory, *Trends Neurosci* (1998) **21**:294–9.
49. Izquierdo I, Medina JH, Memory formation: the sequence of biochemical events in the hippocampus and its connection to activity in other brain structures, *Neurobiol Learn Mem* (1997) **68**:285–316.
50. Squire LR, Zola SM, Episodic memory, semantic memory, and amnesia, *Hippocampus* (1998) **8**:205–11.
51. Hamann SB, Cahill L, Squire LR, Emotional perception and memory in amnesia, *Neuropsychology* (1997) **11**:104–13.
52. Hamann SB, Ely TD, Grafton ST, Kilts CD, Amygdala activity related to enhanced memory for pleasant and aversive stimuli, *Nat Neurosci* (1999) 2:289–93.
53. Akirav I, Richter-Levin G, Biphasic modulation of hippocampal plasticity by behavioral stress and basolateral amygdala stimulation in the rat, *J Neurosci* (1999) **19**:10530–5.
54. Gaffan D, Episodic and semantic memory and the role of the not-hippocampus, *Trends Cog Neurosci* (1997) 1:246–8.
55. Bechara A, Tranel D, Damasio H et al, Double dissociation of conditioning and declarative knowledge relative to the amygdala and hippocampus in humans, *Science* (1995) **269**:1115–18.
56. Morris JS, Ohman A, Dolan RJ, Conscious and unconscious emotional learning in the human amygdala, *Nature* (1998) **393**:467–70.
57. Attias J, Bleich A, Furman V, Zinger Y, Event-related potentials in post-traumatic stress disorder of combat origin, *Biol Psychiatry* (1996) **40**:373–81.
58. Blomhoff S, Reinvang I, Malt UF, Event-related potentials to stimuli with emotional impact in posttraumatic stress patients, *Biol Psychiatry* (1998) 44:1045–53.
59. McFarlane AC, Weber DL, Clark CR, Abnormal stimulus processing in posttraumatic stress disorder, *Biol Psychiatry* (1993) **34**:311–20.

60. Metzger LJ, Orr SP, Lasko NB, Pitman RK, Auditory event-related potentials to tone stimuli in combat-related posttraumatic stress disorder, *Biol Psychiatry* (1997) **42**:1006–15.
61. Basar E, Basar-Eroglu C, Karakas S, Schurmann M, Are cognitive processes manifested in event-related gamma, alpha, theta and delta oscillations in the EEG? *Neurosci Lett* (1999) **259**:165–8.
62. Bremner JD, Brett E, Trauma-related dissociative states and long-term psychopathology in posttraumatic stress disorder, *J Trauma Stress* (1997) **10**:37–49.
63. Shalev AY, Freedman S, Peri T et al, Prospective study of posttraumatic stress disorder and depression following trauma, *Am J Psychiatry* (1998) **155**:630–7.
64. Stein MB, Koverola C, Hanna C et al, Hippocampal volume in women victimized by childhood sexual abuse, *Psychol Med* (1997) **27**:951–9.
65. Post R, Weiss S, Ma S, Sensitization and kindling implications for the evolving neural substrates of post-traumatic stress disorder. In: Friedman M, Charnet D, Ay D, eds, *Neurobiological and Clinical Consequences of Stress: From Normal Adaptation to PTSD* (Lippincott-Raven: Philadelphia, 1995) 203–24.
66. Francis D, Caldji C, Champagne F et al, The role of corticotropin-releasing factor–norepinephrine systems in mediating the effects of early experience on the development of behavioral and endocrine responses to stress, *Biol Psychiatry* (1999) **46**:1153–66.
67. Heim C, Nemeroff C, The impact of early adverse experiences on brain systems involved in the pathophysiology of anxiety and affective disorders, *Biol Psychiatry* (1999) **46**:1509–22.
68. Robbins TW, Arousal systems and attentional processes, *Biol Psychol* (1997) **45**:57–71.
69. Dringenberg HC, Vanderwolf CH, Involvement of direct and indirect pathways in electrocorticographic activation, *Neurosci Biobehav Rev* (1998) **22**:243–57.
70. Hefez A, Metz L, Lavie P, Long-term effects of extreme situational stress on sleep and dreaming, *Am J Psychiatry* (1987) **144**:344–7.
71. Hurwitz TD, Mahowald MW, Kuskowski M, Engdahl BE, Polysomnographic sleep is not clinically impaired in Vietnam combat veterans with chronic posttraumatic stress disorder, *Biol Psychiatry* (1998) **44**:1066–73.
72. Lavie P, Hefez A, Halperin G, Enoch D, Long-term effects of traumatic war-related events on sleep, *Am J Psychiatry* (1979) **136**:175–8.
73. Mellman TA, Kulick-Bell R, Ashlock LE, Nolan B, Sleep events among veterans with combat-related posttraumatic stress disorder, *Am J Psychiatry* (1995) **152**:110–15.
74. Ross RJ, Ball WA, Dinges DF et al, Rapid eye movement sleep disturbance in posttraumatic stress disorder, *Biol Psychiatry* (1994) **35**:195–202.
75. Ross RJ, Ball WA, Sanford LD et al, Rapid eye movement sleep changes during the adaptation night in combat veterans with posttraumatic stress disorder, *Biol Psychiatry* (1999) **45**:938–41.
76. Dagan Y, Lavie P, Bleich A, Elevated awakening thresholds in sleep stage 3–4 in war-related post-traumatic stress disorder, *Biol Psychiatry* (1991) **30**:618–22.
77. Lavie P, Katz N, Pillar G, Zinger Y, Elevated awaking thresholds during sleep: characteristics of chronic war-related posttraumatic stress disorder patients, *Biol Psychiatry* (1998) **44**:1060–5.
78. Glod CA, Teicher MH, Hartman CR, Harakal T, Increased nocturnal activity and impaired sleep maintenance in abused children, *J Am Acad Child Adolesc Psychiatry* (1997) **36**:1236–43.
79. Foa EB, Feske U, Murdock TB et al, Processing of threat-related information in rape victims, *J Abnorm Psychol* (1991) **100**:156–62.
80. McNally RJ, Kaspi SP, Riemann BC, Zeitlin SB, Selective processing of threat cues in posttraumatic stress disorder, *J Abnorm Psychol* (1990) **99**:398–402.
81. Zeitlin SB, McNally RJ, Implicit and explicit memory bias for threat in post-traumatic stress disorder, *Behav Res Ther* (1991) **29**:451–7.
82. Steckler T, Holsboer F, Corticotropin-releasing hormone receptor subtypes and emotion, *Biol Psychiatry* (1999) **46**:1480–508.
83. Van Bockstaele E, Peoples J, Valentino R, A.E. Bennett Research Award. Anatomic basis for differential regulation of the rostrolateral peri-locus coeruleus region by limbic afferents, *Biol Psychiatry* (1999) **46**:1352–63.
84. Van Bockstaele EJ, Colago EE, Valentino RJ, Amygdaloid corticotropin-releasing factor targets locus coeruleus dendrites: substrate for the co-ordination of emotional and cognitive limbs of the stress response, *J Neuroendocrinol* (1998) **10**:743–57.

85. Makino S, Shibasaki T, Yamauchi N et al, Psychological stress increased corticotropin-releasing hormone mRNA and content in the central nucleus of the amygdala but not in the hypothalamic paraventricular nucleus in the rat, *Brain Res* (1999) **850**:136–43.
86. Davis M, Are different parts of the extended amygdala involved in fear versus anxiety? *Biol Psychiatry* (1998) **44**:1239–47.
86a. Richter RM, Weiss F, In vivo CRF release in rat amygdala is increased during cocaine withdrawal in self-administering rats, *Synapse* (1999) **32**:254–61.
87. Sarnyai Z, Neurobiology of stress and cocaine addiction. Studies on corticotropin-releasing factor in rats, monkeys, and humans, *Ann N Y Acad Sci* (1998) **851**:371–87.
88. Schulkin J, Gold PW, McEwen BS, Induction of corticotropin-releasing hormone gene expression by glucocorticoids: implication for understanding the states of fear and anxiety and allostatic load, *Psychoneuroendocrinology* (1998) **23**:219–43.
89. Baker DG, West SA, Nicholson WE et al, Serial CSF corticotropin-releasing hormone levels and adrenocortical activity in combat veterans with posttraumatic stress disorder [published erratum appears in *Am J Psychiatry* (1999) **156**:986], *Am J Psychiatry* (1999) **156**:585–8.
90. Bremner JD, Licinio J, Darnell A et al, Elevated CSF corticotropin-releasing factor concentrations in posttraumatic stress disorder, *Am J Psychiatry* (1997) **154**:624–9.
91. Adamec RE, Evidence that NMDA-dependent limbic neural plasticity in the right hemisphere mediates pharmacological stressor (FG-7142)-induced lasting increases in anxiety-like behavior. Study 2 – The effects on behavior of block of NMDA receptors prior to injection of FG-7142, *J Psychopharmacol* (1998) **12**:129–36.
92. Moghaddam B, Bolinao ML, Stein-Behrens B, Sapolsky R, Glucocorticoids mediate the stress-induced extracellular accumulation of glutamate, *Brain Res* (1994) **655**:251–4.
93. Moghaddam B, Adams B, Verma A, Daly D, Activation of glutamatergic neurotransmission by ketamine: a novel step in the pathway from NMDA receptor blockade to dopaminergic and cognitive disruptions associated with the prefrontal cortex, *J Neurosci* (1997) **17**:2921–7.
94. McEwen BS, Stress and hippocampal plasticity, *Ann Rev Neurosci* (1999) **22**:105–22.
95. Nicoletti F, Magri G, Ingrao F et al, Excitatory amino acids stimulate inositol phospholipid hydrolysis and reduce proliferation in cultured astrocytes, *J Neurochem* (1990) **54**:771–7.
96. Gould E, Reeves A, Graziano M, Gross C, Neurogenesis in the neocortex of adult primates, *Science* (1999) **286**:548–52.
97. Hertzberg M, Butterfield MI, Feldman ME et al, A preliminary study of lamotrigine for the treatment of posttraumatic stress disorder, *Biol Psychiatry* (1999) **45**:1226–9.
98. Rabow LE, Russek SJ, Farb DH, From ion currents to genomic analysis: recent advances in GABA-A receptor research, *Synapse* (1995) **21**:189–274.
99. Graeff FG, Neuroanatomy and neurotransmitter regulation of defensive behaviors and related emotions in mammals, *Braz J Med Biol Res* (1994) **27**:811–29.
100. Deutsch SI, Rosse RB, Mastropaolo J, Environmental stress-induced functional modification of the central benzodiazepine binding site, *Clin Neuropharmacol* (1994) **17**:205–28.
101. Anisman H, Zaharia MD, Meaney MJ, Merali Z, Do early-life events permanently alter behavioral and hormonal responses to stressors? *Int J Dev Neurosci* (1998) **16**:149–64.
102. Hode Y, Ratomponirina C, Gobaille S et al, Hypoexpression of benzodiazepine receptors in the amygdala of neophobic BALB/c mice compared to C57BL/6 mice, *Pharmacol Biochem Behav* (2000) **65**:35–8.
103. Patchev VK, Montkowski A, Rouskova D et al, Neonatal treatment of rats with the neuroactive steroid tetrahydrodeoxycorticosterone (THDOC) abolishes the behavioral and neuroendocrine consequences of adverse early life events, *J Clin Invest* (1997) **99**:962–6.
104. Nutt DJ, The pharmacology of human anxiety, *Pharmacol Ther* (1990) **470**:233–66.
105. Dorow R, Horowski R, Paschelke G et al, Severe anxiety induced by FG 7142, a beta-carboline ligand for benzodiazepine receptors, *Lancet* (1983) **2**:98–9.
106. Abi-Dargham A, Krystal JH, Anjilvel S et al, Alterations of benzodiazepine receptors in type II alcoholic subjects measured with SPECT and [123I]iomazenil, *Am J Psychiatry* (1998) **155**:1550–5.
107. Shalev AY, Bloch M, Peri T, Bonne O, Alprazolam reduces response to loud tones in

panic disorder but not in posttraumatic stress disorder, *Biol Psychiatry* (1998) 44:64–8.
108. Coupland NJ, Lillywhite A, Bell C et al, A pilot study of the effects of flumazenil in posttraumatic stress disorder, *Biol Psychiatry* (1997) 41:988–90.
109. Randall PK, Bremner JD, Krystal JH et al, Effects of the benzodiazepine antagonist flumazenil in posttraumatic stress disorder, *Biol Psychiatry* (1995) **38**:319–24.
110. Aston-Jones G, Rajkowski J, Cohen J, Role of locus coeruleus in attention and behavioral flexibility, *Biol Psychiatry* (1999) **46**:1309–1320.
111. Oyamada Y, Andrzejewski M, Muckenhoff K et al, Locus coeruleus neurones in vitro: pH-sensitive oscillations of membrane potential in an electrically coupled network, *Respir Physiol* (1999) **118**:131–47.
112. Arnsten A, Catecholamine modulation of prefrontal cortical function, *Trends Cog Neurosci* (1998) 2:436–47.
113. O'Carroll R, Drysdale E, Cahill L et al, Stimulation of the noradrenergic system enhances and blockade reduces memory for emotional material in man, *Psychol Med* (1999) **29**:1083–8.
114. O'Carroll R, Drysdale E, Cahill L et al, Memory for emotional material: a comparison of central versus peripheral beta blockade, *J Psychopharmacol* (1999) **13**:32–9.
115. van Stegeren AH, Everaerd W, Cahill L et al, Memory for emotional events: differential effects of centrally versus peripherally acting beta-blocking agents, *Psychopharmacology* (1998) **138**:305–10.
116. Przybyslawski J, Roullet P, Sara SJ, Attenuation of emotional and nonemotional memories after their reactivation: role of beta adrenergic receptors, *J Neurosci* (1999) **19**:6623–8.
117. Valentino RJ, Chen S, Zhu Y, Aston-Jones G, Evidence for divergent projections to the brain noradrenergic system and the spinal parasympathetic system from Barrington's nucleus, *Brain Res* (1996) **732**:1–15.
118. Ennis M, Shipley MT, Aston-Jones G, Williams JT, Afferent control of nucleus locus ceruleus: differential regulation by 'shell' and 'core' inputs, *Adv Pharmacol* (1998) **42**:767–71.
119. Conti LH, Foote SL, Reciprocal cross-desensitization of locus coeruleus electrophysiological responsivity to corticotropin-releasing factor and stress, *Brain Res* (1996) **722**:19–29.
120. Curtis A, Pavcovich L, Valentino R, Long-term regulation of locus ceruleus sensitivity to corticotropin-releasing factor by swim stress, *J Pharmacol Exp Ther* (1999) **289**:1211–19.
121. Curtis AL, Lechner SM, Pavcovich LA, Valentino RJ, Activation of the locus coeruleus noradrenergic system by intracoerulear microinfusion of corticotropin-releasing factor: effects on discharge rate, cortical norepinephrine levels and cortical electroencephalographic activity, *J Pharmacol Exp Ther* (1997) **281**:163–72.
122. Zigmond M, Finlay J, Sved A, Neurochemical studies of central noradrenergic responses to acute and chronic stress. In: Friedman M, Charnet D, Ay D, eds, *Neurobiological and Clinical Consequences of Stress: From Normal Adaptation to PTSD* (Lippincott-Raven: Philadelphia, 1995) 45–60.
123. Esler M, Clinical application of noradrenaline spillover methodology: delineation of regional human sympathetic nervous responses, *Pharmacol Toxicol* (1993) **73**:243–53.
124. Southwick S, Bremner J, Rasmusson A et al, Role of norepinephrine in the pathophysiology and treatment of posttraumatic stress disorder, *Biol Psychiatry* (1999) **46**:1192–204.
125. Dinan TG, Barry S, Yatham LN et al, A pilot study of a neuroendocrine test battery in posttraumatic stress disorder, *Biol Psychiatry* (1990) **28**:665–72.
126. Morgan CA, Grillon G, Southwick SM et al, Yohimbine facilitated accoustic startle in combat veterans with post-traumatic stress disorder, *Psychopharmacology* (1995) **117**:466–71.
127. Southwick SM, Krystal JH, Bremner JD et al, Noradrenergic and serotonergic function in posttraumatic stress disorder, *Arch Gen Psychiatry* (1997) **54**:749–58.
128. Southwick SM, Krystal JH, Morgan A et al, Abnormal noradrenergic function in posttraumatic stress disorder, *Arch Gen Psychiatry* (1993) **50**:266–74.
129. Bremner JD, Innis RB, Ng CK et al, Positron emission tomography measurement of cerebral metabolic correlates of yohimbine administration in combat-related posttraumatic stress disorder, *Arch Gen Psychiatry* (1997) **54**:246–54.
130. Moore H, West A, Grace A, The regulation of forebrain dopamine transmission: relevance to the pathophysiology and psychopathology of schizophrenia, *Biol Psychiatry* (1999) **46**:40–55.

131. Redgrave P, Prescott T, Gurney K, Is the short latency dopamine response too short to signal reward error? *Trends Neurosci* (1999) **22**:146–51.
132. Schultz W, Predictive reward signal of dopamine neurons, *J Neurophysiol* (1998) **80**:1–27.
133. Wilkinson L, Humby T, Killcross A et al, Dissociations in dopamine release in medial prefrontal cortex and ventral striatum during the acquisition and extinction of classical aversive conditioning in the rat, *Eur J Neurosci* (1998) **10**:1019–26.
134. Rosenkranz J, Grace A, Modulation of basolateral amygdala neuronal firing and afferent drive by dopamine receptor activation in vivo, *J Neurosci* (1999) **19**:11027–39.
135. Nader K, Ledoux J, Inhibition of the mesoamygdala dopaminergic pathway impairs the retrieval of conditioned fear associations, *Behav Neurosci* (1999) **113**:891–901.
136. Goldstein LE, Rasmusson AM, Bunney BS, Roth RH, Role of the amygdala in the coordination of behavioral, neuroendocrine, and prefrontal cortical monoamine responses to psychological stress in the rat, *J Neurosci* (1996) **16**:4787–98.
137. Sarter M, Bruno J, Cortical cholinergic inputs mediating a rousal, attentional processing and dreaming: afferent regulation of the basal forebrain by telencephalic and brainstem afferents, *Neuroscience* (2000) **95**:933–52.
138. Berridge KC, Robinson TE, What is the role of dopamine in reward: hedonic impact, reward learning, or incentive salience? *Brain Res Rev* (1998) **28**:309–69.
139. Laruelle M, Imaging dopamine transmission in schizophrenia. A review and meta-analysis, *Q J Nucl Med* (1998) **42**:211–21.
140. Hamner MB, Frueh BC, Ulmer HG, Arana GW, Psychotic features and illness severity in combat veterans with chronic posttraumatic stress disorder, *Biol Psychiatry* (1999) **45**:846–52.
141. Ivezic S, Oruc L, Bell P, Psychotic symptoms in post-traumatic stress disorder, *Mil Med* (1999) **164**:73–5.
142. Everitt BJ, Robbins TW, Central cholinergic systems and cognition, *Ann Rev Psychol* (1997) **48**:649–84.
143. Acquas E, Wilson C, Fibiger HC, Conditioned and unconditioned stimuli increase frontal cortical and hippocampal acetylcholine release: effects of novelty, habituation, and fear, *J Neurosci* (1996) **16**:3089–96.
144. Kaufer D, Friedman A, Seidman S, Soreq H, Acute stress facilitates long-lasting changes in cholinergic gene expression, *Nature* (1998) **393**:373–7.
145. Perry E, Walker M, Grace J, Perry R, Acetylcholine in mind: a neurotransmitter correlate of consciousness? *Trends Neurosci* (1999) **22**:273–80.
146. Sarter M, Bruno JP, Abnormal regulation of corticopetal cholinergic neurons and impaired information processing in neuropsychiatric disorders, *Trends Neurosci* (1999) **22**:67–74.
147. Yokoyama K, Araki S, Murata K et al, Chronic neurobehavioral and central and autonomic nervous system effects of Tokyo subway sarin poisoning, *J Physiol Paris* (1998) **92**:317–23.
148. Shen ZX, Pyridostigmine bromide and Gulf War syndrome, *Med Hypotheses* (1998) **51**:235–7.
149. Johnston D, A series of cases of dementia presenting with PTSD symptoms in World War II combat veterans, *J Am Geriatr Soc* (2000) **48**:70–2.
150. Handley SL, 5-hydroxytryptamine pathways in anxiety and its treatment, *Pharmacol Ther* (1995) **66**:103–48.
151. Morris JS, Smith KA, Cowen PJ et al, Covariation of activity in habenula and dorsal raphe nuclei following tryptophan depletion, *Neuroimage* (1999) **10**:163–72.
152. Jacobs BL, Fornal CA, Activity of serotonergic neurons in behaving animals, *Neuropsychopharmacology* (1999) **21**:9S–15S.
153. Meneses A, Physiological, pathophysiological and therapeutic roles of 5-HT systems in learning and memory, *Rev Neurosci* (1998) **9**:275–89.
154. Kirby L, Rice K, Valentino R, Effects of corticotropin-releasing factor on neuronal activity in the serotonergic dorsal raphe nucleus, *Neuropsychopharmacology* (2000) **22**:148–62.
155. Barnes N, Sharp T, A review of central 5-HT receptors and their function, *Neuropharmacology* (1999) **38**:1083–152.
156. Stutzmann GE, McEwen BS, LeDoux JE, Serotonin modulation of sensory inputs to the lateral amygdala: dependency on corticosterone, *J Neurosci* (1998) **18**:9529–38.
157. Davis M, Pharmacological analysis of fear-potentiated startle, *Braz J Med Biol Res* (1993) **26**:235–60.

158. Beckett S, Marsden CA, The effect of central and systemic injection of the 5-HT1A receptor agonist 8-OHDPAT and the 5-HT1A receptor antagonist WAY100635 on periaqueductal grey-induced defence behaviour, *J Psychopharmacol* (1997) 11:35–40.
159. Jenck F, Moreau J-L, Martin JR, Dorsal periaqueductal gray-induced aversion as a simulation of panic anxiety: elements of face and predictive validity, *Psychiatry Res* (1995) **57**:181–91.
160. Azmitia EC, Serotonin neurons, neuroplasticity, and homeostasis of neural tissue, *Neuropsychopharmacology* (1999) **21**:33S–45S.
161. Evenden J, Impulsivity: a discussion of clinical and experimental findings, *J Psychopharmacol* (1999) **13**:180–92.
162. Mann JJ, Role of the serotonergic system in the pathogenesis of major depression and suicidal behavior, *Neuropsychopharmacology* (1999) 21:99S–105S.
163. Young SN, Pihl RO, Benkelfat C et al, The effect of low brain serotonin on mood and aggression in humans. Influence of baseline mood and genetic factors, *Adv Exp Med Biol* (1996) **398**:45–50.
164. Rogers R, Everitt B, Baldacchino A et al, Dissociable deficits in the decision-making cognition of chronic amphetamine abusers, opiate abusers, patients with focal damage to prefrontal cortex, and tryptophan-depleted normal volunteers: evidence for monoaminergic mechanisms, *Neuropsychopharmacology* (1999) **20**:322–39.
165. Mann JJ, Malone KM, Diehl DJ et al, Positron emission tomographic imaging of serotonin activation effects on prefrontal cortex in healthy volunteers, *J Cereb Blood Flow Metab* (1996) **16**:418–26.
166. Siever L, Buchsbaum M, New A et al, d,l-fenfluramine response in impulsive personality disorder assessed with [18F]fluorodeoxyglucose positron emission tomography, *Neuropsychopharmacology* (1999) **20**:413–23.
167. Brodsky BS, Malone KM, Ellis SP et al, Characteristics of borderline personality disorder associated with suicidal behavior, *Am J Psychiatry* (1997) **154**:1715–9.
168. Southwick SM, Yehuda R, Giller EL Jr, Personality disorders in treatment-seeking combat veterans with posttraumatic stress disorder, *Am J Psychiatry* (1993) **150**:1020–3.
169. Leyton M, Okazawa H, Diksic M et al, Measuring brain serotonin synthesis with PET and alpha[11C]-methyl-L-tryptophan. Presented at the Twenty-first Annual Canadian College of Neuropsychopharmacology Meeting, Montreal, 14–17 June 1998.
170. Manuck SB, Flory JD, McCaffery JM et al, Aggression, impulsivity, and central nervous system serotonergic responsivity in a nonpatient sample, *Neuropsychopharmacology* (1998) **19**:287–99.
171. Davis LL, Clark DM, Kramer GL et al, D-fenfluramine challenge in posttraumatic stress disorder, *Biol Psychiatry* (1999) **45**:928–30.
172. Price LH, Goddard AW, Barr LC, Goodman WK, Pharmacological challenges in anxiety disorders. In: Bloom FE, Kupfer DJ, eds, *Psychopharmacology: The Fourth Generation of Progress*, 1st edn (Raven: New York, 1995) 1311–24.
173. Fichtner CG, O'Connor FL, Yeoh HC et al, Hypodensity of platelet serotonin uptake sites in posttraumatic stress disorder: associated clinical features, *Life Sci* (1995) **57**:PL37–44.
174. Maes M, Lin AH, Verkerk R et al, Serotonergic and noradrenergic markers of post-traumatic stress disorder with and without major depression, *Neuropsychopharmacology* (1999) **20**:188–97.
175. Mellman TA, Kumar AM, Platelet serotonin measures in posttraumatic stress disorder, *Psychiatry Res* (1994) **53**:99–101.
176. Weizman R, Laor N, Schujovitsky A et al, Platelet imipramine binding in patients with posttraumatic stress disorder before and after phenelzine treatment, *Psychiatry Res* (1996) **63**:143–50.
177. Manuck SB, Flory JD, Ferrell RE et al, Aggression and anger-related traits associated with a polymorphism of the tryptophan hydroxylase gene, *Biol Psychiatry* (1999) **45**:603–14.
178. Fanselow MS, Conditioned fear-induced opiate analgesia: a competing motivational state theory of stress analgesia, *Ann N Y Acad Sci* (1986) **467**:40–54.
179. Rubinstein M, Mogil JS, Japon M et al, Absence of opioid stress-induced analgesia in mice lacking beta-endorphin by site-directed mutagenesis, *Proc Natl Acad Sci U S A* (1996) **93**:3995–4000.
180. Charney DS, Heninger GR, Alpha 2-adrenergic and opiate receptor blockade. Synergistic effects on anxiety in healthy subjects, *Arch Gen Psychiatry* (1986) **43**:1037–41.

181. Pitman RK, van der Kolk BA, Orr SP, Greenberg MS, Naloxone-reversible analgesic response to combat-related stimuli in posttraumatic stress disorder. A pilot study, *Arch Gen Psychiatry* (1990) 47:541–4.

182. Baker DG, West SA, Orth DN et al, Cerebrospinal fluid and plasma beta-endorphin in combat veterans with post-traumatic stress disorder, *Psychoneuroendocrinology* (1997) 22:517–29.

183. Hoffman L, Burges Watson P et al, Low plasma beta-endorphin in post-traumatic stress disorder, *Aust N Z J Psychiatry* (1989) 23:269–73.

184. Van der Kolk BA, Greenberg MS, Orr SP, Endogenous opioids, stress induced analgesia, and post traumatic stress disorder, *Psychopharmacol Bull* (1989) 25:417–21.

185. Nijenhuis ER, Vanderlinden J, Spinhoven P, Animal defensive reactions as a model for trauma-induced dissociative reactions, *J Trauma Stress* (1998) 11:243–60.

186. de Vries GJ, Miller MA, Anatomy and function of extrahypothalamic vasopressin systems in the brain, *Prog Brain Res* (1998) 119:3–20.

187. Diaz Brinton R, Vasopressin in the mammalian brain: the neurobiology of a mnemonic peptide, *Prog Brain Res* (1998) 119:177–99.

188. Born J, Pietrowsky R, Fehm HL, Neuropsychological effects of vasopressin in healthy humans, *Prog Brain Res* (1998) 119:619–43.

189. Kellner M, Wiedemann K, Yassouridis A et al, Behavioral and endocrine response to cholecystokinin tetrapeptide in patients with posttraumatic stress disorder, *Biol Psychiatry* (2000) 47:107–11.

190. De Felipe C, Herrero JF, O'Brien JA et al, Altered nociception, analgesia and aggression in mice lacking the receptor for substance P, *Nature* (1998) 392:394–7.

191. Hahn M, Bannon M, Stress-induced C-fos expression in the rat locus coeruleus is dependent on neurokinin 1 receptor activation, *Neuroscience* (1999) 94:1183–8.

192. Mongeau R, De Oca BM, Fanselow MS, Marsden CA, Differential effects of neurokinin-1 receptor activation in subregions of the periaqueductal gray matter on conditional and unconditional fear behaviors in rats, *Behav Neurosci* (1998) 112:1125–35.

193. Duman R, Malberg J, Thome J, Neural plasticity to stress and antidepressant treatment, *Biol Psychiatry* (1999) 46:1181–91.

194. Aurer A, Aurer-Kozelj J, Stavljenic-Rukavina A et al, Inflammatory mediators in saliva of patients with rapidly progressive periodontitis during war stress induced incidence increase, *Coll Antropol* (1999) 23:117–24.

195. Maes M, Lin AH, Delmeire L et al, Elevated serum interleukin-6 (IL-6) and IL-6 receptor concentrations in posttraumatic stress disorder following accidental man-made traumatic events, *Biol Psychiatry* (1999) 45:833–9.

196. Spivak B, Shohat B, Mester R et al, Elevated levels of serum interleukin-1 beta in combat-related posttraumatic stress disorder, *Biol Psychiatry* (1997) 42:345–8.

7

Psychosocial treatments of post-traumatic stress disorder

Barbara O Rothbaum

Impressive advances in treating post-traumatic stress disorder (PTSD) have been made in the past decade with respect to group psychotherapy, individual psychodynamically oriented therapy, and cognitive-behavioral therapy. This chapter summarizes the literature on psychosocial interventions for PTSD, beginning with a brief review of traditional therapies. We then examine the larger literature on the efficacy of cognitive-behavioral procedures with PTSD.

Traditional interventions

Hypnotherapy

Hypnosis has been advocated in the treatment of trauma since it was introduced by Freud to attain the abreaction and catharsis he deemed necessary to resolve a psychic conflict (see Spiegel[1] for a review) and continues to be used to treat trauma survivors. Spiegel noted that hypnosis may be useful in treating PTSD because hypnotic phenomena such as dissociation are common in coping with trauma as it occurs and in its sequelae, and hypnosis may facilitate the recall of traumatic events that were encoded in a dissociative state and that therefore are not available to conscious recollection.

A number of case studies have reported that hypnosis was useful in treating post-trauma disturbances following a variety of traumas, but most of these lack methodological rigor and thus cannot allow strong conclusions to be drawn.

In the one controlled study[2] of 112 trauma victims, the relative efficacies of hypnosis, desensitization, and psychodynamic psychotherapy were compared against a waiting list control group. The participants were victims of a variety of traumas who all met symptom criteria for PTSD; the majority did not directly experience the trauma but had lost a loved one. The results indicated that participants in all three treatment conditions were more improved than those in the waiting list condition, but no differences across the three treatments were observed. Inspection of the pre- and post-treatment means indicated 29% improvement on the Impact of Event Scale (IES)[3] for those in psychodynamic therapy, 34% for hypnotherapy, and 41% for desensitization, compared to about 10% improvement in the waiting list condition. The results suggest that hypnotherapy, as well as desensitization and psychodynamic therapy, may offer some help for post-trauma suffering.

Psychodynamic treatments

Treatment by dynamic psychotherapy has often been advocated as a final component of crisis intervention.[4–6] However, empirical investigations of their efficacy are scarce, and those that do exist are not usually well controlled.

In an attempt to account for post-trauma reactions, psychodynamic theorists (for example Horowitz[7]) emphasize concepts such as denial, abreaction, catharsis, and stages of recovery from trauma. The target of Horowitz's brief psychodynamic therapy is the resolution of intrapsychic conflict arising from a traumatic experience, rather than specific symptom reduction. Other psychodynamic theorists focus largely on group process.[8] Several studies have suggested that psychodynamic treatments may be useful in the treatment of PTSD, while others have not found them effective.

Psychodynamic psychotherapy was not found useful in the treatment of a traumatized Vietnam veteran.[9] After 19 months of no progress with psychodynamic psychotherapy, therapy by imagery was introduced. The therapist presented a trauma-related scene and allowed the client to develop it spontaneously through associations rather than by plan. The use of the imagery technique was not planned in advance, but rather it was introduced at appropriate times in the context of a session. The client moved on to other trauma-related scenes when he was ready. Avoidance was addressed through psychodynamic techniques of dealing with transference and resistance. Ten sessions of this imagery therapy were effective in ameliorating the client's PTSD as observed by the therapist and reported by the client. Although constrained by the limitations of a single case report and unsystematic measures, this report suggests that traditional 'talking' therapy was not helpful for PTSD, whereas behaviorally oriented techniques appeared to be effective.

Using psychoanalytic-oriented therapy, Bart[10] reported that trauma victims worsened following treatment. On the other hand, short-term dynamic group therapy for 9 rape victims was determined to be somewhat helpful.[11] Fear and hostility decreased significantly from pre- to post-treatment, but 3 of the 7 victims who completed the study reported only slight change in their overall level of distress. Unfortunately, no control group was included and the content of the therapy sessions was not specified.

Twenty-eight victims of the Beverly Hills Supper Club fire were treated with individual short-term (6–12 sessions) psychodynamic psychotherapy.[12] Diagnoses included PTSD, complicated bereavement, major depressive disorder, and adjustment disorder. Patients who completed treatment showed more improvement than patients with interrupted treatment. Lindy et al[12] subsequently observed that all treated patients 'improved to a subclinical level two years after the fire' (p. 602).

As mentioned above in the section on hypnotherapy, Brom et al[2] conducted a controlled study of Horowitz's brief psychodynamic therapy, comparing this treatment with hypnosis, desensitization, and a waiting list control group. Although the authors found no differences among the three active treatment conditions, inspection of the means on the IES suggested that psychodynamic therapy in this study yielded inferior outcome compared to desensitization (29% vs 41% mean pre–post reduction).

The efficacy of a brief psychodynamic treatment based upon Horowitz's[7] model for bereavement was investigated in 61 women who had lost their husbands.[13] Patients were randomly assigned either to 12 weekly sessions of brief dynamic therapy or to a mutual help group led by a nonclinician. Although many of the participants in this study reported symptoms of PTSD, death of a husband does not necessarily qualify as a DSM criterion A trauma. Results indicated that patients in both conditions improved slightly on both interview and self-report ratings of PTSD symptoms, but there were no group differences.

Using a quasi-experimental design, interpersonal process group therapy (IPGT) was compared with a naturally occurring waiting list control in 43 female childhood sexual abuse survivors.[14] The IPGT treatment was based on the treatment guidelines established by Courtois[15] and Yalom.[8] History of abuse was the only specified inclusion criterion. Results indicated that IPGT patients improved on several measures including PTSD diagnostic status. At pre-treatment, 91% of the IPGT group and 85% of the control group met DSM criteria for PTSD; at post-treatment, only 39% of the IPGT group v 83% of the control group met criteria for PTSD. The IPGT group showed greater symptom reduction than did the control group on some measures (for example, self-report measure of intrusion), whereas both groups evidenced similar symptom reduction on other measures (for example, depression, dissociation).

In summary, most studies of psychodynamic psychotherapy were plagued by methodological flaws, including lack of controls, lack of adequate assessment of outcome, and vaguely described treatments. Thus, the information about the efficacy of traditional interventions with PTSD from these studies is quite limited and is open to various interpretations.

Cognitive-behavioral therapy

Cognitive-behavior therapy (CBT) includes a variety of treatment programs, including exposure procedures, cognitive restructuring procedures, anxiety management programs, and their combinations. Reviews of the extant literature on the treatment of PTSD are quite positive regarding CBT.[16–18] A recent meta-analysis found the largest treatment effects for cognitive-behavioral techniques and selective serotonin reuptake inhibitor (SSRI) medications.[18] One form of CBT employed with PTSD sufferers is exposure treatment, which assists patients in confronting their feared memories and situations. A very recent comprehensive review of CBT studies for PTSD found the strongest evidence for exposure therapy.[16]

Both exposure in imagination and exposure in real life to trauma-related events appear to be therapeutic. The exposure treatment that has been developed by Foa and Rothbaum[19] and their colleagues typically incorporates imaginal exposure that has the patient recall the traumatic memories in the therapist's office. The patient is asked to go back in his or her mind to the time of the trauma and to relive it in his or her imagination. He or she is asked to close his or her eyes and to describe it out loud in the present tense, as if it were happening now. Very often, this narrative is tape-recorded (audiotaped) and that tape is sent home with the patient so that he or she may practice imaginal exposure daily at home between therapy sessions. Although this reliving is often painful for the patient initially, it quickly becomes less painful as exposure is repeated. The idea behind this type of treatment is that the trauma needs to be emotionally processed, or digested, so that it can become less painful.[20,21] Also, many victims with PTSD mistakenly view the process of remembering their trauma as dangerous and therefore devote much effort to avoiding thinking about or processing the trauma. Imaginal reliving serves to disconfirm this mistaken belief.

Other forms of exposure involve repeatedly confronting realistically safe situations, places, or objects that are reminders of the trauma (called in vivo, or in real life, exposure) until they no longer elicit such strong emotions. Some therapists have patients write repeatedly about the trauma as a form of exposure.[22] In systematic desensitization (SD), the patient is taught how to relax, then presented with reminders of the trauma gradually, working up a hierarchy from the least disturbing to the most disturbing. If they become very anxious or upset, they stop the trauma imagery, relax themselves, then go back to the material for exposure, until they can encounter all memories or situations without becoming upset.

Another CBT approach, anxiety management training (AMT), involves teaching patients skills to control their anxiety, and has also been helpful with PTSD. Stress inoculation training (SIT), the AMT program that has received the most attention, was developed for victims who remained highly fearful 3 months after being raped.[23] SIT typically consists of education and training of coping skills. These skills include deep muscle relaxation training, breathing control, role-playing, covert modeling, thought-stopping, and guided self-dialogue following SIT. The idea is that sufferers of PTSD experience a great deal of anxiety in their lives because they are frequently reminded of the trauma. Very often, when they become anxious, this is a cue for them to feel they are in danger and thus to become even more scared. SIT aims to teach skills to help decrease this anxiety in many different situations, to help 'take the edge off'.

Exposure therapy

The efficacy of exposure treatment for PTSD was first demonstrated with several case reports on war veterans.[24–26] Both flooding in imagination[27] and flooding in vivo to trauma-related events[25] appeared to be therapeutic. Most of these treatments also included additional techniques, such as anger control or relaxation training.

Only three controlled studies have examined the utility of prolonged imaginal exposure (PE) for reducing PTSD and related pathology in male Vietnam veterans. Treatment was conducted over 6–16 sessions. In one study, all patients received the 'standard' PTSD treatment (weekly individual and group therapies) in addition to exposure.[28] In the second study,[27] PE was compared to a waiting list control group. During each session, patients were initially instructed to relax. The patients subsequently received 45 minutes of imaginal flooding, followed by relaxation. In the third study, all patients received a group treatment milieu program; one-half received additional PE and the remaining patients received weekly individual traditional psychotherapy.[29,30]

All three studies found some benefit from the PE compared to the control groups, but the effects were small. In the Cooper and Clum[28] study, PE improved the PTSD symptoms, but had little effect on depression or trait anxiety. A mixed picture emerged from the Keane et al[27] study: therapists rated exposure patients as more improved on PTSD symptoms than control subjects, but on self-report measures of these symptoms, no differences were detected. However, exposure patients did rate themselves as more improved on general psychopathology measures than did those in the wait list control. Boudewyns and Hyer[29] found no group differences on psychophysiological measures, but at the 3-month follow-up, the exposure group improved more on the Veterans Adjustment Scale (VAS). Regardless of treatment, a positive relationship was found between psychophysiological reduction to combat-related stimuli following treatment and improvement on the VAS. In further analysis of the data with additional patients, a slight superiority emerged for the exposure group. A higher percentage of the exposure-treated patients were classified as successes when compared with those receiving traditional therapy.[30] An uncontrolled report found that flooding benefited Vietnam veterans with PTSD only on avoidance symptoms as measured by the IES and self-recorded number of daily intrusions.[31]

The first controlled study of the treatment of PTSD in rape victims randomly assigned PTSD rape victims to one of four conditions: stress inoculation training (SIT), prolonged exposure (PE), supportive counseling (SC), or waiting list control (WL). Exposure treatment consisted of nine biweekly individual sessions. The first two sessions were devoted to information-gathering, explaining the treatment rationale, and treatment-planning including the construction of a hierarchy of feared situations for in vivo exposure. During the remaining sessions, victims were instructed to relive in imagination their traumatic experiences and describe it aloud 'as if it were happening now'. Exposure continued for about 60 minutes and was tape-recorded so that victims could practice imaginal exposure as homework by listening to the tape. Also for homework, victims were instructed to approach feared situations or objects that were realistically safe. Detailed instructions for conducting exposure therapy with PTSD patients can be found in Foa and Rothbaum.[19]

SIT began with information regarding the assault and the victim's history gathered in session 1, followed by brief breathing retraining to alleviate anxiety aroused by the discussion of the assault. The rationale for treatment was explained in session 2, and coping skills were taught in sessions 3–9. Skills were applied first to a non-assault-related example, and then to an assault-related example. Supportive counseling focused on assisting patients in solving daily problems which may or may not be assault-related. Discussion of the assault itself was largely avoided because such discussions were viewed as a form of exposure. Patients were redirected to 'here and now' issues when they began discussing the assault. Patients were taught problem-solving, and therapists engaged in active listening and support. Victims in the waiting list condition were assessed at the same 5-week intervals as the treated victims and were contacted by phone in between to maintain contact.

Treatments were delivered in nine biweekly 90-minute individual sessions. All conditions produced improvement on all measures immediately post-treatment and at follow-up. SIT produced significantly more improvement on PTSD symptoms than WL immediately following treatment. At follow-up, PE produced superior outcome on PTSD symptoms. Clients who received PE continued to improve after treatment termination, whereas clients in the SIT and SC conditions evidenced no change between post-treatment and follow-up.[32] The exposure technique studied has proven successful even in cases complicated by other diagnoses such as conversion mutism.[33]

A second study compared PE, SIT, the combination of SIT and PE, and a waiting list control group.[34] All three active treatments showed significant improvement in PTSD symptoms and depressive symptoms at post-test, and the waiting list group did not improve. These treatment effects were maintained at 6-month follow-up. On most outcome measures PE was more effective than the other two treatments, although this difference did not always reach significance. An examination of patients who achieved good end-state functioning showed that 21% of patients in SIT, 46% of patients in PE, and 32% of patients in SIT/PE achieved this goal at post-treatment. At 6-month follow-up, 75% of patients in PE, 68% of patients in SIT, and 50% of patients in SIT/PE lost the PTSD diagnosis, whereas all waiting list patients retained the diagnosis. The hypothesis that the combined treatment would be superior was not supported. The authors suggested that these results may be due to the fact the clients in that condition actually received less prolonged imaginal exposure and SIT training than participants in the individual treatments as treatment sessions were all equal in length. In a third study,[35] 9–12 weekly sessions of PE alone were compared to PE combined with cognitive restructuring. Preliminary results indicated that both treatments were highly effective, but PE alone was more efficient. More than half the clients in that group achieved over 70% improvement on PTSD symptoms after 9 sessions; only 15% of the combined group achieved that status after 9 sessions, the remaining required 3 additional sessions to arrive at the same outcome.[35] Versions of the PE program have been helpful in preventing the development of chronic PTSD following rape[36] and in treating PTSD in abused children.[37]

Additional studies also provide support for the efficacy of exposure treatment for PTSD in samples heterogeneous with regard to their traumas. Richards et al[38] treated 14 participants with PTSD with either four sessions of imaginal exposure followed by four sessions of in vivo exposure, or in vivo followed by imaginal exposure. Patients in both treatment conditions improved considerably. The authors noted that the percentage of symptom reduction of 65–80% seen in this study is much higher than those of most treatment studies for other anxiety disorders. Also, at post-treatment and at 1-year follow-up, no patients met criteria for PTSD. The only notable difference between the two exposure types was in the area of phobic avoidance, on which in vivo exposure appeared to be more effective regardless of the order in which it was presented. In another study of outpatients with PTSD resulting from a variety of traumas,[39] exposure, cognitive therapy, and exposure plus cognitive therapy combination were all equally successful in reducing PTSD at post-treatment and 6-month follow-up. All three treatments were more effective than relaxation.

Exposure treatment was efficacious in an open trial of eight weekly sessions of imaginal and in vivo exposure with 23 traumatized individuals with PTSD.[40] Participants improved significantly on a variety of measures at post-treatment, with reductions of 42% on the IES, 61% on a measure of general health (General Health Questionnaire), 38% on a general symptom checklist (the Symptom Checklist-90, or SCL-90), and 35% on the Clinician-Administered PTSD Scale (CAPS).

Exposure therapy was compared to cognitive therapy in a mixed sample of trauma survivors.[41] Type of trauma included crime

(52%), accident (34%), and other (15%). There was a significant improvement on all measures at post-treatment, which was maintained at follow-up for both treatments, with no significant differences between the two treatments.

A new medium for conducting exposure therapy has been introduced. Virtual reality exposure (VRE) presents the user with a computer-generated view of a virtual world that changes in a natural way with head motion. During VRE sessions patients wear the head-mounted display with stereo earphones that provide visual and audio cues consistent with being in a 'virtual Vietnam'. Patients in one investigation are exposed to two virtual environments, a virtual Huey helicopter flying over a virtual Vietnam and a clearing surrounded by jungle. In this way, patients are repeatedly exposed to their most traumatic memories but immersed in Vietnam stimuli. The results of the first patient to complete the virtual Vietnam treatment indicate preliminary success.[42] The subject was an unemployed 50-year-old Caucasian male on 100% Veterans Administration (VA) compensation who served in Vietnam 26 years prior to the onset of this study as a helicopter pilot. He met criteria for current PTSD, current major depressive disorder, and past alcohol abuse. Treatment was delivered in 14 90-minute individual sessions conducted twice weekly over 7 weeks. Scores on all measures decreased from pre- to post-treatment. No statistical analyses were incorporated since this was a single subject. The following symptom measures decreased at least 30%: CAPS total (34%), CAPS reexperiencing (61%), CAPS arousal (36%), IES total (45%), IES intrusion (42%), IES avoidance (50%), and Spielberger-state anger (63%).

The results from the studies discussed above consistently support the efficacy of imaginal and in vivo exposure for the treatment of PTSD resulting from a variety of traumas. These results are even more impressive given the methodological precision that was applied to many of these studies.

Anxiety management techniques (AMT)

Of the various AMT programs, stress inoculation training (SIT),[43] developed for rape victims with chronic fear and anxiety, has received the most attention. The efficacy of SIT has been supported by several reports from Veronen, Kilpatrick and their colleagues and others.[32,44]

In an uncontrolled investigation, a clear treatment effect emerged on rape-related fear, anxiety, phobic anxiety, tension, and depression in female rape victims who showed elevated fear and avoidance to phobic stimuli 3 months post-rape.[23] A later study was designed to compare 10 sessions each of SIT, peer counseling and SD.[23] Victims were permitted to select their treatment and the vast majority opted for SIT, few chose peer counseling, and none chose SD, which precluded statistical analyses. The authors reported noticeable improvement from pre- to post-treatment on most measures for the SIT completers. Case studies of rape victims treated with SIT or its variant also indicated positive results.[45]

In a controlled study, the efficacy of six 2-hour sessions of three types of group therapy for rape-related fear and anxiety were compared to a naturally occurring waiting list control group, including SIT, assertion training, or supportive psychotherapy plus information.[44] SIT was similar to that described by Kilpatrick et al[43] with two exceptions: (a) cognitive restructuring, assertiveness training, and role-play were excluded since they were used in the comparative treatment; and (b) exposure in vivo was added to the application phase. Results indicated that all three treatments were highly effective in reducing rape-related fears, intrusion, and avoidance symptoms, with no group differences evident, whereas no improvements were found in the waiting list control group. Improvement was maintained at 6-month follow-up on rape-related fear measures, but not on depression, self-esteem, and social fears.

A controlled study compared three different forms of relaxation for 90 Vietnam veterans.[46] Relaxation, relaxation plus deep breathing exercises, and relaxation plus deep breathing plus biofeedback were equally, but only mildly, effective in leading to improvement. The effects of cognitive therapy and systematic desensitization (SD) were studied in rape victims, some of whom entered treatment an average of 2 weeks after their assault.[47,48] Ratings of fear, anxiety, depression, and social adjustment all showed significant gains for both cognitive therapy and SD.

In summary, SIT has received the most support for PTSD. Other AMTs such as relaxation or cognitive therapy are best viewed as treatment components of a comprehensive treatment package.

Systematic desensitization

Some of the earliest studies of behavioral treatments for PTSD adopted the systematic desensitization (SD) technique pioneered by Wolpe.[49] Although participants in these studies showed improvement in post-trauma symptoms, methodological problems plagued each of these studies, rendering the results inconclusive. An exception was the Brom et al[2] study described in detail in the section on hypnotherapy and psychodynamic therapy. In this study, patients in the desensitization condition showed a mean improvement of 41% on the IES, which was higher than the other treatments examined, although the difference did not reach statistical significance. In light of the methodological problems with the resulting lack of strong conclusions to be drawn, SD will be reviewed very briefly below.

The successful outcome of SD compared to a no-treatment control group was demonstrated in two studies with war veterans using psychophysiological measures (electromyography and heart rate),[50,51] but the treatment required a large number of sessions over an extended period of time and PTSD was not assessed. Thirteen to 18 sessions of SD with the last two sessions spent in in vivo exposure were used successfully with three automobile accident victims.[52] Several uncontrolled studies demonstrated that SD was effective with rape victims in reducing fear, anxiety, depression, and social maladjustment.[48,53,54] However, SD alone was not successful in one case study of a rape victim.[55]

In summary, several studies examined the effects of SD with a variety of trauma victims, most showing some beneficial results. However, the lack of adequate control conditions and/or the absence of PTSD diagnoses and measures in some of the studies limit the conclusions that can be drawn from them. With the empirical finding that relaxation during confrontation with feared material was not necessary, and with evidence for the inferiority of SD to flooding in most anxiety disorders, the use of SD for anxiety disorders including PTSD was largely abandoned. In its place, researchers and clinicians have used a variety of imaginal and in vivo exposure techniques.

Combined treatment programs

A modified version of Foa et al's SIT/PE combination program was adopted to treat 10 motor vehicle accident (MVA) victims.[56] The modification consisted of the addition of pleasurable activity scheduling and discussion of existential issues. Results of this study suggest that the nine to 12 sessions of combined treatment reduced PTSD symptoms by 68% on the CAPS.

A comprehensive treatment package was studied in an uncontrolled investigation.[57] The treatment, trauma management therapy, consisted of education, individual exposure therapy including the 'core fear', programmed practice of the exposure, and social and emotional rehabilitation (SER). SER was conducted in a group format and consisted of social skills training, anger management, and veterans' issues management. Fifteen male Vietnam combat veterans with PTSD were entered, and 11 completed 29 treatment sessions over 17 weeks. Results indicated significant improvements from pre- to post-treatment on the Clinical Global Impressions (CGI), Hamilton Rating Scale for Anxiety, heart rate reactivity to traumatic cues, total hours of sleep, number of social activities, frequency of nightmares, and trends towards significant improvement on the CAPS and flashbacks. There was no significant improvement noted on self-report measures including the Beck Depression Inventory, Social Phobia and Anxiety Inventory, or the Spielberger Anger Expression Inventory.

A quasi-experimental design tested a combination therapy for rape victims with PTSD.[58] Nineteen female sexual assault survivors received cognitive processing therapy (CPT) over 12 weekly sessions in a group format. CPT includes education, exposure via writing about the assault and sharing it in a group, and cognitive restructuring components and is based on an information processing theory of PTSD. Treated participants were not randomly assigned but rather were compared to a naturally occurring waiting list control group. Results were very encouraging for the efficacy of CPT in this population. CPT subjects improved significantly from pre- to post-treatment on PTSD and depression ratings and maintained their improvement throughout the 6-month follow-up period. The waiting list subjects evidenced no change during a comparable 12-week period.

In a later report with a larger sample, Resick[59] reported that of the 66 women who completed CPT, 97% met full criteria for PTSD at pre-treatment, and of these only 12% met criteria for PTSD at post-treatment. Fifty-three women completed a 6-month follow-up and only 11% met criteria for PTSD. At pre-treatment, 52% met criteria for major depression. At post-treatment, only 12.5% were still depressed. At the 6-month follow-up, 8% were depressed.

In a preliminary report of a controlled trial comparing CPT, PE, and waiting list control groups, Resick et al[60] reported that female sexual assault survivors who received CPT (n=29) or PE (n=26) were significantly more improved than the waiting list control (n= 29) group from pre- to post-treatment on PTSD and depressive symptomatology. CPT and PE were equally effective in reducing PTSD.

Another study testing a combination treatment approach compared self-exposure plus cognitive restructuring to progressive relaxation training in 20 female sexual assault survivors.[61] Results indicated a superiority at post-treatment and follow-up for the participants treated with exposure plus cognitive restructuring.

Eye movement desensitization and reprocessing

Eye movement desensitization and reprocessing (EMDR)[62] is a form of exposure (desensitization) accompanied by saccadic eye movements. Briefly, the technique involves the patient's imagining a scene from the trauma, focusing on the accompanying cognition and arousal, while the therapist waves two fingers across the client's visual field and instructs the client to track the fingers. The sequence is repeated until anxiety decreases, at which point the patient is instructed to generate a more adaptive thought and to associate it with the scene while moving his/her eyes. After each session patients indicate their subjective units of discomfort (SUDS) level and their degree of belief in a positive cognition (validity of cognition; VOC).

A number of case studies have reported positive findings with EMDR (for a comprehensive review, see Lohr et al[63]). In the first study of EMDR, Shapiro[64] randomly assigned trauma victims to either one session of EMDR or an exposure control condition (EMDR without the eye movements). The results showed that clients who received EMDR reported lower SUDS ratings after the one session of EMDR than did clients in the exposure control condition, but lack of methodological rigor makes this finding difficult to interpret.

Combat veterans were randomly assigned to two 90-minute EMDR sessions, an exposure control (EC; EMDR without the eye movements), both as an adjunct to standard milieu treatment for veterans with PTSD, or standard milieu treatment alone.[65] SUDS ratings to traumatic stimuli were lower in the EMDR group and therapists rated more patients as responders in the EMDR versus EC group. However, the three groups did not differ in their lack of response as seen on standardized self-report measures, interviews of PTSD, or on physiological responses. Jensen[66] randomly assigned 74 veterans with PTSD to either three sessions of EMDR conducted over 10 days or to a control condition of standard VA services. Neither group improved on the PTSD severity measure. SUDS ratings decreased in the EMDR group but not in controls. Silver et al[67] compared standard milieu treatment with milieu treatment plus EMDR, biofeedback, or group relaxation training in a sample of 100 veterans with PTSD. Results indicated that EMDR led to greater reduction of symptoms relative to the control and the biofeedback groups, but as the study was uncontrolled, the strength of the findings is limited.

In a study addressing the role of eye movement, Pitman et al[68] compared EMDR with and without the eye movement component in a crossover design with 17 male veterans diagnosed with PTSD. Patients were randomly assigned to the two conditions. The results of this methodologically vigorous study indicated that both treatments effected modest improvement in symptoms as measured by the IES, but not on the independent assessment. In contrast to expectations, on the IES, there was slightly more improvement in the eyes-fixed condition than from EMDR.

Twenty-three trauma victims received either standard EMDR or one of two variations: an EMDR analog in which eye movements were induced by a flashing light rather than a waving finger, and an analog in which a light blinked only in the center of the visual field.[69] The groups did not differ on physiological measures, SUDS or the VOC. No analyses on PTSD severity were reported, but following treatment, only five of the 23 participants met criteria for PTSD. Using a sample of 36 victims of heterogeneous traumas, Vaughan et al[70] compared EMDR with imagery habituation training (IHT), a procedure that involved repeated presentation of traumatic stimuli in the form of an oral scenario, and applied muscle relaxation training. The authors concluded that all three groups were equally improved on the independent assessors' rating of PTSD. Wilson et al[71] compared EMDR to a delayed-treatment condition in a mixed sample of traumatized individuals, about half of whom had PTSD. Overall, patients in the EMDR group reported decreases in presenting complaints and in anxiety, and increases in positive cognitions at post-treatment, whereas the waiting list group reported no improvement.

A well-controlled study on the efficacy of EMDR was conducted by Rothbaum,[72] who randomized 21 female victims of rape to either EMDR or a waiting list control group. Measures consisted of standardized self-report and interview instruments, with the interviews conducted by a blind evaluator. Treatment consisted of four weekly sessions conducted by a well-trained clinician, and treatment adherence was monitored and deemed acceptable by an independent evaluator designated by EMDR's originator. EMDR led to improvement on PTSD symptoms on both interview (57% reduction in symptom severity) and IES (74% reduction), and gains were maintained at a 3-month follow-up. These reductions were significantly different from the control group, who evidenced no change in symptoms.

In a comparison study, participants were randomly assigned to either routine clinical care, 12 sessions of biofeedback-assisted relaxation, or 12 sessions of EMDR.[73] At post-treatment and at a 3-month follow-up, the EMDR-treated participants were more improved on self-report, psychometric, and standardized measures. However, there were no differences on psychophysiological measures. EMDR was compared to general outpatient treatment in a managed care organization (HMO).[74] On measures of PTSD, depression, and anxiety, EMDR was superior.

In one of the best-controlled studies involving EMDR to date, a course of nine sessions of EMDR was compared to nine sessions of a CBT treatment consisting of prolonged imaginal exposure, stress inoculation training, and cognitive therapy.[75] The results indicated that CBT was superior to EMDR at post-treatment and 1-year follow-up.

In summary, several studies report beneficial effects of EMDR, although other studies report equivocal findings with EMDR not resulting in significant improvements over control conditions or comparison treatments, especially on blind standardized PTSD measures.

Summary and conclusions

Reports on the efficacy of psychodynamic interventions on post-trauma problems are equivocal: some report negative results, and others are more optimistic, but the majority of the reports are not well controlled. In view of the fact that these interventions are widely employed with trauma victims, it is imperative that their efficacy will be examined in well-controlled studies.

Overall, the most controlled studies have been conducted on cognitive behavioral treatments. These studies demonstrate that techniques such as prolonged exposure procedures, stress inoculation training, and cognitive processing therapy are effective in reducing symptoms of PTSD. Systematic desensitization has largely been abandoned in favor of pure exposure techniques. Relaxation and cognitive therapy are best viewed as treatment components rather than stand-alone treatments. Many of the studies examining EMDR have methodological flaws and the results are mixed. Contrary to clinical intuition, there is no evidence indicating the superiority of programs that combine different cognitive behavioral techniques.

References

1. Spiegel, D, Hypnosis in the treatment of victims of sexual abuse, *Psychiatr Clin North Am* (1989) 12:295–305.
2. Brom D, Kleber RJ, Defares PB, Brief psychotherapy for posttraumatic stress disorders, *J Consult Clin Psychol* (1989) 57:607–12.
3. Horowitz MJ, Wilner N, Alvarez W, Impact of event scale: a measure of subjective distress, *Psychosom Med* (1979) 41:207–18.
4. Burgess AW, Holmstrom LL, The rape trauma syndrome, *Am J Psychiatry* (1974) 131:981–6.
5. Evans HI, Psychotherapy for the rape victim: some treatment models, *Hosp Community Psychiatry* (1978) 29:309–12.
6. Fox SS, Scherl DJ, Crisis intervention with victims of rape, *Soc Work* (1972) 17:37–42.
7. Horowitz MJ, *Stress-Response Syndromes* (Jason Aronson: Northvale, NJ, 1976).
8. Yalom I, *The Theory and Practice of Group Psychotherapy*, 4th edn (Basic: New York, 1995).
9. Grigsby JP, The use of imagery in the treatment of posttraumatic stress disorder, *J Nerv Ment Dis* (1987) 175:55–9.
10. Bart P, Unalienating abortion, demystifying depression, and restoring rape victims. Paper presented at the 128th Annual Meeting of the American Psychiatric Association, Anaheim, CA, May 1975.
11. Cryer L, Beutler L, Group therapy: an alternative treatment approach for rape victims, *J Sex Marital Ther* (1980) 6:40–6.
12. Lindy JD, Green BL, Grace M, Titchener J, Psychotherapy with survivors of the Beverly Hills Supper Club fire, *Am J Psychother* (1983) 4:593–610.
13. Marmar CR, Horowitz MJ, Weiss DS et al, A controlled trial of brief psychotherapy and mutual-help group treatment of conjugal bereavement, *Am J Psychiatry* (1998) 145:209–209.
14. Scarvalone P, Cloitre M, Difede J, Interpersonal process therapy for incest survivors: preliminary outcome data. Paper presented at the Society for Psychotherapy Research, Vancouver, British Columbia, 1995.
15. Courtois C, *Healing the Incest Wound: Adult Survivors in Therapy* (W.W. Norton: New York, 1988).
16. Rothbaum BO, Meadows EA, Resick P, Foy DW, Cognitive-behavioral treatment position paper for the ISTSS Treatment Guidelines Committee, unpublished manuscript.
17. Solomon SD, Gerrity ET, Muff AM, Efficacy of treatments for posttraumatic stress disorder, *JAMA* (1992) 268:633–8.
18. Van Etten ML, Taylor S, Comparative efficacy of treatments for posttraumatic stress disorder: a meta-analysis, *Clin Psychol Psychother* (1998)5:126–45.
19. Foa EB, Rothbaum BO, *Treating the Trauma of Rape: A Cognitive-Behavioral Therapy for PTSD* (Guilford: New York, 1998).
20. Foa EB, Kozak MJ, Emotional processing of fear: exposure to corrective information, *Psychol Bull* (1986) 99:20–35.
21. Foa EB, Steketee G, Rothbaum BO, Behavioral/cognitive conceptualizations of post-traumatic stress disorder, *Behavior Therapy* (1989) 20:155–76.
22. Resick PA, Schnicke MK, *Cognitive Processing Therapy for Rape Victims: A Treatment Manual* (Sage: Newbury Park, 1993).
23. Veronen LJ, Kilpatrick DG, Stress management for rape victims. In: Meichenbaum D, Jaremko ME, eds, *Stress Reduction and Prevention* (Plenum: New York, 1983).
24. Fairbank JA, Gross RT, Keane TM, Treatment of posttraumatic stress disorder: evaluation of outcome with a behavioral code, *Behav Modif* (1983) 7:557–68.
25. Johnson CH, Gilmore JD, Shenoy RZ, Use of a feeding procedure in the treatment of a stress-related anxiety disorder, *J Behav Ther Exp Psychiatry* (1982) 13:235–7.
26. Keane TM, Kaloupek DG, Imaginal flooding in the treatment of post-traumatic stress disorder, *J Consult Clin Psychol* (1982) 50:138–40.
27. Keane TM, Fairbank JA, Caddell JM, Zimering RT, Implosive (flooding) therapy reduces symptoms of PTSD in Vietnam combat veterans, *Behavior Therapy*, (1989) 20:245–60.
28. Cooper NA, Clum GA, Imaginal flooding as a supplementary treatment for PTSD in combat veterans: a controlled study, *Behavior Therapy* (1989) 3:381–91.
29. Boudewyns PA, Hyer L, Physiological response to combat memories and preliminary treatment outcome in Vietnam veterans PTSD patients treated with direct therapeutic exposure, *Behavior Therapy* (1990) 21:63–87.

30. Boudewyns PA, Hyer, L, Woods MG et al, PTSD among Vietnam veterans: an early look at treatment outcome using direct therapeutic exposure, *J Trauma Stress* (1990) 3:359–68.
31. Pitman RK, Orr SP, Altman B, Longpre RE, Emotional processing and outcome of imaginal flooding therapy in Vietnam veterans with chronic posttraumatic stress disorder, *Compr Psychiatry* (1996) 37:409–18.
32. Foa EB, Rothbaum BO, Riggs D, Murdock T, Treatment of post-traumatic stress disorder in rape victims: a comparison between cognitive-behavioral procedures and counseling, *J Consult Clin Psychol* (1991) 59:715–23.
33. Rothbaum BO, Foa EB, Exposure treatment of PTSD concomitant with conversion mutism: a case study, *Behavior Therapy* (1991) 22:449–56.
34. Foa EB, Dancu CV, Hembree EA, et al A comparison of Exposure therapy, stress inoculation training and their combination in ameliorating PTSD in female assault victims *J Consult Clin Psychol* (1999)67:194–200.
35. Foa 1998 (personal communication)
36. Foa EB, Hearst-Ikeda D, Perry KJ, Evaluation of a brief cognitive-behavioral program for the prevention of chronic PTSD in recent assault victims, *J Consult Clin Psychol* (1995) 63:948–55.
37. Deblinger E, McLeer SV, Henry D, Cognitive behavioral treatment for sexually abused children suffering from post-traumatic stress: preliminary findings, *J Am Acad Child Adolesc Psychiatry* (1990) 29.747–52.
38. Richards DA, Lovell K, Marks IM, Post-traumatic stress disorder: evaluation of a behavioral treatment program, *J Trauma Stress* (1994) 7:669–80.
39. Marks I, Lovell K, Noshirvani H et al, Treatment of post-traumatic stress disorder by exposure and/or cognitive restructuring: a controlled study, *Arch Gen Psychiatry* (1998) 55:317–25.
40. Thompson JA, Charlton PFC, Kerry R et al, An open trial of exposure therapy based on deconditioning for post-traumatic stress disorder, *Br J Clin Psychol* (1995) 34:407–16.
41. Tarrier N, Pilgrim H, Sommerfield C et al, A randomised trial of cognitive therapy and imaginal exposure in the treatment of chronic post traumatic stress disorder, *J Consult Clin Psychol* (1999)67:13–18.
42. Rothbaum, BO, Hodges L, Alarcon R et al, Virtual Vietnam: a virtual environment for the treatment of Vietnam war veterans with post-traumatic stress disorder. Paper presented at the Lake George Research Conference on Posttraumatic Stress Disorder, Lake George, NY, 1998.
43. Kilpatrick DG, Veronen LJ, Resick PA, Psychological sequelae to rape: assessment and treatment strategies. In: Dolays DM, Meredith RL, eds, *Behavioral Medicine: Assessment and Treatment Strategies* (Plenum: New York, 1982) 473–97.
44. Resick PA, Jordan CG, Girelli, SA et al, A comparative victim study of behavioral group therapy for sexual assault victims, *Behavior Therapy* (1988) 19:385–401.
45. Pearson MA, Poquette BM, Wasden RE, Stress inoculation and the treatment of post-rape trauma: a case report, *The Behavior Therapist* (1983) 6:58–9.
46. Watson CG, Tuorila JR, Vickers KS et al, The efficacies of three relaxation regiments in the treatment of PTSD in Vietnam war veterans, *J Clin Psychol* (1997) 53:917–23.
47. Frank E, Anderson B, Stewart BD et al, Efficacy of cognitive behavior therapy and systematic desensitization in the treatment of rape trauma, *Behavior Therapy* (1988) 19:403–20.
48. Frank E, Stewart BD, Depressive symptoms in rape victims, *J Affect Disord* (1984) 1:269–77.
49. Wolpe J, *Psychotherapy by Reciprocal Inhibition* (Stanford University Press: Stanford, CA, 1988).
50. Bowen GR, Lambert JA, Systematic desensitization therapy with post-traumatic stress disorder cases. In: Figley CR, ed, *Trauma and its Wake*, vol 2 (Brunner/Mazel: New York, 1986) 280–91.
51. Peniston EG, EMG biofeedback-assisted desensitization treatment for Vietnam combat veterans' post-traumatic stress disorder, *Clinical Biofeedback Health* (1986) 9:35–41.
52. Muse M, Stress-related, posttraumatic chronic pain syndrome: behavioral treatment approach, *Pain* (1986) 25:389–94.
53. Frank E, Stewart BD, Treating depression in victims of rape, *The Clinical Psychologist* (1983) 8:65–74.
54. Turner SM, Systematic desensitization of fears and anxiety in rape victims. Paper presented at the Association for the Advancement of Behavior Therapy, San Francisco, CA, 1979.
55. Becker JV, Abel GG, Behavioral treatment of victims of sexual assault. In: Turner SM, Calhoun KS, Adams HE, eds, *Handbook of Clinical Behavior Therapy* (Wiley: New York, 1981) 347–79.

56. Hickling EJ, Blanchard EB, The private practice psychologist and manual-based treatments: post-traumatic stress disorder secondary to motor vehicle accidents, *Behav Res Ther* (1997) 35:191–203.
57. Frueh BC, Turner SM, Beidel DC, et al, Trauma management therapy: a preliminary evaluation of a multicomponent behavioral treatment for chronic combat-related PTSD, *Behav Res Ther* (1996) 34:533–43.
58. Resick PA, Schnicke MK, Cognitive processing therapy for sexual assault victims, *J Consult Clin Psychol* (1992) **60**:748–56.
59. Resick PA (1994, September). Does prior history of victimization affect rape therapy outcome? Paper presented at the Research Workshop on Violence in the Lives of Women: Impact and Treatment. NIMH, Washington, DC.
60. Resick PA, Nishith P, Astin M, A controlled trial comparing cognitive processing therapy and prolonged exposure: preliminary findings. Paper presented at the Lake George Research Conference on Posttraumatic Stress Disorder, Lake George, NY, March 1998.
61. Echeburua E, de Corral P, Zubizarreta I, Sarasua B, Psychological treatment of chronic posttraumatic stress disorder in victims of sexual aggression, *Behav Modif* (1997) **21**:433–56.
62. Shapiro F, *Eye Movement Desensitization and Reprocessing: Basic Protocols, Principles, and Procedures* (Guilford: New York, 1996).
63. Lohr JM, Tolin DF, Lilienfeld SO, Efficacy of eye movement desensitization and reprocessing: implications for behavior therapy, *Behavior Therapy* (1998) **29**:123–56.
64. Shapiro F, Efficacy of the eye movement desensitization procedure in the treatment of traumatic memories, *J Trauma Stress* (1989) 2:199–223.
65. Boudewyns PA, Stwertka SA, Hyer, LA et al, Eye movement desensitization for PTSD of combat: a treatment outcome pilot study, *The Behavior Therapist* (1993) **16**:29–33.
66. Jensen JA, An investigation of eye movement desensitization and reprocessing (EMD/R) as a treatment for posttraumatic stress disorder (PTSD) symptoms of Vietnam combat veterans, *Behav Ther* **25**:311–25.
67. Silver SM, Brooks A, Obenchain J, Treatment of Vietnam war veterans with PTSD: a comparison of eye movement desensitization and reprocessing, biofeedback, and relaxation training, *J Trauma Stress* (1995) **8**:337–42.
68. Pitman RK, Orr SP, Altman B et al Emotional processing during eye movement desensitization and reprocessing (EMDR) therapy of Vietnam veterans with post-traumatic stress disorder. *Compr Psych* (1996) 37: 419–29.
69. Renfrey G, Spates CR, Eye movement desensitization and reprocessing: a partial dismantling procedure, *J Behav Ther Exp Psychiatry* (1994) **25**:231–9.
70. Vaughan K, Armstrong MF, Gold, R et al, A trial of eye movement desensitization compared to image habituation training and applied muscle relaxation in post-traumatic stress disorder, *J Behav Ther Exp Psychiatry* (1995) **25**:283–91.
71. Wilson SA, Becker, LA, Tinker RH, Eye movement desensitization and reprocessing (EMDR) treatment for psychologically traumatized individuals, *J Consult Clin Psychol* (1995) **63**:928–37.
72. Rothbaum BO, A controlled study of eye movement desensitization and reprocessing in the treatment of posttraumatic stress disordered sexual assault victims, *Bull Menninger Clin* (1997)**61**:317–34.
73. Carlson JG, Chemtob CM, Rusnak K et al, Eye movement desensitization and reprocessing (EMDR) treatment for combat-related Posttraumatic Stress Disorder, *J Trauma Stress*, (1998) **11**:3–24.
74. Marcus SV, Marquis P, Sakai C, Controlled study of treatment of PTSD using EMDR in an HMO setting, *Psychotherapy* (1997) **34**:307–15.
75. Devilly GJ, Spence SH, The relative efficacy and treatment distress of EMDR and a cognitive behavioral treatment protocol in the amelioration of Post Traumatic Stress Disorder, *J Anxiety Disord* (1999)**13**:131–57.

8

Psychological debriefing

Martin Deahl

A variety of techniques have been employed to reduce the incidence of post-traumatic stress disorder (PTSD). *Primary prevention* includes the selection, preparation and training of individuals likely to be exposed to potentially traumatizing events. These strategies are described in the disparate literature and language of several different medical and non-medical disciplines but lack a credible evidence-base to support their effectiveness. *Secondary prevention* comprises a variety of brief psychological techniques immediately or shortly after traumatizing life events. Secondary preventative strategies are widely employed in civilian and military practice and comprise various forms of brief counselling as well as more specific psychological interventions of which the most widely known is psychological debriefing (PD) or 'critical incident stress debriefing' (CISD).[1,2] *Tertiary* interventions are the treatments of establihed PTSD. These are far from satisfactory, particularly once the disorder has become chronic, and a variety of psychological and pharmacological interventions used separately or in combination often produce only partial symptom relief.[3–5] Less attention has been paid to the effectiveness of secondary strategies designed to prevent or minimize post-traumatic morbidity which have only relatively recently been subject to critical evaluation.

More than two-thirds of the population at some point in their lives are exposed to potentially traumatizing events of sufficient severity to meet the 'stressor' criterion for current PTSD diagnostic criteria.[6] The point prevalence of clinically significant PTSD in the general population is at least 1–2%.[7] The victims of accidents, terrorist outrage,[8] disasters[9,10] and personal tragedy such as torture or rape[11] are all equally vulnerable to PTSD. Unfortunately, many of these receive little or no psychological support, particularly when serious physical injuries are also present, since these deflect attention from psychological problems and take precedence, particularly on a busy trauma unit.

Certain 'high-risk' occupations are also associated with an increased incidence of serious and sometimes disabling psychological and psychiatric symptoms, including PTSD, although it is only recently that employers (often only following the threat of litigation) have taken an interest in providing psychological support to their workforce. In combat veterans the prevalence of PTSD has been reported to exceed 31%.[12] Following serious accidents and disasters PTSD prevalence figures as high as 30% or more have been reported in observers and rescuers alike.[9,10,13] The handling and identification of human remains is particularly likely to be associated with subsequent psychological morbidity[14,15] and is recognized as a stressor that 'can make victims of rescuers' (Figure 8.1).[16] Significant psychological morbidity has also been reported in 'second-line' support workers such as administrators, control room and reception staff, switchboard operators, hospital ancillary and volunteer workers, as well as the families of servicemen and emergency service personnel.[17] The witnesses of conflict and disaster including aid workers, journalists and other members of the media all suffer from a high incidence of PTSD, yet frequently receive little or no psychological support following traumatic events.

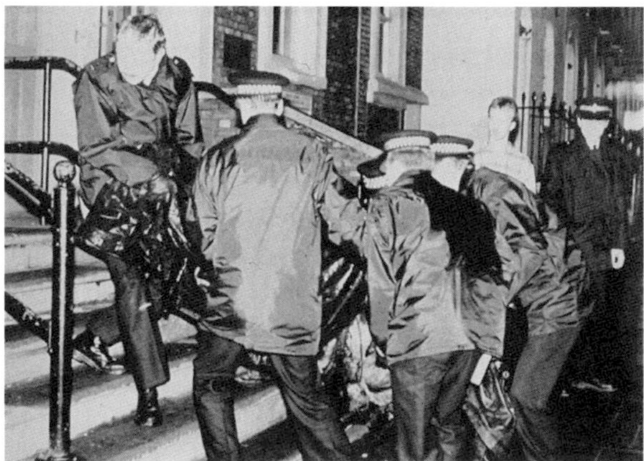

Figure 8.1. Body handling is a stressor that can make victims of rescuers.

Preventing PTSD in these 'high-risk' groups has important implications for employers and occupational health physicians. Organizations which routinely send their employees into potentially traumatizing situations have a statutory 'duty of care' to protect the health of employees and minimize the impact of occupational health hazards to which employees may be exposed. Identifying effective techniques to minimize long-term psychological sequelae is an important but neglected area of occupational medicine which improves the health of the workforce as well as discharging the employer's duty of care under occupational health legislation. Recent litigation has arisen not because workers have suffered PTSD per se, but because their employers have been negligent in failing to minimize the risk of exposure to trauma and to detect or offer treatment for psychiatric disorder which has developed as a result of workplace exposure.

The importance of debriefing

Efforts to minimize long-term psychiatric morbidity following traumatic events have resulted in calls for the routine provision of early psychological intervention for the victims of trauma. These calls are based on the assumption that the earlier intervention occurs the less opportunity there is for maladaptive and disruptive cognitive and behavioural patterns to become established.[18] Early interventions are intuitively appealing and a response to perceived need, but whether or not they work is unclear.

The place of preventive strategies, particularly in disaster planning, has become extrememly controversial. Moreover, psychological trauma is newsworthy. The media regularly expose the public to the images of accident, disaster and conflict, as well as often controversial litigation in which victims and rescuers seek compensation following traumatic events. Disaster entertains and media attention is heightened by public curiosity and a fascination with the 'human interest' story. When disaster strikes it has become a matter of routine for the media to report that 'trained counsellors have arrived at the scene to counsel the survivors'. But who are these people? What training have they received and what exactly do they say to traumatized victims? Does it do any good? Does it matter? Can it even do harm? Victims and therapists alike are viewed with ambivalence and at times suspicion and downright hostility. Stigma and fear born of ignorance and discrimination pervade public attitudes to the victims of psychological trauma and reflect attitudes to psychiatry in general. Patients are frequently portrayed as skrimshankers and malingerers, and counsellors and therapists as quacks and charlatans. These negative perceptions have been fuelled by contentious litigation and a number of high-profile compensation cases.

Disaster projects psychiatrists and other mental health workers into the media spotlight and their attitudes, conduct and effectiveness are an important 'showcase' for the mental health professions. Psychiatry generally only receives media attention in the wake of a tragedy when things have gone wrong. Interest in the psychological aftermath of traumatic events affords a rare opportunity to educate the public. By delivering timely, effective interventions and ensuring that the work of mental health professionals is reported in a positive light, a powerful positive influence can be exerted on public opinion and attitudes to victims and psychiatrists.

Psychological trauma raises important theoretical as well as numerous practical issues and challenges. National health policy places increasing emphasis on preventive medicine. Considering the high prevalence of mental illness and the resulting social and economic burden to society, psychiatry has little to offer by way of preventive mental health strategies. PTSD is a common and potentially disabling disorder, its epidemiology well known following traumatic events, and the 'at-risk' population and the interventions used can be well defined. No other area of mental health lends itself so well to preventive research. The complexities of methodology and experimental design encountered in trauma research should serve as an exemplar for preventive work in other areas of mental health.

Psychological trauma also provides important insights into neuroscience and a unique opportunity to explore the relationship between external events, brain biology and mental phenomena. Exploring how psychological techniques modify these associations enables the development of heuristic models to explore similar phenomena in other areas of psychiatry. A number of biological abnormalities in PTSD have been well described and demonstrating the impact of psychological therapies on these challenges the 'mind–body' dualism that pervades and still hampers research in psychology and other neurosciences.

The effectiveness of interventions to prevent PTSD or other long-term psychological sequelae has become increasingly politicized and more than a matter of science. The interpretation of a number of recent randomized controlled clinical trials (RCTs) is keenly contested. Many workers in the field of psychological trauma clearly have a vested interest in demonstrating the efficacy of techniques such as PD, indeed their research grants and livelihood may depend on it! The past decade has witnessed the emergence of a 'disaster industry'. Diverse groups both from statutory organizations and the voluntary sector, such as lay counsellors, psychologists, social workers and psychiatrists, have at times uncritically promoted these techniques in order to establish a role for themselves following traumatic incidents.[19] Although intuitively appealing and a response to perceived need, demonstrating the effectiveness of early intervention has been extremely difficult,[20] and it is only recently that PD has been subject to RCTs.

The 'anti-therapy' movement (both from within psychiatry and outside) have also taken an interest in debriefing and have been quick to draw parallels (unfairly, in my opinion) between PD, psychotherapy and counselling in general. The (essentially negative) results of RCTs of preventive interventions, particularly psychological debriefing, have been used as a 'stick' with which to beat and challenge the evidence-base of psychotherapy and the counselling industry. Debriefing however, is not psychotherapy nor is it counselling. Its clients are not ill, nor are they seeking help. Debriefing aims to minimize the adverse effects of the normal stress response; it is primarily educational and instructive in content rather than a psychotherapeutic process. Generalizing the findings of PD research to the psychological treatment of established disorder and disparate forms of counselling in diverse settings such as marital breakdown, bereavement, rape and sexual abuse is both nonsensical and unfair.

Research into PD and other techniques raises important questions about the ethics and nature of evidence-based medicine (EBM). PD was designed for groups of emergency service workers following traumatic events. Conducting a methodologically rigorous RCT of group debriefing would be extremely difficult given that group trauma generally only occurs in unpredictable and often chaotic circumstances such as war or disaster. In emergency situations such as these the operational imperative is paramount and investigators must do the best they can with the available material under difficult and at times extremely fraught circumstances. Irrespective of whether or not PD reduces long-term morbidity, many individuals find it subjectively helpful at the time.[20] Under these circumstances can it therefore be ethically justifiable to employ 'non-intervention' controls, denying individuals short-term support whatever the long-term outcome? In conflict, or following disaster or accident, naturalistic studies, often conducted opportunistically, remain useful. These have considerable heuristic value, despite methodological shortcomings particularly relating to sample selection and randomization to different treatment conditions. Applying the stringent CONSORT[21] criteria demanded by evidence based medicine to trials of preventive interventions not only means that useful work may go unpublished, but that researchers may forsake such methodologically challenging research entirely in favour of more biologically oriented research where variables can be more easily controlled, confounding factors minimized and publishable outcomes virtually guaranteed. Trauma and debriefing research which may not meet CONSORT criteria illustrates that there are other types of evidence with intrinsic value. Recognizing the contribution of such studies to evidence-based medicine has important implications for social psychiatry and empirical science in general.

What is psychological debriefing?

Jeffrey Mitchell, an American psychologist, initially described 'critical incident stress debriefing' (CISD) with ambulance personnel in 1983.[2] Having developed CISD during his long-standing association with the emergency services, he formalized the process to help ambulancemen come to terms with and consider the psychological aspects of the traumatic events they confronted during the course of their work. CISD has been modified and expanded by others, including Dyregrov, who coined the term PD.[1] Other refinements to Mitchell's basic model have been described.[22–24] PD has been used with those directly involved in traumatic events, emergency service workers and the providers of psychological aftercare. PD has now become the most widely practised form of early intervention aimed at everyone involved in a trauma, irrespective of whether they suffer an acute stress reaction or not (Box 8.1).

Box 8.1. The goals of psychological debriefing.

- Insure participants' basic needs are met and adequate information provided.
- Explore the symbolic meaning of loss.
- Normalize feelings and reduce the sense of uniqueness of the individual.
- Provide group supports, enhance peer social support and improve group cohesion.
- Explain normal and abnormal stress reactions.
- Encourage, teach and reinforce coping skills.
- Teach anxiety reduction techniques.
- Facilitate return to pre-incident functioning and routine.
- Identify 'high risk' participants with acute stress reactions. Ensure follow-up and refer for professional assistance where necessary.

A PD is a structured intervention designed to promote the emotional processing of traumatic events through the ventilation and normalization of reactions and preparation for possible future experiences. PD is based on the principles of rapid outreach and intervention, a focus on the present and 'here and now', and the mobilization of existing internal and external resources. Debriefing is thought to allow victims of psychological trauma to be able to cognitively and emotionally process their experience. PD is believed to reduce the opportunity for maladaptive and disruptive cognitive and behavioural patterns to become established.[18] Trauma psychology suggests that the majority of victims of severe trauma will experience some distressing phenomena as they assimilate their experience. Horowitz's information-processing model[25] predicts alternating intrusive and avoidant symptoms which decrease in magnitude with time and which form an integral part of the normal stress response. It is only when these symptoms become excessive in duration, frequency or intensity that the reaction is considered pathological. Although intuitively appealing and a response to perceived need, demonstrating the effectiveness of PD and other early interventions has been extremely difficult,[20] and it is only recently that PD has been subject to RCTs. Although initially designed as one element of a critical incident stress management package (CISM) for use in groups, debriefing has increasingly come to be used in isolation as a 'stand-alone' technique. It has also been used with individuals, couples and families. PD generally takes place 48–72 hours after the trauma as a single meeting in groups lasting approximately 2 hours. Ideally, group PD is led by two debriefers working together. PD should be regarded as a preventative measure as opposed to a formal therapy (Box 8.2).

Seven stages are passed through during PD. A brief introduction stressing the focus of the intervention and its confidentiality is followed by a chronological description of the facts of what happened from the varied perspectives of each of the group members. The expectations, thoughts and impressions of those involved are then discussed. By this stage of the PD a detailed reconstruction of what happened will have occurred, and, at least in theory, led to the open expression of associated emotions including guilt and anger. These are considered in depth and normalized as far as is reasonably possible. Group processes such as universality and peer support are mobilized during group PD, which helps with the acceptance of experienced emotions. The emphasis remains on normalization throughout and this is discussed formally towards the end of the PD. In conclusion the debriefer or debriefers prepare the participants for future symptoms and reactions, should they occur, and give guidelines as to when further help should be sought and where it can be found. These points are often reinforced with written infor-

Box 8.2. The stages of debriefing.

1. Introduction.
   Purpose of the meeting, confidentiality, ground rules, etc.
2. Facts.
   Chronological account of events by each group member.
3. Perception and thoughts.
   Sights, smells, other sensory impressions and thoughts about what happened.
4. Emotional reactions.
   Feelings, regard of self, victims, colleagues and managers during and after trauma.
5. Symptoms.
   Review symptoms and signs of distress.
   Description of the normal trauma response demonstrating universality and normalizing the feelings of group members.
   Challenge inappropriate feelings of guilt and responsibility.
6. Education.
   How to deal with similar situations in the future, going home and coping with family and friends. Coping strategies to deal with post-traumatic psychological symptoms.
   When, where, how and under what circumstances to get further help if necessary. Supplement with written information.
7. Re-entry and disengagement.
   Summarize, discuss outstanding issues, give additional advice where appropriate.

mation distributed to the participants before they leave.

A number of variations on the basic Dyregrov model have been developed. At one extreme, debriefing packages have been developed which are primarily educational, pragmatic and supportive, often conducted by peers or line managers. This model is often employed in organizations such as the military, where the prevailing culture inhibits the open expression of emotion and tends to be rejecting of outsiders and mental health professionals. Other models, generally employed with victims in civilian settings, have been developed with a more psychodynamic emphasis highlighting the importance of group processes and the relationship between group members and facilitators (Box 8.3).[26]

Box 8.3. Individual factors influencing the debriefing process.

- Trauma exposure
  - Multiple (type II) vs single (type I)
  - Perceived life threat
  - Concomitant physical injuries
  - Losses
- Participants
  - Training, experience and acceptability of debriefers
  - Prior trauma exposure
  - Support networks
  - Gender
- Group factors
  - Group cohesion
  - Size
  - Debriefing environment
  - Timing of debriefing after trauma

How effective is psychological debriefing?

There are numerous anecdotal reports suggesting that providing PD for everyone involved in a traumatic experience reduces subsequent psychological morbidity.[1,22] The acceptance of such claims has led to the widespread use of PD following traumatic events. Indeed it is now used routinely in Scandinavia and in a number of commercial organizations following traumatic events such as bank robberies. Unfortunately, there is little other than anecdotal evidence to demonstrate the effectiveness of PD and the vast majority of published data suffer from serious methodological difficulties (Box 8.4).

Methodological shortcomings

The lack of methodologically rigorous research concerning PD and other early psychological

Box 8.4. Common methodological shortcomings in psychological debriefing research.

- Not prospective.
- Small sample sizes.
- Lack of baseline data.
- Absence of randomized control groups.
- Comparison of single v multiple debriefing.
- Varying trauma exposure.
- Other confounding variables ignored.
- Low response rates.
- Failure of 'intent to treat analysis'.
- Sampling bias.
- Lack of uniformity of psychological debriefing.
- Timing variance.
- Questionnaire vs interview results.
- Differences between outcome measures at baseline.
- Adjunctive therapy, counselling, practical support.

interventions is striking. Most importantly, the majority of studies lack a prospective controlled design and random allocation to treatment groups. Studies should employ a controlled design with pre- and post-treatment measures.[27] Several other important deficits reduce the validity of much of the published data. Studies generally lack any pre-PD data on their subjects and rely on questionnaire results as opposed to validated interview data.

No two traumatic events are the same and comparing one incident with another is problematic. Unfortunately, standard measures of the dimensions of the trauma are rarely recorded and comparisons are often made between relatively minor traumatic events and major disasters.[28] Similar problems arise when single-event trauma is compared with sustained or repetitive traumatic events. Other factors known to influence psychological outcome should also be considered. These include the context in which an event occurs as well as personal factors such as past psychiatric history, coping mechanisms and the presence of an acute stress reaction at the time of the trauma. The true effectiveness of PD can only be assessed in well-controlled studies taking factors such as these into account.

Another common problem in the literature is low response rates resulting in sample bias. Lindy[29] described the 'trauma membrane' which needs to be penetrated. If a group of individuals is sceptical about the value of any psychological intervention, it is unlikely to co-operate or sanction 'experimentation' with colleagues or loved ones. In the outreach programme following the Beverly Hills Supper Club fire, only 5% of those involved 'engaged' despite extensive publicity and personal invitations to attend. The prevailing culture in the armed forces and emergency services, with its emphasis on psychological 'tough-mindedness', creates particular difficulties in studying these groups.

A further major confounding factor is the lack of detailed description of the content of the PD; those that are described frequently vary considerably. As the term becomes more widely used, so its actual content seems to vary more. Perhaps the most complicated PD is that advocated by Hayman and Scaturo,[23] who suggested a 10-session PD for American Army Gulf veterans. This seems excessive and as a preventative intervention is longer than many treatment techniques.

The timing of the PD also varies greatly in reported studies. Immediate debriefing is often neither possible nor desirable. Following serious trauma individuals are often extremely fatigued and in poor physical health needing food, rest and medical attention before PD can take place. Similarly, many individuals experience emotional 'numbing' during and immediately following traumatic events and do not benefit from immediate debriefing. Dyregrov himself[1] suggests that debriefing should take place 48–72 hours after the incident, although some authors have reported on PDs several months after the incident.[30] Owing to logistical problems, especially with wide dispersal of victims, as in the King's Cross fire,[31] delays of up to a few weeks may be inevitable. The advocates of PD believe that whilst immediacy is important, delayed PDs can still help.[32] Comparison between studies is difficult given such discrepancies.

Uncontrolled studies

Early data-containing studies lack any control or comparison group. Sloan described 30 survivors of a non-fatal plane crash who received PD.[33] All of them initially experienced distressing symptoms, the intensity of which decreased rapidly over the first 8 weeks and thereafter more slowly. Robinson and Mitchell[34] assessed the efficacy of PD amongst 172 emergency workers in Australia. Of these, 60% completed questionnaires 2 weeks after the PD: overall the respondents found the PD to be of 'considerable value' and the majority believed it had helped to reduce their stress-related symptoms. Very few criticisms were voiced, although some participants complained that it was 'too political' and gave them a sense of 'lack of control'.

Flannery et al[35] described the debriefing of psychiatric staff members who had been assaulted by patients. This occurred immediately after the incident and was followed up by further contact at 3 and 10 days. Over the 90-day study period there were 67 assaults and debriefing was offered to the victims of 62 of these. Five victims refused to participate. Some 69% were reported as 'regaining a sense of control' within 10 days and only seven required further support, which was offered in the form of a group.

Searle and Bisson described eight soldiers severely traumatized during the Gulf War who received PD within 5 days of the trauma.[36] Six of them satisfied the DSM-III-R criteria for PTSD at 5 weeks and five of them required prolonged treatment before their symptoms improved. Perhaps after the multiple and often sustained trauma of warfare, a more limited but realistic goal of PD would be to encourage effective processing and to promote earlier presentation for further help if necessary.

The absence of a control group in these four studies makes interpretation of the results impossible because of the natural diminution in symptoms (akin to a normal bereavement reaction), irrespective of whether or not subjects received PD. These studies are also difficult to compare due to the varying degrees of trauma experienced. It is unfortunate that many studies in the area of traumatic stress do not take the natural history of post-traumatic stress reactions into account.

Comparison studies

Comparison studies consider a group of individuals involved in a traumatic event or events and then compare them according to whether or not PD was received. Their findings are weakened by the absence of random allocation to intervention or non-intervention groups: the reasons that determine whether or not individuals attend PD may be extremely important and result in considerable sample bias, markedly affecting the outcome.

McFarlane followed up 469 firefighters involved in a series of Australian bushfires.[17] Although this was not the main focus of the paper, he found that those who received PD shortly after the incident were less likely to develop an acute post-traumatic stress reaction than those who were not debriefed. However, the effectiveness of the debriefing process was thrown into doubt by his finding that individuals who developed a delayed-onset post-traumatic stress reaction were more likely to have attended a debriefing than those who had suffered no psychological disorder at any time during the follow-up period. This led McFarlane to comment that PD may have immediate protective value but have little effect in the longer term.

Deahl et al[37] considered the effectiveness of PD in soldiers who acted as grave-diggers during the Gulf War. Seventy-four soldiers took part in the study, of whom 55 received a PD soon after completing their duties. Nine months later 50% of the group showed evidence of PTSD. Debriefing made no difference to the incidence of PTSD. Soldiers who developed PTSD were more likely to have experienced an acute stress reaction or believe their lives were in danger. Interestingly, soldiers experiencing relationship difficulties with partners were also more likely to develop PTSD. Hyton and Hasle[38] similarly questioned the effectiveness of PD as a result of their study of 58 non-professional firefighters exposed to dead bodies following a major hotel fire in Norway. They found no difference in psychological symptoms 2 weeks later between those formally debriefed and those who had talked with colleagues.

Where individuals have an adequate support network PD may be redundant. Joseph et al[39] found that survivors of the Jupiter incident who received more 'crisis support' from family and friends suffered fewer avoidance symptoms at 18 months, although similar levels of intrusion to the comparison group. They argued that individuals without such support could be identified and offered more help. The identification of 'high-risk' groups seems sensible, particularly when resources are scarce.

Controlled studies

There have been few adequate prospective controlled studies involving random subject allocation to PD or no intervention. Bunn and Clarke[40] assessed the use of a 20-minute 'supportive interview' with a psychologist as opposed to no intervention in the relatives of severely ill or injured patients admitted to an emergency ward. Those interviewed were less anxious immediately after the interview but unfortunately there was no follow-up to assess its effectiveness even in the short term.

In the wake of these disappointing results four subsequent RCTs have been conducted which have largely confirmed these findings, failing to demonstrate any benefit of PD in preventing subsequent PTSD and other psychiatric disorders. These studies have randomized individuals following disparate traumatizing events of varying severity. Debriefing has generally followed the Dyregov model, although the timing of the intervention has varied both within and between studies. Hobbs and Adshead[41] conducted two RCTs, one studying 42 victims of various traumas, the other a follow-up study of 86 road traffic accident victims.[41] In both these studies debriefing was carried out within 24 hours of the traumatic event. Lee et al[42] studied 39 women 2 weeks following miscarriage. Bisson et al[43] studied 110 burn victims; the treatment group received debriefing on average 6 days following their injury. In this study the debriefed group actually had a worse outcome, although it was suggested that they had a greater pre-incident vulnerability. Although debriefing was designed for groups of emergency service workers, there have been few adequate RCTs of group debriefing to date.

Although PD is sometimes used in isolation, many clinicians employ PD as one element of a comprehensive CISM and evaluating PD as a 'stand-alone' intervention may not be valid. Moreover, PD was originally devised for groups of ambulance workers attached to the emergency services, and carrying out RCTs of PD in individuals disregards the complex group dynamics which develops amongst a cohesive close-knit group who have shared a common trauma. In a recent RCT of group debriefing carried out amongst a group of soldiers returning from United Nations peacekeeping duties in Bosnia, debriefing appeared to make no differences to PTSD or affective symptomology.[44] However CAGE scores (a widely used measure of alcohol misuse) were significantly reduced in the debriefed group 6 months and 1 year later. These findings suggest that debriefing may have an effect but that a broader range of outcome measures should be used, including substance misuse and social dysfunction (both common behavioural sequelae of PTSD), to monitor outcome.

Few studies have compared debriefing with any other form of practical support. Bordow and Porritt[45] studied 70 male road trauma victims who were hospitalized for at least 1 week. The 30 individuals in group A received no intervention. The 10 in group B were 'reviewed' (an intervention similar to PD with detailed discussion of the trauma) soon after their admission but received no further intervention. The remaining 30 (group C) received the 'immediate review' and then between 2 and 10 hours of formal intervention from a social worker looking at practical, social and emotional levels of support depending on their apparent needs. Follow-up 3–4 months later revealed that group C suffered significantly fewer psychological sequelae than group B, who in turn fared better than Group A.

More complex early interventions

Bordow and Porritt's study[45] suggests that more complex preventative interventions following traumatic events may be more effective than PD alone. A number of workers argue that a CIS model is too simplistic and have suggested that a 'loss and bereavement' model is more appropriate. Mitchell himself acknowledges that 'not everyone in every instance will benefit from a CISD.[46] Many times they will need more help than a debriefing alone can provide.' Robinson and Mitchell[34] emphasized the important fact that PD should be one element of a comprehensive management plan following trauma and the British Psychological Society working party[19] concluded that single methods of support in isolation following traumatic events are unlikely to be effective unless combined with other measures. There are several studies describing more complex interventions after various traumatic events, including the extensive literature on crisis intervention in psychiatry.[47]

Some of the best data on the effectiveness of early interventions come from Israeli studies on combat stress reaction (CSR) sufferers during the Lebanon War. Solomon and Benbenishty[48] looked at the functions of the principles of proximity (to the battlefield), immediacy (of treatment) and expectancy (of return to duty) in the outcome of CSR victims. Where all three principles were employed, 60% returned to duty and 40% had developed PTSD 1 year later. Where none of the principles were employed only 22% returned to duty and 71% were suffering with PTSD after 1 year. Although it is important to appreciate that these individuals were unwell and therefore unlike the recipients of PD, the study nevertheless seems to confirm the impression that early intervention may help to reduce psychological sequelae in this vulnerable group, but not actually prevent them. It is interesting to compare the incidence of PTSD in these CSR victims with the 14% incidence of PTSD amongst veterans who had not suffered CSR.[49] Perhaps the presence or absence of an acute stress reaction has more effect on outcome than the presence or absence of early psychological intervention (Figure 8.2).

Civilian studies have focused on other types of trauma. Raphael[50] evaluated the effectiveness of an intervention in 30 'high-risk' widows compared with a control group of 30 widows felt to be at a similarly high risk of suffering problematic grief reactions. The intervention comprised an average of four sessions in the first 3 months post-bereavement. Widows receiving the intervention

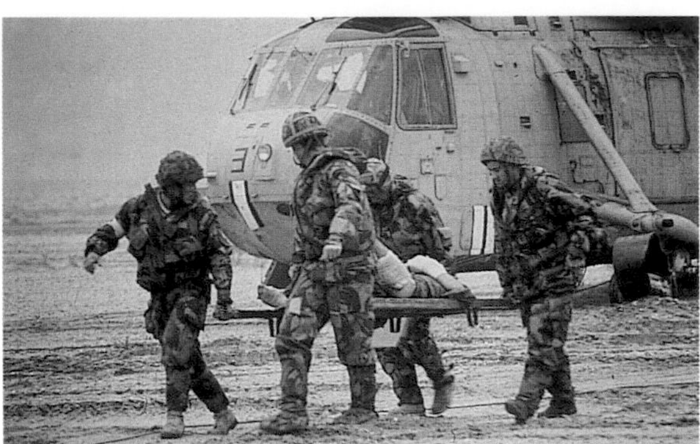

Figure 8.2. Combat veterans are often the subjects of trauma research, but are the findings applicable to civilian populations?

suffered significantly fewer psychological symptoms than controls as determined by questionnaire follow-up at 13 months. Duckworth reported a non-controlled study of policemen involved in the Bradford football stadium fire in 1985.[9] A total of 234 policemen completed the General Health Questionnaire (GHQ) 1 month after the incident; of those the 55 who scored above a cut-off of 12 were offered brief therapy with a cognitive, rational–emotive and problem-solving basis. Thirty-four policemen received the therapy and all had GHQ scores below 12 after treatment and reported themselves as 'feeling better' at 9-month telephone follow-up.

A more recently reported intervention failed to demonstrate any difference at 1- and 6-month follow-up between a group of 68 road traffic accident victims who received a preventative counselling programme and 83 who did not.[51] Ten per cent satisfied the criteria for PTSD in both the intervention and control groups. It is interesting to note that in common with Robinson and Mitchell's PD findings,[34] those who received the intervention said they found it useful. This perceived usefulness does not always seem to be detectable with the research tools employed in the studies.

Risks of psychological debriefing

It has become increasingly recognized that there may be risks associated with PD and other forms of early psychological intervention. The provision of such services results in 'helpers' being exposed to the expression of powerful emotions by the victims of the trauma. This can make the work extremely difficult and stressful. An unfortunate corollary is the recognition that the service providers may themselves become secondary victims.[52–54]

Another risk is the possibility of passive participation and resentment engendered by mandatory PD.[35] A good example of enforced early intervention is the case of the Americans held hostage in Iran in the late 1970s.[55] Many of the hostages felt 'ready to fly home immediately' but instead spent a 4-day period of seclusion and gradual reintroduction in Germany before being reunited with their families. Although 'nearly all' acknowledged that their initial feelings were 'overly optimistic', no comment was made on the feelings of those who were forced to undergo this process against their will (Box 8.5).

Another danger of early intervention discussed by McFarlane is that overenthusiasm for primary preventative methods might delay the institution of diagnosis and effective treatment for those who do suffer psychological sequelae.[56] He argues that 'clear definition of the limitations of the crisis intervention approach and the point at which more formal treatment is required' is needed. His concerns were fuelled by his finding that many individ-

Box 8.5. What not to do in debriefing.

- Enforce mandatory debriefing on unwilling subjects.
- Use outside debriefers alien to the group (especially mental health workers).
- Be complacent – fail to make efforts to detect subsequent psychopathology in group members.
- Fail to arrange adequate follow-up and inform primary care physicians that patient has been a victim of trauma and a recipient of debriefing.

uals with psychiatric disorders arising out of the Australian bushfires presented late due to other professionals' fears that labelling would occur following referral to a psychiatrist.[57] Such fears must be overcome if the victims of trauma are to receive the treatment they often need. If PD is employed following traumatic events some form of follow-up is important. This facilitates the identification of those who go on to develop serious psychological sequelae and ensures that they are offered adequate treatment.

Conclusions

Whether or not debriefing reduces the incidence of long-term psychological morbidity following trauma remains uncertain. The data available from mostly methodologically flawed studies suggest that at best PD affords some protection against later sequelae and, at worst, makes no difference or may even make some individuals worse. Certainly individuals receiving PD are not immune to developing long-term psychological sequelae. Therefore, regardless of whether PD is employed following traumatic events, formal follow-up to identify individuals who do go on to develop serious psychological sequelae is vital (Box 8.6).

Before recommending its widespread use and committing substantial resources to PD, it is crucial unequivocally to demonstrate clinical effectiveness. The function of PD must also be clearly defined. Despite a lack of adequate data supporting the long-term efficacy of PD, it may have short-term benefit and have an (as yet untested) role in sustaining individuals in emergency operations and helping emergency workers suffering from acute stress reactions return to duty. Clinical experience suggests that many individuals value the opportunity to express feelings of anger and guilt and derive comfort from the realization that these are a normal emotional response to trauma. Many of the feelings expressed during PD, particularly those associated with guilt and anger, are intensely personal, and disaster workers and victims often experience difficulty in confiding in, and indeed tend to be suspicious of, 'outsiders', especially mental health professionals. If PD is

Box 8.6. Elements of successful debriefing.

- Cohesive group with shared experience.
- Experienced debriefers accepted by group.
- Proximity.
- Immediacy (48–72 hours).
- Expectancy (of full recovery).
- Simplicity.
- Combination of debriefing with practical support and adequate follow-up.

to be effective it should be carried out as locally as possible and preferably within a few days of the trauma. It should be a task for military commanders, managers within the emergency services and primary health care workers. The primary role of mental health professionals should be directed towards educating these groups rather than trying to deliver a service themselves.

It is clear that the presence or absence of other factors, for example the nature of the event itself, an acute stress reaction, personality, past psychiatric history and adequate social support, may all have a much greater influence than the presence or absence of PD in determining the psychological outcome of individuals involved in traumatic events. Indeed, when individuals have an adequate support network and do not have other vulnerability factors, a PD may be redundant.

At present PD falls into that group of psychological interventions discussed by Fahy and Wessely as urgently requiring proper evaluation.[58] The role of PD within a comprehensive intervention package must be defined. Who should deliver PD, when, and what form it should take are all important unresolved issues. The answers to these questions should give a clearer indication as to whether PD should be routinely offered to everyone involved in traumatic events, be restricted to 'high-risk' individuals or those suffering from an acute stress reaction, or be abandoned. Whatever the outcome of such research, overenthusiasm for preventative methods must not be allowed to delay diagnosis and effective treatment for those who do suffer psychological sequelae. Whatever the putative benefits of PD, it is clear that PD by itself is inadequate and indeed may even do harm.[59] Future research should seek to identify other measures which may effectively reduce morbidity following trauma, including primary preventative measures such as more careful recruit selection, realistic training, stress inoculation and operational stress training packages. Outcome measures employed in PD trials have focused on PTSD symptomology such as intrusive (nightmares, flashbacks, etc.) or avoidance phenomena. Although the symptoms of PTSD are an important consequence of psychological trauma, they should not be used as the sole measure of outcome in studies of treatment or epidemiology. A variety of adjustment, affective and other anxiety disorders as well as enduring personality changes are all recognized but much less well understood following trauma. The efficacy of PD in preventing other trauma-related disorders is unknown. Debriefing clearly has an educational role in informing individuals what symptoms they might anticipate following psychological trauma and when and where to seek help. Broader outcome measures such as social functioning and substance misuse have not been studied. These are both important behavioural sequelae of PTSD and often the patient's presenting complaint. Future studies should employ a wider range of outcome measures than hitherto and assess social and occupational function, personality, substance misuse and a broader range of psychopathology as well as the symptoms of PTSD.

In the aftermath of traumatic events rescuers typically feel helpless and impotent. The desire to 'do something' is a powerful human instinct. Psychiatrists and other mental health professionals have a duty to resist 'knee-jerk' responses, do no harm and provide credible interventions underpinned by a sound evidence-base. In a field so subject to public scrutiny we must eschew instinctive responses and apply clinically effective techniques for the sake of victims and psychiatry alike.

References

1. Dyregrov A, Caring for helpers in disaster situations: psychological debriefing, *Disaster Management* (1989) 2:25–30.
2. Mitchell JT, When disaster strikes . . . the critical incident debriefing process, *J Emerg Med Serv* (1983)8: 36–9.
3. Blake DD, Treatment outcome research on PTSD, *NCP Clinical Newsletter* (1993) 3:14–17.
4. Marks I, Lovell K, Treatment of post-traumatic stress disorder by exposure and/or cognitive restructuring. *Arch Gen Psychiatry* (1988) 55:317–325.
5. Solomon SD, Gerrity ED, Muff AM, Efficacy of treatments for posttraumatic stress disorder: an empirical review, *JAMA* (1992) 268:633–8.
6. Green BL. Psychosocial research in traumatic stress: an update, *J Trauma Stress* (1994) 7:341–62.
7. Helzer JE, Robins LN, McEvoy L, Post-traumatic stress disorder in the general population, *N Engl J Med* (1987) 317:1630–4.
8. Curran PS, Psychiatric aspects of terrorist violence: Northern Ireland 1969–87, *Br J Psychiatry* (1988) 153:470–5.
9. Duckworth DH, Psychological problems arising from disaster work, *Stress Medicine* (1986) 2:315–23.
10. Cobb S, Lindemann E, Neuropsychiatric observations after the coconut grove fire. *Ann Surg* (1943) 117:814–24.
11. Mezey GC, Taylor PJ, Psychological reactions of women who have been raped: a descriptive and comparative study, *Br J Psychiatry* (1988) 152:330–9.
12. Kulka RA, Schlenger WE, Fairbank JA et al, Brunner Mazel Psychosocial stress series No. 18, Trauma and the Vietnam War Generation: Report of Findings from the National Vietnam Veterans Readjustment Study. (Brunner Mazel: New York, 1990)
13. McFarlane AC, The longitudinal course of post-traumatic morbidity: the range of outcomes and their predictors, *J Nerv Ment Dis* (1988) 176:30–9.
14. Taylor AJW, Frazer AG, The stress of post-disaster body handling and victim identification work, *J Human Stress* (1982) 8:4–12.
15. Jones DJ, Secondary disaster victims: the emotional effects of identifying and recovering human remains, *Am J Psychiatry* (1985) 142:303–7.
16. Ursano RJ, McCarroll JE, The nature of a post-traumatic stressor: handling dead bodies, *J Nerv Ment Dis* (1990) 178:396–8.
17. McFarlane AC, The longitudinal course of post-traumatic morbidity: the range of outcomes and their predictors, *J Nerv Ment Dis* (1988) 176:30–9.
18. Rachman S, Emotional processing, *Therapy* (1980) 18:51–60.
19. British Psychological Society Working Party, *Psychological Aspects of Disaster* (The British Psychological Society: Leicester, 1990).
20. Bisson JI, Deahl MP, Psychological debriefing and preventing post traumatic stress, *Br J Psychiatry* (1994) 165:717–20.
21. Moher, D, CONSORT: an evolving tool to help improve the quality of reports of randomized controlled trials. Consolidated Standards of Reporting Trials, *JAMA* (1998) 279:1489–91.
22. Armstrong K, O'Callahan W, Marmar CR, Debriefing Red Cross disaster personnel: the multiple stressor debriefing model, *J Trauma Stress* (1991) 4:581–93.
23. Hayman PM, Scaturo DJ, Psychological debriefing of returning military personnel: a protocol for post combat intervention. Paper presented at the Twenty-fifth International Congress of Psychology, Brussels, 1992.
24. Talbot A, Manton M, Dunn PJ, Debriefing the debriefers: an intervention strategy to assist psychologists after a crisis, *J Trauma Stress* (1992) 5:45–62.
25. Horowitz MJ, Stress response syndromes: character style and dynamic psychotherapy, *Arch Gen Psychiatry* (1974) 31:768–81.
26. Dyregrov A, The process in psychological debriefing, *J Trauma Stress* (1997) 10:589–605.
27. Fairbank JA, Nicholson RA, Theoretical and empirical issues in the treatment of post-traumatic stress disorder in Vietnam veterans, *J Clin Psychol* (1987) 43:44–55.
28. Green BL, Grace MC, Lindy JD et al, Levels of functional impairment following a civilian disaster: the Beverly Hills Supper Club fire, *J Consult Clin Psychol* (1983) 51:573–80.
29. Lindy JD, Grace MC, Green BL, Survivors: outreach to a reluctant population, *Am J Orthopsychiatry* (1981) 51:468–78.
30. Stallard P, Law F, Screening and psychological debriefing of adolescent survivors of life-threatening events, *Br J Psychiatry* (1993) 163:660–5.

31. Turner SW, Thompson JA, Rosser RM, King's Cross fire: planning a 'phase two' psychosocial response, *Disaster Management* (1989) 2:31–7.
32. Jimmerman C, Critical incident stress debriefing, *J Emerg Nurs* (1988) 14:43–5.
33. Sloan P, Post traumatic stress in survivors of an airplane crash-landing, *J Trauma Stress* (1988) 1:211–29.
34. Robinson RC, Mitchell JT, Evaluation of psychological debriefings, *J Trauma Stress* (1993) 6:367–82.
35. Flannery RB, Fulton P, Tausch J, DeLoffi AY, A program to help staff cope with psychological sequelae of assaults by patients, *Hosp Community Psychiatry* (1991) 42:935–8.
36. Searle MM, Bisson JI, Psychological sequelae of friendly fire. Proceedings of Military Psychiatry conference 'Stress Psychiatry and War', Paris, 1992.
37. Deahl MP, Gillham AB, Thomas J et al, Psychological sequelae following the Gulf War: factors associated with subsequent morbidity and the effectiveness of psychological debriefing, *Br J Psychiatry* (1994) 165:60–5.
38. Hyton K, Hasle A, Fire fighters: a study of stress and coping, *Acta Psychiatr Scand* (1989) **80**: Supplementum 355.
39. Joseph S, Yule W, Williams R, Andrews B, Crisis support in the aftermath of disaster: a longitudinal perspective, *Br J Clin Psychol* (1993) 32:177–85.
40. Bunn TA, Clarke AM, Crisis intervention: an experimental study of the effects of a brief period of counselling on the anxiety of relatives of seriously injured or ill hospital patients, *Br J Med Psychol* (1979) 52:191–5.
41. Hobbs M, Adshead G, Preventive psychological intervention for road crash survivors. In: Mitchell, M, ed, *The Aftermath of Road Accidents: Psychological, Social and Legal Perspectives* (Routledge: London, 1996) 159–71.
42. Lee C, Slade P, Lygo V, The influence of psychological debriefing on emotional adaptation in females following early miscarriage, *Br J Med Psychol* (1996) 69:47–58.
43. Bisson JI, Jenkins PL, Alexander J, Bannister C, Randomised controlled trial of psychological debriefing for victims of acute burn trauma, *Br J Psychiatry* (1997) 171:78–81.
44. Deahl M, Srinivasan M, Jones N et al, Preventing psychological trauma in soldiers. The role of operational stress training and psychological debriefing, *Br J Med Psychol*, (2000) 73:77–85.
45. Bordow S, Porritt D, An experimental evaluation of crisis intervention, *Psychol Bull* (1979) 84:1189–217.
46. Mitchell JT, The history, status and future of critical incident stress debriefings, *J Emerg Med Serv* (1988) 13:47–52.
47. Szmukler GI, The place of crisis intervention in psychiatry, *Aust N Z J Psychiatry* (1987) 21:24–34.
48. Solomon Z, Benbenishty R, The role of proximity, immediacy and expectancy in front-line treatment of combat-stress reaction among Israelis in the Lebanon war, *Am J Psychiatry* (1986) 143:613–17.
49. Solomon Z, Weisenberg M, Schwarzwald J, Mikulincer M, Post-traumatic stress disorder among frontline soldiers with combat stress reaction: the 1982 Israeli experience, *Am J Psychiatry* (1989) 144:448–54.
50. Raphael B, Preventive intervention with the recently bereaved, *Arch Gen Psychiatry* (1977) 34:1450–4.
51. Brom D, Kleber RJ, Hofman MC, Victims of traffic accidents: incidence and prevention of post-traumatic stress disorder, *J Clin Psychol* (1993) 49:131–40.
52. Talbot A, The importance of parallel process in debriefing crisis counsellors, *J Trauma Stress* (1990) 3:265–77.
53. Berah EF, Jones HJ, Valent P, The experience of a mental health team involved in the early phase of a disaster, *Aust N Z J Psychiatry* (1984) 18:354–8.
54. Raphael B, *When Disaster Strikes* (Hutchinson: London, 1986).
55. Rahe RH, Karson S, Howard NS et al, Psychological and physiological assessments on American hostages freed from captivity in Iran, *Psychosom Med* (1990) 52:1–16.
56. McFarlane AC, The treatment of post-traumatic stress disorder, *Br J Med Psychol* (1989) 62:81–90.
57. McFarlane AC, The Ash Wednesday bushfires in South Australia: implications for planning for future post-disaster services, *Med J Aust* (1984) 141:286–91.
58. Fahy T, Wesseley S, Should purchasers pay for psychotherapy? *BMJ* (1993) 307:576–7.
59. McFarlane AC, The prevention and management of the psychiatric morbidity of natural disasters: an Australian experience, *Stress Medicine* (1989) 5:29–36.

9

Pharmacotherapy of post-traumatic stress disorder

Dan J Stein, Soraya Seedat, Geoffrey van der Linden and Debra Kaminer

In the past decade or so, the study of post-traumatic stress has undergone an exciting paradigm shift. Post-traumatic stress has long been considered a normal response to abnormal events, a primarily psychological phenomenon involving various defenses, for which a psychotherapeutic intervention focusing on 'working through' of the trauma is indicated. In this traditional view, the role of pharmacotherapy is restricted, although in the past it has been suggested that denial and psychological defenses can exert a strong suppressive effect on the hypothalamic–pituitary–adrenal (HPA) axis,[1] and that barbiturates and similar agents may be useful insofar as they facilitate the process of anamnesis.[2]

In contrast, the modern concept of post-traumatic stress emphasizes that this is a disorder (PTSD) – a psychobiological phenomenon involving neurobiological dysregulation and psychological dysfunction, which may be reversed by specific pharmacotherapeutic and psychotherapeutic interventions. In this view, advances in the neurobiology of PTSD provide clinicians the hope of developing more specific and more effective pharmacotherapeutic interventions for the treatment of PTSD.

In clinical practice, this paradigm shift arguably remains incomplete. Our understanding of the specific psychobiological abnormalities that characterize PTSD, although steadily advancing, remains incomplete. Similarly, while preclinical models of stress and biological studies of PTSD provide some rationale for particular pharmacotherapeutic interventions, clinical treatment studies are the more convincing source of data. This chapter reviews the exciting developments in the pharmacotherapy of PTSD, as well as some of the important uncertainties that remain.

Diagnosis and assessment

The diagnosis and assessment of PTSD have been covered in previous chapters in this book. From the perspective of the psychopharmacologist, a number of issues deserve particular emphasis.

First, there is the question of principal and comorbid diagnoses. As will become apparent in this chapter, there is a relatively limited database of clinical trials on PTSD in comparison to the wealth of available information on major depression and other anxiety disorders. Indeed, one rationale for the use of antidepressant medication in PTSD is the high prevalence of comorbid major depression and panic disorder. Certainly, it is crucial for the clinician to begin by assessing the range of comorbid diagnostic disorders that may be present in a given patient with PTSD.

Second, there are questions about the phenomenology of the traumatic event and of the PTSD response. Was this a single event, or were there multiple events? Did the event take place in a civilian or a combat setting? Did the PTSD begin immediately afterward, or was it delayed? How long has the duration of the PTSD been? How severe has it been? Has the patient previously failed to respond to a trial of medication? Presumably such phenomenological differences are mediated by different neurobiological mechanisms, with implications for pharmacotherapy. While there are relatively few data about these underlying mechanisms, we return to these questions later in the chapter.

Third, there is the issue of symptom subtypes and associated features. It is possible that different symptom clusters in PTSD, for example, are mediated by different neurobiological systems and therefore respond to different psychotropic agents. Again, the limited number of trials in PTSD makes it difficult to base this assertion on empirical data. Nevertheless, it is certainly worth considering what the chief target symptoms are, and what their underlying neurobiology might be. Associated features may respond directly to pharmacotherapy or may respond indirectly via a facilitating effect of pharmacotherapy on psychotherapy.

Fourth, there is the question of which PTSD symptom scales are most useful in the context of pharmacotherapy. The comprehensiveness and reliability of the Clinician-Administered PTSD Scale (CAPS) has made it a gold standard in clinical trials. However, the Treatment Outcome PTSD Scale (TOP-8) is much less time-consuming and possibly equally reliable, and may therefore be the symptom scale of choice for the busy clinician. The self-rated Duke Trauma Scale (DTS) also appears sensitive to treatment effects. The Clinical Global Impressions (CGI) scale appears to provide particularly robust drug–placebo differences.[3]

The meaning of medication

Kleinman[4] has drawn a useful distinction between disease and illness. Disease refers to the underlying psychobiology of a disorder; in the case of PTSD, certain universal biological dysregulations and psychological dysfunctions are apparent in these patients. Illness refers to the patient's subjective experience of the disorder; in the case of PTSD, psychological and cultural views of trauma and trauma response will influence the particular way in which symptoms are experienced and expressed.

The freedom fighter who has succeeded in his or her political objectives and who has told comrades openly about PTSD symptoms may have an entirely different perspective on pharmacotherapy, for example, from the survivor of a rape who has been encouraged by family not to report the incident and who is concerned about being allowed to communicate symptoms. Shay[5] has explored historical trauma narratives, arguing that these kinds of psychosocial factors have long contributed to the healing or maintenance of PTSD symptoms. Current empirical research continues to demonstrate the importance of social support in predicting symptoms.

From a practical perspective, it is important for the clinician to ask about the patient's explanatory model of PTSD symptoms, and similarly to inquire about the meaning of medication. The combat veteran who regards medication from a Veterans Administration (VA) psychiatrist as another example of government-inflicted injury or a rape victim who views the 'necessity' of medication as another example of trauma caused her by her rapist will need to establish a relationship of trust before medication can begin to be considered. Elucidating the patient's explanatory model is a useful first step prior to psychoeducation.

Such considerations are, of course, important in any medical or psychiatric encounter. However, they are perhaps particularly important in the case of PTSD, where medical intervention may be subject to a wide range of possible interpretations,[6] depending on the patients' particular experience of trauma, developmental history, and current perspective.

It may be useful for the clinician to present a layperson's view of the modern paradigm of PTSD, describing PTSD as an alarm that is set off by a traumatic event, but that is then triggered unnecessarily (a false alarm) because of trauma-induced psychobiological changes. Medication can be useful in switching off this false alarm. A negotiation can then take place between the explanatory model of the patient and this clinical model, with ongoing exploration of the patient's perspective. Such steps may well increase treatment acceptability and compliance.

Preclinical and clinical neurobiology

The neurobiology of PTSD has been discussed in previous chapters of this book. What are the main issues here from the perspective of psychopharmacology? In this section, we discuss the basis for using noradrenergic medications, serotonergic medications, and dopaminergic agents. These are amongst the most widely used pharmacological interventions in PTSD.

Preclinical studies demonstrate that the noradrenergic system plays a key role in focusing attention on to salient events in threatening situations. Furthermore, there is clinical evidence of noradrenergic sensitization in PTSD, with increased sympathetic nervous system activity and reactivity. It may be postulated that this system is particularly important in mediating the hyperarousal cluster of symptoms in PTSD. Selective noradrenergic reuptake inhibitors have not been studied in PTSD to date. However, we review the use of the tricyclic antidepressants and other noradrenergic agents below.

There are several studies documenting serotonergic involvement in PTSD. First, preclinical studies demonstrate that serotonergic pathways project to a range of areas and systems that are crucial in co-ordinating fear responses; these include the amygdala, the hypothalamus (and the HPA axis) and the brain stem (and the noradrenergic system).[7] The serotonin agonist m-chlorophenylpipcrazine (mCPP) can provoke PTSD symptoms.[8] Third, there are platelet paroxetine binding abnormalities in PTSD.[9] These appear to correlate with PTSD symptom level[9] and to predict response to treatment with the selective serotonin reuptake inhibitors (SSRIs).[10] The serotonin system may be postulated to play a role in a wide range of PTSD symptoms, including intrusive ones. We review the growing database of studies on SSRIs in PTSD below.

Dopaminergic involvement in PTSD is again supported by a range of studies. Preclinical studies suggest that dopamine agonists and environmental stressors act as cross-sensitizers of one another.[11] The dopamine and serotonin systems have significant interactions with one another. Dopamine may be hypothesized to be particularly important in paranoid and other psychotic symptoms in PTSD.

A wide range of other systems are possibly involved in the mediation of PTSD. These include the glutamatergic, opioid, thyroid and HPA systems. Nevertheless, while it is theoretically possible to employ pharmacological agents to affect these systems, to date clinical pharmacotherapy studies with such psychotropics are very few in number.

Studies of pharmacotherapy of PTSD

Studies of the pharmacotherapy of PTSD have focused primarily on the antidepressants. The first studies were of tricyclic antidepressants and monoamine oxidase inhibitors; more recent studies have investigated the SSRIs and serotonin antagonists and reuptake inhibitors (see below). Most recently, the value of newly introduced antidepressants such as mirtazapine in PTSD has been explored.

It is important to note the methodological problems associated with the early body of work on PTSD. First, there are very few controlled studies (Table 9.1). Second, sample sizes have been relatively small, and most have focused on American and Israeli combat veterans rather than on subjects with other experiences of trauma. Third, the duration of treatment in most studies has been limited; current recommendations are that clinical trials last for 8–12 weeks. Fourth, early studies relied on the patient-rated Impact of Events Scale (IES) rather than on reliable clinician-rated scales such as the CAPS.

Tricyclics and monoamine oxidase inhibitors (MAOIs)

Early uncontrolled studies suggested the value of tricyclic antidepressants[12–16] and MAOIs[17–19] in the treatment of PTSD. More recently, an open trial indicated that the reversible MAOI, moclobemide, may also be useful in PTSD.[20]

Reist and colleagues[21] undertook a crossover trial with 4 weeks each of desipramine and placebo in 27 inpatients (18 completers) with DSM-III PTSD. All patients were combat veterans. Patients with comorbid disorders were not excluded, and many had mood or substance use disorders. Maximum dose was 200 mg/day, with mean dose 165 mg. In completers there appeared to be some response of depressive symptoms to desipramine, but PTSD symptoms as measured by the IES did not respond to the treatments. These data are limited by the short trial duration.

Davidson and colleagues[22] undertook an 8-week placebo-controlled trial of amitriptyline in 46 patients (33 completers) with chronic DSM-III PTSD. All patients were veterans, and 31 had comorbid diagnoses (including major depression). Amitriptyline was increased up to 300 mg/day. In the total group, amitriptyline was significantly superior to placebo for depressive symptoms, but not for PTSD symptoms. However, in completers, desipramine was superior to placebo on the

Table 9.1 Controlled studies of pharmacotherapy for post-traumatic stress disorder

Authors	Medication	Subjects details (completers)	Response rate (medication vs placebo)	Effect size (scale)
Baker et al 1995 (27)	Brofaromine up to 150 mg/d	118 DSM-III-R PTSD (83), PTSD>6 mos, CAPS>45, 60% combat-related, MADRS<23	60% vs 40%	–
Braun et al 1990 (71)	Alprazolam crossover up to 6 mg/d for 5 wks	16 DSM-III PTSD (10), treatment-refractory, combat-related and non-combat, two with comorbid MDE	–	0.23 (IES)
Davidson et al 1990 (22)	Amitriptyline up to 300 mg/d for 8 wks	46 DSM-III PTSD (33), combat-related, comorbid MDE allowed	50% vs 17%	1.32 (IES)
Kaplan et al 1996 (72)	Inositol 12 g/d for 4 wks	17 DSM-III-R PTSD (13), combat-related and non-combat, little comorbidity	–	0.22 (IES)
Katz et al 1994 (26)	Brofaromine up to 150 mg/d for 12 wks	64 DSM-III-R PTSD (45), CAPS>36, majority non-combat, HAM-D<22	52% vs 29%	0.46 (CAPS)
Kosten et al 1991 (25)	Imipramine up to 300 mg/d	60 DSM-III PTSD (31),	65% vs 28%	0.26 (IES)
	Phenelzine up to 75mg/d for 8 wks	Vietnam veterans, no comorbid MDE	68% vs 28%	0.95 (IES)
Nagy et al 1996 (46)	Fluoxetine up to 80 mg/d for 10 wks	22 PTSD (15), combat-related, comorbid MDE allowed	–	

CAPS, Clinician – Administered PTSD Scale; IES, Intrusive Experiences Scale; MDE, Major Depressive Episode: MADRS, Montgomery-Asberg Depression Rating Scale.

Table 9.1 Continued

Authors	Medication details (completers)	Subjects	Response rate (medication vs placebo)	Effect size (scale)
Reist et al 1989 (21)	Desipramine up to 200 mg/d for 4 wks	27 DSM-III PTSD (18), combat-related, comorbid MDE allowed	–	0.10 (IES)
Shestatzky et al 1988 (24)	Phenelzine crossover up to 90 mg/d for 5 wks	13 DSM-III PTSD (13), combat-related and non-combat, two with MDE	–	0.09 (IES) 0.25 (IES)
van der Kolk et al 1994 (45)	Fluoxetine crossover up to 60 mg/d for 5 wks	64 DSM-III-R PTSD (48), combat-related and non-combat, comorbid MDE allowed	–	

Note: Response rates in the Baker et al (27) and Katz et al (26) studies are taken from Davidson et al (1997).

CGI scale (severity item) and on the Impact of Events Scale (especially avoidance).

In an analysis of a larger database from the same study, Davidson and colleagues[23] focused on predictors of treatment response. They found that prior degree of combat intensity, current levels of PTSD, several items in the avoidant cluster of the IES, levels of depressive and anxiety symptoms, the symptom of guilt and the personality trait of neuroticism all predicted poor response to amitriptyline. Such findings differ from those in depression, where severity and guilt are good predictors of response to medication.

Shestatzky and colleagues[24] undertook a crossover trial with 5 weeks each of phenelzine and placebo in 13 patients (all of whom were completers) with chronic DSM-III PTSD. Patients had suffered various kinds of trauma (civilian and combat-related), and two had comorbid major depression. Target dose was 90 mg/day. There was a significantly higher dropout rate with phenelzine than with placebo, and phenelzine did not significantly differ from placebo in effects on PTSD, as assessed by scales including the CGI (severity item) scale and the IES. Improvement was, however, seen over time on these scales, possibly suggesting that a longer trial may have yielded greater efficacy.

Kosten and colleagues[25] undertook a comparison of imipramine, phenelzine and placebo in an 8-week trial in 60 patients (31 completers) with chronic DSM-III PTSD. All patients were Vietnam veterans, and none had comorbid major depression, although 57% had a history of past substance abuse. Target doses for imipramine were 200–300 mg/day, and for phenelzine 60–75 mg/day. By week 5, both imipramine and phenelzine significantly reduced PTSD symptoms on the IES. Phenelzine appeared superior to imipramine in terms of treatment retention, degree of improvement and range of improvement (phenelzine improved both intrusion and avoidance symptoms, whereas imipramine improved only intrusion symptoms). This study was important in showing that PTSD response was not dependent on patients having comorbid major depression.

Katz and colleagues[26] undertook a 14-week European multicentre placebo-controlled trial of brofaromine in 64 patients (45 completers) with DSM-III-R PTSD. Patients had a minimal score of 36 on the CAPS and none had comorbid major depression. The majority of subjects were civilians rather than combat veterans. Brofaromine, which is a reversible selective monoamine oxidase (MAO) type A inhibitor and serotonin reuptake inhibitor, was increased to a maximum of 150 mg/day. There was no significant benefit for brofaromine over placebo on PTSD symptoms as assessed by the CAPS. However, brofaromine was significantly superior to placebo on the CGI scale (severity item), and a subanalysis of 45 patients with PTSD symptoms lasting 1 year or longer demonstrated superiority for the active agent on the CAPS and CGI score. This trial is notable for representing the first large multicentre trial of PTSD.

A second, 12-week, multicentre placebo-controlled study of brofaromine was conducted, this time in the United States, in 146 patients (83 completers) with DSM-III-R PTSD of at least 6 months' duration.[27] Patients had a minimum score of 45 on the CAPS and a maximum score of 22 on the Montgomery-Asberg Depression Rating Scale (MADRS). In contrast to the first study of brofaromine, in this cohort 60% had combat-related trauma. Brofaromine was increased up to 150 mg/day. There was no significant drug-placebo difference on PTSD symptoms, as assessed by the CAPS and the CGI scale. Unfortunately, in both brofaromine studies there was a higher placebo response rate than in early PTSD studies.[21,22,25] Baker et al[27] suggested that this might reflect repeated patient–rater interactions because of multiple administrations of the lengthy CAPS interview. However, they also noted a high response rate during the single-blind placebo run-in. In sum, however, data on the value of this agent (which is not likely to reach the market) in PTSD are conflicting.

Selective serotonin reuptake inhibitors (SSRIs)

Several open studies investigating the role of the SSRIs and of the serotonin antagonist and reuptake inhibitors (SARIs) in the treatment of PTSD have been published in the past decade.[28–44]

In one of the largest open trials in combat-related trauma, for example, De Boer et al[34] studied fluvoxamine in 24 Dutch resistance fighters with chronic DSM-III-R PTSD or partial PTSD. Overall analysis indicated only modest improvement on a PTSD self-rating scale, but five of 11 completers reported a substantial improvement of their general condition, and particularly of sleep quality. These subjects insisted on continued use of fluvoxamine. Changes were most marked for re-experiencing and hyperarousal symptoms, rather than avoidance. Also interesting was a decrease in survivor guilt. Marmar et al[38] also studied fluvoxamine in combat veterans, but this time in the United States. There was substantial improvement in all three symptom clusters. Interestingly, however, hostility did not improve. Finally, fluvoxamine appeared effective in a civilian population.[31]

Marshall et al[39] completed one of the largest open trials in a non-combat population, in which they demonstrated efficacy for paroxetine in chronic DSM-III-R PTSD. Paroxetine was increased up to 60 mg over 12 weeks. The study was particularly interesting insofar as a careful analysis of the time course of response across different symptom clusters was undertaken. Most of the improvement in hyperarousal, and much of the improvement in avoidance, occurred within the first 8 weeks. However, re-experiencing symptoms improved more gradually throughout the 12 weeks of the study. All endpoint responders were responders by week 8, but PTSD symptom reduction continued steadily to reach 48% reduction by 12 weeks. Another interesting finding was that cumulative childhood trauma was significantly and negatively correlated with response.

In an open trial in six combat veterans with PTSD, trazodone at doses up to 400 mg/day was only modestly helpful in decreasing PTSD symptoms on the CAPS, but did increase sleep quality and duration.[35] Subsequently, this group reported that in a 12-week study of nefazodone, at doses increased up to 600 mg/day, 10 of 10 combat veterans with DSM-IV chronic PTSD (seven with comorbid major depression) demonstrated a clinical response on the CGI change item.[36] The authors emphasized the improvement of both sleep and anger symptoms. Also of interest, re-experiencing symptoms did not improve by week 12, but did show improvement in a follow-up appointment at week 16. These preliminary findings are supported by a number of other open studies in different populations,[32,33] and by an open study indicating that nefazodone was useful in 18 combat veterans who had proved refractory to multiple medication trials.[44]

Van der Kolk and colleagues[45] undertook a placebo-controlled 5-week trial of fluoxetine in 64 patients (48 completers) with DSM-III-R PTSD. Of these 31 were veterans, and 33 had experienced non-combat trauma; 54% had current MDE. Fluoxetine was increased to a maximum of 60 mg/day. Fluoxetine was significantly superior to placebo on the CAPS. However, in the VA subgroup, a significant difference was seen only on depression symptoms. Although VA patients had more severe PTSD symptoms at baseline, in the non-combat patients severity predicted good outcome. Changes were most marked in hyperarousal and numbing symptoms. Interestingly, on the Disorders of Extreme Stress Inventory, fluoxetine had a significant positive effect on several associated features of PTSD including affect dysregulation, distorted relationships with others and lack of sustaining beliefs (but not in hostility or dissociation). Also of note was that a placebo response was present in the non-combat group. Nevertheless, it may be argued that although PTSD placebo-responders can be identified, the magnitude of their response on the CGI falls below that associated with medication.[3]

Nagy et al[46] and Davidson et al[3] have also reported no benefit of fluoxetine in placebo-controlled trials in combat veterans. However, in a 12-week placebo-controlled study of PTSD in 53 civilians, Davidson et al[3] reported a significant effect for fluoxetine in all symptom clusters. Patients who failed to respond by week 4 were unlikely to respond by week 12. Notably, there was also a significant improvement on quality of life indicators in this trial.

Two large multisite placebo-controlled trials of sertraline have recently been undertaken.[47] Preliminary presentations of this work suggest that this agent is both safe and effective in PTSD. There is also ongoing work on fluoxetine, paroxetine and nefazodone.

Other agents

Several other agents have been suggested as useful in case reports or small open-label trials. Propranolol and clonidine, both of which effectively suppress noradrenergic activity, have been described as useful in a number of open case series.[48–51] There is also a case report suggesting the efficacy of the alpha-agonist guanfacine in a young girl.[52] Although preliminary, these data are certainly consistent with hypotheses which emphasize the role of noradrenergic dysfunction in PTSD.

Serotonergic agents other than the antidepressants have also been suggested to be useful in cases of PTSD. There is some work, for example, on buspirone.[53–55] Fichtner and Crayton[56] suggest that doses of 60 mg/day or higher are effective, particularly for hyperarousal symptoms. In addition, cyproheptadine (up to 12 mg at bedtime) has been reported valuable for relieving nightmares in small case series of patients with PTSD.[57,58]

Dopamine blockers have occasionally been reported useful in some cases of PTSD.[13,59] The introduction of the novel atypical antipsychotics with their relatively favourable side effect profile and serotonergic effects raises the question of their role in PTSD. Leyba and Wampler[60] recently reported the use of risperidone in four cases of PTSD characterized by vivid flashbacks and nightmares. Controlled studies of these novel agents seem warranted.

Preclinical data and pharmacological challenge studies provide some evidence that the opioid system plays a role in mediating PTSD symptoms.[11] Interestingly, Glover[61] reported that eight of 18 veterans responded to the opiate antagonist nalmefene. Similarly, naltrexone (50 mg/day) was reported to be effective in reducing flashbacks in two patients with PTSD.[62] However, there are no controlled studies of opioid agents in PTSD.

There are several reports of the value of thymoleptics – lithium,[63–65] carbamazepine[66–68] and valproate[69] – in PTSD. This work is of particular theoretical interest in view of the hypothesis that neuronal kindling may play a role in the mediation of PTSD symptoms.[64] Lipper et al[66] reported that seven of 10 combat veterans responded to carbamazepine. Interestingly, there was a decrease not only in intrusive symptoms, but also in hostility; this is certainly consistent with the effects of these agents in other disorders. In Wolf and colleagues' study,[67] carbamazepine was effective in eight of 10 of patients, with a particular decrease in impulsivity. Fesler[69] found that 10 of 16 combat veterans without comorbid major depression responded when valproate was initiated or added to an ongoing medication regime. Hyperarousal and avoidant symptoms were particularly responsive.

The use of benzodiazepines in PTSD has been described by a number of authors.[64,70] Clonazepam might seem promising insofar as it has a relatively long duration of action as well as serotonergic effects, but there are no controlled trials of this agent in PTSD. Braun and colleagues[71] undertook a crossover trial of 5 weeks each of alprazolam and placebo in 16 patients (10 completers) with chronic DSM-III PTSD. Patients had suffered various kinds of trauma (civilian and combat-related), and only two had comorbid major depression. However, the group was characterized as 'treatment-refractory', having failed to respond to a number of different antidepressants. Alprazolam was increased up to 6 mg/day. Improvement in anxiety symptoms was significantly greater with alprazolam than with placebo, but modest in extent. Furthermore, there was no significant benefit of alprazolam over placebo on PTSD symptoms, as assessed by scales including the IES.

Inositol (12 g/day) was studied in 17 patients (13 were completers) with DSM-III-R PTSD in a 4-week placebo-controlled crossover design study.[72] Patients had suffered various kinds of trauma (civilian and combat-related), but had relatively little comorbidity. Reduction in scores on the IES did not significantly differ between inositol and placebo. Even considering the methodological limitations of the study, the results were somewhat disappointing in view of the apparent efficacy of inositol in controlled studies of major depression and panic disorder.

Summary

There is stronger evidence for the use of antidepressants than for any other class of agent in PTSD. A recommendation to use antidepressants seems particularly reasonable given the comorbidity of PTSD, which frequently includes major depression and other anxiety disorders for which the antidepressants are effective. Although there is a paucity of controlled trials comparing different antidepressants, the SSRIs may be argued to be the agents of choice in view of their safety and tolerability, and in view of the possibility that serotonergic agents may be particularly effective in PTSD. The choice of an SSRI with proven efficacy across a range of anxiety disorders would seem sensible.

Indeed, according to a meta-analysis of six controlled trials of PTSD by Penava et al,[73] there is evidence of a correlation between greater serotonergic activity and higher effect size. In Table 9.1, we provide our own calculations of CGI response rate and of PTSD symptom scale effect sizes. Effect sizes of 0.5–0.8 are considered moderate, while effective sizes of greater than 0.8 are strong. Although effect sizes from ongoing multicentre trials of the SSRIs in PTSD are not yet published, on the basis of preliminary analyses Davidson et al[3] have indicated that effect sizes may be moderate to strong.

Similarly, in a retrospective chart assessment of CGI scores after at least 1 month of medication in 72 patients with PTSD and comorbid depression, Dow and Kline[74] found that serotonergic antidepressants were associated with better outcomes than noradrenergic ones. Success rates of greater than 30% were obtained for fluoxetine, sertraline, imipramine and phenelzine, while success rates of less than 10% were obtained with several agents including desipramine, amitriptyline, nortriptyline and bupropion.

Is there any evidence that particular subsymptoms of PTSD will respond to particular agents? One suggestion might be that noradrenergic tricyclics are particularly useful for re-experiencing symptoms, serotonergic agents are particularly useful for numbing symptoms, while addition of benzodiazepines and other agents can be considered for any non-responsive hyperarousal symptoms.[45,75] Nevertheless, over time the SSRIs may also decrease intrusive symptoms (much as is the case in obsessive-compulsive disorder),[39] supporting the case for initiating pharmacotherapy with these agents.

Agents other than the SSRIs may, however, be useful in a number of circumstances. MAOIs, for example, may have a role in the management of treatment-refractory cases.[18,76] Noradrenergic agents may be posited to be useful for hyperarousal, thymoleptics for hostility and impulse dysregulation and atypical neuroleptics for paranoid or other psychotic symptoms.[77] Nevertheless, these are extremely rough guidelines which remain to be demonstrated conclusively by empirical studies. In the interim, such agents should perhaps be primarily considered in the augmentation of refractory patients (see below). In contrast, there are several reasons to be cautious about the use of benzodiazepines, including lack of efficacy, adverse effects including sexual dysfunction,[78] possible depressogenic and paradoxical effects, and well-documented severe withdrawal problems.[79] Nevertheless, these agents may be considered for such symptoms of hyperarousal as insomnia, on a time-limited basis.

Is it possible to predict which PTSD patients will respond to medication? Van der Kolk et al[45] found that PTSD in civilians is more likely to respond to SSRIs than is combat PTSD. However, this finding may reflect any number of factors that differ between these two populations (including a history of multiple failed treatments in veterans). Indeed, an overall examination of studies in combat and non-combat populations suggests that drug response rates may in fact be similar[3] (see also Table 9.1). In a combat population, Davidson et al[23] found that severity of PTSD symptoms was a negative predictor of response to medication. However, in a non-combat population, van der Kolk et al[45] found severity of PTSD symptoms to be a positive predictor. Increased childhood abuse may be a negative predictor of response to medication.[39]

Augmentation strategies

There is growing acknowledgement that in major depression and many anxiety disorders, not all patients respond to treatment with a first- or even second-line agent. It is possible that in refractory patients, multiple systems are involved, requiring the use of medications with different actions.

Of course, before making the determination that a patient is refractory, it is important to return to basic principles. Is the diagnosis correct? Has a comorbid substance use disorder or underlying general medical disorder been missed? Has medication been used at appropriate doses and durations?

Unfortunately, the number of studies of augmentation in PTSD is extremely limited. Imipramine with clonidine has been described in Cambodian refugees.[50] As noted earlier there are also reports of the successful addition of anticonvulsants.[69]

An open study of buspirone augmentation (30–60 mg/day) of antidepressant agents (mostly SSRIs) was undertaken in 15 Vietnam veterans with chronic DSM-IV PTSD (14 with comorbid major depression).[80] The authors found that nine of 14 completers were responders on the CGI scale (change item). Improvement was seen in all PTSD symptom subtypes as well as in depression. These data are consistent with a range of studies of buspirone augmentation in depression.

Conclusion

The outlines of an algorithm for the pharmacotherapy of PTSD are presented in Figure 9.1. It should be emphasized, however, that this algorithm is based on an extremely limited number of studies. Nevertheless, as noted earlier, we think that there is reasonable evidence for choosing an antidepressant, and an SSRI in particular, as a first-line agent in the pharmacotherapy of most patients with PTSD. Of course, each patient must be assessed individually, and choice will vary accordingly, particularly if there are complications. SSRIs may, however, be useful in certain complicated patients, for example, those with comorbid substance abuse.[28]

The time to onset of a drug vs placebo difference appears longer for some medications than others.[3] In the case of a robust agent such as fluoxetine, any improvement on the CGI by

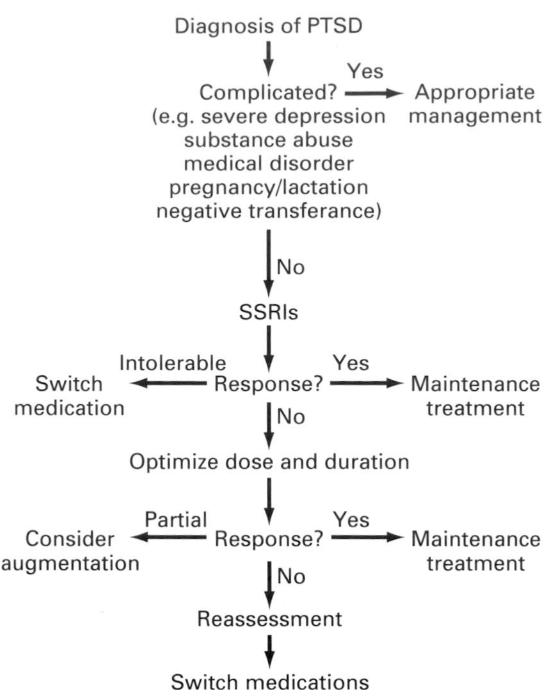

Figure 9.1. Algorithm for the pharmacotherapy of post-traumatic stress disorder (PTSD). (SSRIs, selective serotonic reuptake inhibitors.)

week 2 may be a good predictor of clinical response at week 12.[3] Similarly, patients on paroxetine appear to respond before 8 weeks if at all.[39] Nevertheless, up to 12 weeks of treatment may be necessary to determine accurately the extent of possible symptomatic benefit. Similarly, although standard antidepressant doses of the SSRIs can be effective in PTSD,[45] our tendency is to use maximum recommended doses if these are tolerated.

The treatment of refractory patients is poorly explored, although there is anecdotal evidence that agents such as phenelzine may be useful.[18] Despite the lack of a good empirical database, augmentation of SSRIs with a range of agents, including tricyclic antidepressants,[29] noradrenergic agents, thymoleptics or atypical neuroleptics, can be considered. Similarly, on the basis of studies of major depression, it may be suggested that switching SSRIs, or switching antidepressant classes, may be useful. The classical MAOIs should certainly be borne in mind. Ultimately, the roles of a range of other somatic interventions, such as transcranial magnetic stimulation, also deserve further exploration in PTSD.

There are several areas which call out for further research. Large multicentre studies continue to be warranted. These are needed not only to determine optimal dose and duration of agents, but also to ascertain differential response of patients with different traumas (combat vs civilian, single vs multiple), different symptoms (intrusive vs avoidant), and different subtypes of PTSD (for example, delayed onset) to pharmacotherapy and to better delineate other predictors (such as comorbidity) of pharmacotherapy response. Similarities and differences between drug and placebo response characteristics[3] deserve further scrutiny. Finally, pharmacoeconomic and quality of life issues require further exploration.

The pharmacotherapy of children and adolescents with PTSD is an area in which there has been particularly little work. Published case reports and open trials have focused primarily on noradrenergic agents; beta-blockers,[48] clonidine[49] and guanfacine.[52] There is also preliminary work on the efficacy of carbamazepine.[63] Nevertheless, our impression is that the SSRIs also have a particularly useful role in the treatment of PTSD in younger patients.[81]

There is relatively little work on patients with acute stress disorder or with partial PTSD,[34] so that questions of how long to wait before beginning treatment or of the minimum criteria for treatment cannot be answered with certainty using extant data. Furthermore, despite an animal literature suggesting that early pharmacological intervention may prevent traumatic stress responses, there is no evidence as yet for the efficacy of such interventions in humans. In one study, 13 trauma survivors were treated within 2–18 days of the trauma with clonazepam or alprazolam for up to 6 months,[82] but subjects fared no better in terms of PTSD symptoms on the IES and other scales at 6 months than a matched untreated group. This parallels findings in the psychotherapy literature which raise questions about the value of early intervention. Ongoing work may, however, provide new insights in this area. Certainly, there is already some evidence that neurobiological markers in the aftermath of trauma can be used to predict the later development of PTSD.

Maintenance pharmacotherapy and antidepressant discontinuation in PTSD have not been well studied. Given that structural changes have been associated with PTSD, it might be hypothesized that a cautious approach, with patients receiving at least a year of treatment before discontinuation, should be suggested. Similarly, it would seem prudent to ensure that psychosocial factors (including support) are optimal at the time of discontinuation. Again, despite the lack of rigorous data, a slow taper of medication would seem advisable.

Research comparing pharmacotherapy with other modalities of treatment and with the combination of pharmacotherapy and psychotherapy is also needed. There is anecdotal evidence that pharmacotherapy may facilitate psychotherapy.[13,17,18] Theoretically, reduction of anxiety may optimize cognitive-affective reprocessing of the traumatic event.[6] Certainly, meta-analytic studies have been positive about the effect size of certain psychotherapies in PTSD. Nevertheless, there is a lack of studies directly comparing pharmacotherapy and psychotherapy in PTSD.

The integration of pharmacotherapy studies with other biological research is also an important area for further investigation. A study showing that abnormal platelet 3H-paroxetine binding predicted positive response to fluoxetine,[10] for example, is one of the few in which biological markers are used in this way. Similarly, there are few studies of the effects of medication on functional brain imaging. There is little question that future studies in this vein will significantly expand our understanding of the neurobiology and pharmacotherapy of this complex disorder.

Acknowledgment

The authors are supported by the Medical Research Council (South Africa).

References

1. Friedman MJ, Toward rational pharmacotherapy for posttraumatic stress disorder: an interim report, *Am J Psychiatry* (1988) 145:281–5.
2. Kolb LC, The place of narcosynthesis in the treatment of chronic and delayed stress reactions of war. In: Sonnenberg SM, Blank AS, Talbott JA, eds, *The Trauma of War Stress and Recovery in Vietnam Veterans* (American Psychiatric Press: Washington, DC, 1985).
3. Davidson JRT, Malik ML, Sutherland SN, Response characteristics to antidepressants and placebo in post-traumatic stress disorder, *Int Clin Psychopharmacol* (1997) 12:291–6.
4. Kleinman A, *Rethinking Psychiatry: From Cultural Category to Personal Experience* (Free Press: New York, 1988).
5. Shay, J, *Achilles in Vietnam: Combat Trauma and the Undoing of Character* (Touchstone: 1995).

6. Southwick SM, Yehuda R, The interaction between pharmacotherapy and psychotherapy in the treatment of posttraumatic stress disorder, *Am J Psychother* (1993) 47:404–10.
7. Kent JM, Coplan JD, Gorman JM, Clinical utility of the selective serotonin reuptake inhibitors in the spectrum of anxiety, *Biol Psychiatry* (1998) 44:812–24.
8. Southwick SM, Krystal JH, Bremner JD et al, Noradrenergic and serotonergic function in posttraumatic stress disorder, *Arch Gen Psychiatry* (1997) 54:749–58.
9. Arora FC, Fichtner CG, O'Connor F, Crayton JW, Paroxetine binding in the blood platelets of post-traumatic stress disorder patients, *Life Sci* (1993) 53:919–28.
10. Fichtner CG, Arora RC, O'Connor FL, Crayton JW, Platelet paroxetine binding and fluoxetine pharmacotherapy in posttraumatic stress disorder: preliminary observations on a possible predictor of clinical treatment response, *Life Sci* (1994) 54:39–44.
11. Charney DS, Deutch AY, Krystal JH et al, Psychobiologic mechanisms of posttraumatic stress disorder, *Arch Gen Psychiatry* (1993) 50:294–306.
12. Blake DJ, Treatment of acute post-traumatic stress disorder with tricyclic antidepressants, *South Med J* (1986) 79:201–4.
13. Bleich A, Siegel B, Garb R et al, Post-traumatic stress disorder following combat exposure: clinical features and psychopharmacological treatment, *Br J Psychiatry* (1986) 149:365–9.
14. Burstein A, Treatment of post-traumatic stress disorder with imipramine, *Psychosomatics* (1984) 25:3681–7.
15. Falcone S, Tricyclics: possible treatment for post-traumatic stress disorder, *J Clin Psychiatry* (1985) 46:385–9.
16. White NS, Post-traumatic stress disorder, *Hosp Community Psychiatry* (1983) 34:1061–2.
17. Davidson J, Walker JI, Kilts C, A pilot study of phenelzine in the treatment of post-traumatic stress disorder, *Br J Psychiatry* (1987) 150:252–5.
18. Hogben GL, Cornfield RB, Treatment of traumatic war neurosis with phenelzine, *Arch Gen Psychiatry* (1981) 38:440–5.
19. Milanes F, Mack C, Phenelzine treatment of post-Vietnam stress syndrome, *VA Practitioner* (1984) 1:40–9.
20. Neal LA, Shapland W, Fox C, An open trial of moclobemide in the treatment of post-traumatic stress disorder, *Int Clin Psychopharmacol* (1997) 12:231–7.
21. Reist C, Kauffman CD, Haier RJ et al, A controlled trial of desipramine in 18 men with posttraumatic stress disorder, *Am J Psychiatry* (1989) 146:513–16.
22. Davidson JRT, Kudler HS, Smith RD et al, Treatment of post-traumatic stress disorder with amitriptyline and placebo, *Arch Gen Psychiatry* (1990) 47:259–66.
23. Davidson JRT, Kudler HS, Saunders WB et al, Predicting response to amitriptyline in posttraumatic stress disorder, *Am J Psychiatry* (1993) 150:1024–9.
24. Shestatzky M, Greenberg D, Lerer B, A controlled trial of phenelzine in post-traumatic stress disorder, *Psychiatry Res* (1988) 24:149–55.
25. Kosten TR, Frank JB, Dan E et al, Pharmacotherapy for posttraumatic stress disorder using phenelzine or imipramine, *J Nerv Ment Dis* (1991) 179:366–70.
26. Katz RJ, Lott MH, Arbus P et al, Pharmacotherapy of post-traumatic stress disorder with a novel psychotropic, *Anxiety* (1995) 1:169–74.
27. Baker DG, Diamond BI, Gillette G et al, A double-blind, randomized placebo-controlled multi-center study of brofaromine in the treatment of post-traumatic stress disorder, *Psychopharmacology* (1995) 122:386–9.
28. Brady KT, Sonne SC, Roberts JM, Sertraline treatment of comorbid posttraumatic stress disorder and alcohol dependence, *J Clin Psychiatry* (1995) 56:502–5.
29. Burdon AP, Sutker PB, Foulks EF et al, Pilot program of treatment for PTSD [letter], *Am J Psychiatry* (1991) 148:1269–70.
30. Davidson J, Roth S, Newman E, Fluoxetine in post-traumatic stress disorder, *J Trauma Stress* (1990) 4:419–23.
31. Davidson JR, Weisler RH, Malik M et al, Fluvoxamine in civilians with posttraumatic stress disorder [letter], *J Clin Psychopharmacol* (1998) 18:93–5.
32. Davidson JRT, Weisler RH, Malik ML, Connor MK, Treatment of posttraumatic stress disorder with nefazodone, *Int Clin Psychopharmacol*, (1998) 13:111–3.
33. Davis L, Nugent A, Murray J et al, Nefazodone treatment for chronic PTSD: an open trial [abstract], *Biol Psychiatry* (1998) 43:57S.

34. De Boer M, Op den Velde W, Falger PJR et al, Fluvoxamine treatment for chronic PTSD: a pilot study, *Psychother Psychosom* (1992) **57**:158–63.
35. Hertzberg MA, Feldman ME, Beckham JC et al, Trial of trazodone for posttraumatic stress disorder using a multiple baseline group design, *J Clin Psychopharmacol* (1996) **16**:294–8.
36. Hertzberg MA, Feldman ME, Beckham JC et al, Open trial of nefazodone for combat-related posttraumatic stress disorder, *J Clin Psychiatry* (1998) **59**:460–4.
37. Kline NA, Dow BM, Brown SA et al, Setraline efficacy in depressed combat veterans with posttraumatic stress disorder [letter], *J Clin Psychopharmacol* (1993) **13**:107–13.
38. Marmar CR, Schoenfeld F, Weiss DS et al, Open trial of fluvoxamine treatment for combat-related posttraumatic stress disorder, *J Clin Psychiatry* (1996) **57S**:66–72.
39. Marshall RD, Schneier FR, Fallon BA et al, An open trial of paroxetine in patients with noncombat-related, chronic posttraumatic stress disorder, *J Clin Psychopharmacol* (1998) **18**:10–18.
40. McDougle CJ, Southwick SM, Charney DS et al, An open trial of fluoxetine in the treatment of posttraumatic stress disorder, *J Clin Psychopharmacol* (1991) **11**:325–7.
41. Nagy LM, Morgan CA, Southwick SM et al, Open prospective trial of fluoxetine for posttraumatic stress disorder, *J Clin Psychopharmacol* (1993) **13**:107–13.
42. Rothbaum BO, Ninan PT, Thomas L, Sertraline in the treatment of rape victims with posttraumatic stress disorder, *J Trauma Stress* (1996) **9**:865–71.
43. Shay J, Fluoxetine reduces explosiveness and elevates mood of Vietnam combat veterans with PTSD, *J Trauma Stress* (1992) **5**:97–101.
44. Zisook S, Chentsova-Dutton Y, Ellenor G et al, Nefazodone in patients with treatment-refractory PTSD. Presented at the Annual Meeting of the American Psychiatric Association, 1999.
45. van der Kolk BA, Dreyfuss D, Michaels B et al, Fluoxetine treatment in posttraumatic stress disorder, *J Clin Psychiatry* (1994) **55**:517–22.
46. Nagy LM, Southwick SM, Charney DS, Placebo-controlled trial of fluoxetine in PTSD. Poster presentation, International Society for Traumatic Stress Studies Twelfth Annual Meeting, San Francisco, CA, 11 November 1996.
47. Rothbaum B, Farfel G, Two multicenter trials evaluating sertraline and placebo for the treatment of PTSD. Presented at the Annual Meeting of the American Psychiatric Association, Washington, DC, 1999.
48. Famularo R, Kinscherff R, Fenton T, Propranolol treatment for childhood post traumatic stress disorder, acute type. A pilot study, *Am J Dis Child* (1988) **142**:1244–7.
49. Harmon RJ, Riggs PD, Clonidine for post-traumatic stress disorder in preschool children, *J Am Acad Child Adolesc Psychiatry* (1996) **35**:1247–9.
50. Kinzie JD, Leung P, Clonidine in Cambodian patients with post-traumatic stress disorder, *J Nerv Ment Dis* (1989) **177**:546–50.
51. Kolb LC, Burris BC, Griffiths S, Propranolol and clonidine in the treatment of post-traumatic stress disorders of war. In: van der Kolk BA, ed, *Post-Traumatic Stress Disorder: Psychological and Biological Sequelae* (American Psychiatric Press: Washington, DC, 1984).
52. Horrigan JP, Guanfacine for PTSD nightmares, *J Am Acad Child Adolesc Psychiatry* (1996) **35**:975–6.
53. Duffy JD, Malloy PF, Efficacy of buspirone in the treatment of post-traumatic stress disorder: an open trial, *Ann Clin Psychiatry* (1994) **6**:33–7.
54. LaPorta LD, Ware MR, Buspirone and the treatment of posttraumatic stress disorder, *J Clin Psychopharmacol* (1992) **12**:133–4.
55. Wells BG, Chu CC, Johnson R et al, Buspirone in the treatment of post-traumatic stress disorder, *Pharmacotherapy* (1991) **11**:340–3.
56. Fichtner CG, Crayton JW, Buspirone in combat-related posttraumatic stress disorder, *J Clin Psychiatry* (1994) **57S8**:66–72.
57. Brophy MH, Cyproheptadine for combat nightmares in posttraumatic stress disorder and dream anxiety disorder, *Mil Med* (1991) **156**:100–1.
58. Gupta S, Popli A, Bathurst E et al, Efficacy of cyproheptadine for nightmares associated with posttraumatic stress disorder, *Compr Psychiatry* (1998) **39**:160–4.
59. Dillard ML, Bendfeldt F, Jernigan P, Use of thioridazine in post-traumatic stress disorder, *South Med J* (1993) **86**:1276–8.
60. Leyba CM, Wampler TP, Risperidone in PTSD [letter], *Psychiatr Serv* (1998) **49**:245–6.
61. Glover H, A preliminary trial of nalmefene for the treatment of emotional numbing in combat veterans with post-traumatic stress disorder, *Isr J Psychiatry Relat Sci* (1993) **30**:255–63.

62. Bills, LJ, Kreisler K, Treatment of flashbacks with naltrexone [letter], *Am J Psychiatry* (1993) **150**:1430.
63. Kitchner I, Greenstein R, Low dose lithium carbonate in the treatment of post traumatic stress disorder: brief communication, *Mil Med* (1985) **150**:378–81.
64. van der Kolk BA, The drug treatment of post-traumatic stress disorder, *J Affect Disord* (1987) **13**:203–13.
65. Forster PL, Schoenfield FB, Marmar CR et al, Lithium for irritability in post-traumatic stress disorder, *J Trauma Stress* (1995) **8**:143–9.
66. Lipper S, Davidson JRT, Grady TA et al, Preliminary study of carbamazepine in post-traumatic stress disorder, *Psychosomatics* (1986) **27**:849–54.
67. Wolf ME, Alavi A, Mosnaim AD, Posttraumatic stress disorder in Vietnam veterans: clinical and EEG findings; possible therapeutic effects of carbamazepine, *Biol Psychiatry* (1988) **23**:642–4.
68. Looff D, Grimley P, Kuller F et al, Carbamazepine for PTSD, *J Am Acad Child Adolesc Psychiatry* (1995) **34**:703–4.
69. Fesler FA, Valproate in combat-related posttraumatic stress disorder, *J Clin Psychiatry* (1991) **52**:361–4.
70. Lowenstein RJ, Hornstein N, Farber B, Open trial of clonazepam in the treatment of post traumatic stress symptoms in multiple personality disorder, *Dissociation* (1988) **1**:3–12.
71. Braun P, Greenberg D, Dasberg H, Lerer B, Core symptoms of posttraumatic stress disorder unimproved by alprazolam treatment, *J Clin Psychiatry* (1990) **51**:236–8.
72. Kaplan Z, Amir M, Swartz M, Levine J, Inositol treatment of post-traumatic stress disorder, *Anxiety* (1996) **2**:51–2.
73. Penava SJ, Otto MW, Pollack MH et al, Current status of pharmacotherapy for PTSD: an effect size analysis of controlled studies, *Depression Anxiety* (1996/1997) **4**:240–2.
74. Dow B, Kline N, Antidepressant treatment of posttraumatic stress disorder and major depression in veterans, *Ann Clin Psychiatry* (1997) **9**:1–5.
75. Sutherland SM, Davidson JRT, Pharmacotherapy for post-traumatic stress disorder, *Psychiatr Clin North Am* (1994) **17**:409–23.
76. Demartino R, Mollica RF, Wilk V, Monoamine oxidase inhibitors in posttraumatic stress disorder, *J Nerv Ment Dis* (1995) **183**:510–15.
77. Hamner MB, Clozapine treatment for a veteran with comorbid psychosis and PTSD [letter], *Am J Psychiatry* (1996) **153**:841.
78. Fossey MD, Hamner MB, Clonazepam-related sexual dysfunction in male veterans with PTSD, *Anxiety* (1994/1995) **1**:233–6.
79. Risse SC, Whitters A, Burke J et al, Severe withdrawal symptoms after discontinuation of alprazolam in eight patients with combat-induced posttraumatic stress disorder, *J Clin Psychiatry* (1990) **51**:206–9.
80. Hamner M, Ulmer H, Horne D, Buspirone potentiation of antidepressants in the treatment of PTSD, *Depression Anxiety* (1997) **5**:137–9.
81. Seedat S, Lockhat R, Zungu-Dirwayi N et al, Preliminary data from an open trial of citalopram in adolescents with PTSD. Presented at Biannual Meeting of the Society of Biological Psychiatrists of South Africa, Stellenbosch, 1999.
82. Gelpin E, Bonne O, Peri T et al, Treatment of recent trauma survivors with benzodiazepines: a prospective study, *J Clin Psychiatry* (1996) **57**:390–4.

10

Traumatic stress disorders in children

John S March, Norah Feeny, Lisa Amaya-Jackson and Edna Foa

Since post-traumatic stress disorder (PTSD) entered the psychiatric lexicon with DSM-III,[1] followed shortly by Terr's pioneering studies of the children of Chowchilla,[2] numerous investigations have confirmed that exposure to life-threatening stressors can lead to serious and often debilitating PTSD in young persons[3] just as in adults.[4] With over 20 years of research on pediatric PTSD in place, child psychiatrists and psychologists have come to appreciate the extent to which children are exposed to traumatic situations, the severity of their acute distress, and the potential serious long-term psychiatric sequelae, and to embed the empirical investigation of traumatic events and their post-traumatic sequelae within a sound developmental framework. In this chapter, we review the epidemiology, diagnosis and assessment, and treatment (psychosocial and medical) of PTSD. Interested readers may wish also to review more in-depth treatments of developmental approaches to PTSD[5] assessment,[6] and treatment.[7]

Epidemiology

Most experts agree that PTSD is common, chronic, underdiagnosed, and undertreated. PTSD is also associated with considerable impairment. In adults, it is estimated that traumatic events are experienced by 70% of the population and are linked etiologically to the development of PTSD.[8] Exposure to high-magnitude trauma also occurs at alarmingly high rates in children. For example, in one study, 40% of adolescents in a community school sample experienced a PTSD-qualifying trauma by age 18.[9] Of over 1000 middle and high school students in Chicago, 35% had witnessed a stabbing, 39% had seen a shooting, and almost 25% had witnessed someone being killed.[10] Nearly half of the victims were known to the child (for example, friends, family members, classmates). Additionally, 46% of these students reported having been a victim of at least one severe violent crime, including armed robbery, rape, and being shot or stabbed.

While the events that cause PTSD are common,[11] there are no epidemiological studies that look specifically at the general population incidence or prevalence of PTSD in young persons. It is quite clear, however, that PTSD is more common in youth exposed to life-threatening events, such as criminal assault,[12] hostage-taking,[13] combat,[14] bone marrow transplantation,[15] severe burns,[16] suicide,[17] and naval disaster.[18,19] Studies across a variety of industrial[20] and natural disasters[21,22] also show elevated rates of post-traumatic stress in disaster victims relative to controls.

Although the variety of events capable of producing PTSD varies somewhat between children and adults, characteristics of the stressor remain primary determinants of psychological reactions within and across a variety of settings.[23] For example, Pynoos and Nader showed that exposure (proximity) was linearly related to the risk for PTSD symptoms,[24] and that children's memory disturbances, indicating distorted cognitive processing during the event, closely followed exposure.[25] Saigh later showed that PTSD could result from direct, witnessed, or verbal exposure to trauma.[26] Aspects of the symptom picture vary with stressor-specific factors.[27–29] Chronic physical and sexual abuse in childhood often results in severe psychopathology that bears little resemblance to the classic PTSD symptom picture.[28] In this regard, Terr makes the clinically useful distinction between type I traumas (sudden, unpredictable single-incident stressor, that may be multiply repeated) and type II traumas (chronic expected repeated stressor, usually childhood physical and/or sexual abuse),[30] with these two broad categories representing differing literatures and sometimes different treatment approaches.[7]

Diagnosis and phenomenology

Four criteria must be met to establish a DSM-IV diagnosis of PTSD:[31]

1. Exposure to a PTSD-magnitude stressor.
2. Subsequent reexperiencing of the event.
3. Consequent avoidance or numbing of general responsiveness.
4. Persistent increased arousal.

Additionally, these difficulties must last more than 1 month and cause clinically significant distress or impairment.

Stressor

As noted above, the stressor criterion specifies PTSD-qualifying traumas, namely, exposure to a life-threatening event; the three latter symptom clusters point to important clinical parameters in the phenomenology of the disorder. Such traumatic experiences inevitably involve intense perceptual experiences and internal moment-to-moment appraisals of the threat and hence meet the DSM-IV criterion requiring terror, horror, or helplessness.[32]

Reexperiencing

Children and adolescents with PTSD typically reexperience the traumatic event in the form of distressing intrusive thoughts or memories, dreams, and less commonly, flashbacks. Reexperiencing may occur spontaneously or in response to reminders that are linked to traumatic moments within the event itself. For example, recurrent intrusive and distressing images, sounds, smells, or impressions often relate directly to moments of extreme horror or helplessness during the traumatic event. Children's traumatic dreams include repetitions of aspects of the experience, depiction of other life-threatening dangers or, over time, more general fearful dreams, for example, in young children, of being pursued by monsters.

Traumatic play and reenactment behaviors are not uncommon manifestations of reexperiencing in traumatized children and adolescents. Traumatic play refers to the repetitive expression in play of elements or themes of the event, for example, scenes of violence, or 'tornado' or 'earthquake' games.[33] Children sometimes involve siblings or peers in their traumatic play, with the incorporation of traumatic elements potentially impeding play's developmentally normative purpose,[34] which may go unnoticed by parents unless overtly distressing, dangerous, violent, suicidal, or sexually precocious. In contrast, reenactment behavior refers to unconscious recreation of some aspect of the traumatic experience.[33,35] In younger children, the behavior may be an 'action memory'. For example, an abused preschool child who had been locked in a closet subsequently repeatedly hid in small spaces, such as boxes or under desks, while consciously avoiding closets. Reenactment behavior in adolescents can be dangerous due to access to guns, automobiles, and drugs.

Avoidance and numbing

Children with PTSD invariably make conscious attempts to avoid traumatic reminders, namely thoughts, feelings, activities, or human behaviors that lead to distressing recollections of the event. Technically, traumatic reminders are conditioned stimuli that provoke conditioned responses directly or indirectly related to the traumatic event itself – including the external circumstances of the event and the internal emotional and physical reactions of the child. Common reminders include the following: circumstances (for example, location, time, preceding activity, clothes worn); precipitating conditions (for example, high winds after a tornado, arguing); other signs of danger (for example, staring eyes); unwanted results of the trauma (for example, fixed and dilated eyes, blood); potentially dangerous objects (for example, trees, broken glass, weapons); and a sense of helplessness (for example, cries for help, crying, fast heart beat, a sinking feeling, ineffectualness or moments of aloneness). Normal school procedures and academic exercises may serve as reminders. For example, a fire drill may evoke the sense of a prior emergency, or a civics class discussion of judicial proceedings may kindle fear and rage over the trial of a father's murderer.

Traumatic avoidance may selectively restrict daily activity or generalize to more phobic behavior. Children who have been exposed to trauma may discontinue pleasurable activities in order to avoid excitement or fear. Diminished activity may represent a preoccupation with intrusive phenomena, a depressive reaction, an avoidance of affect or of traumatic reminders, or an effort to reduce the risk of further trauma. Not surprisingly, children pay a high price for these survival strategies, which often spill over into other domains of functioning. For example, child survivors of trauma may show markedly diminished interest in usually significant activities or elevated somatic/autonomic symptoms.[36] The loss of previously acquired skills may leave a child less verbal, or regressed to behaviors such as thumb-sucking or enuresis. Rather than reporting feeling 'numb', younger children report not wanting to know how they feel, tell of feeling alone with their subjective experience, or describe efforts to keep an emotion from emerging, for example by going to sit alone. Although initial clinical attention suggested a relative absence of major amnesia in children, recent studies have demonstrated a variety of memory disturbances,[37] including microamnesias and temporal or spatial distortions related to proximity, duration, or sequencing of the event. Less commonly, dissociative memory disturbances also occur, especially in response to physical coercion, molestation, or abuse.[38]

Hyperarousal

Sleep disturbances, irritability, difficulty concentrating, hypervigilance, exaggerated startle responses, and outbursts of aggression are evidence that the child is in a state of increased physiological arousal.[39,40] Somatic symptoms of autonomic hyperactivity may be both tonic or phasic in nature, with the latter occurring more often when the child encounters traumatic reminders.[36] The child is 'on alert', ready to respond to any environmental threat.[41] Especially in school age children, physiological reactivity may include somatic symptoms as a form of reexperiencing.[42] Sleep disturbances may be severe and persistent; changes seen in sleep architecture have been noted in adult studies.[43] Sleepwalking and night terrors are not uncommon. These sleep problems can further impair the child's ability to concentrate and attend to important tasks and thus may also adversely impact learning and behavior in school. Hypervigilance and exaggerated startle may alter a child's usual behavior by leading to persistent efforts to ensure personal security or the safety of others.[41,42] Lastly, temporary or chronic difficulty in modulating aggression can make children more irritable and easy to anger, resulting in a reduced tolerance of normal behaviors, of the demands and slights of peers and family members, and in unusual acts of aggression or social withdrawal.[44]

Comorbidity

As in adults,[4] children and adolescents with PTSD also exhibit higher rates of psychiatric comorbidity than those without PTSD. Depressive spectrum conditions, ranging from simple demoralization through melancholic major depression, are among the most common secondary symptoms.[45,46] Giaconia et al[9] reported that more than 41% of adolescents with PTSD met criteria for major depression by age 18, compared to 8% among their peers, and that PTSD was associated with a significantly increased risk for social anxiety (33%), specific phobia (29%), alcohol dependence (46%), and drug dependence (25%). Moreover, for many, the onset of PTSD preceded or co-occurred with the onset of these disorders, suggesting that PTSD triggered their occurrence. In a study of children traumatized by an industrial fire, exposure independent of post-traumatic stress symptoms strongly predicted general anxiety, depression, and externalizing symptoms.[20] Finally, a variety of collateral symptoms important to functional outcomes have also been reported in traumatized children. For example, adolescents with PTSD are at substantially greater risk for suicidal thoughts and attempts, have lower perceived health, greater numbers of sick days per month at school, lower high school grade point averages, and more school-related problems.[9,47]

Assessment

As with all psychiatric disorders, the first step in setting up a program of treatment for PTSD is a careful assessment.[6] Drawing from a recent National Institute of Mental Health (NIMH) consensus conference on assessing PTSD, March recently summarized the variables thought essential in treatment outcome and other studies of PTSD, including PTSD-specific factors as well as non-PTSD outcomes and risk and protective factors,[6] noting that three types of instruments are available for assessing PTSD in youth. These include:

1. Structured interviews that include a PTSD module.
2. PTSD-specific interviews.
3. Self-report checklists.

While semi-structured interviews are *de rigeur* for assessing psychiatric problems in children and adolescents, reliability or validity data regarding the PTSD modules for common instruments are just now becoming available.[48,49] Among PTSD-specific instruments, the most commonly used measure, the Pynoos–Nader version of the Stress-Reaction Index,[24] shows modest empirical support as a semi-structured interview and has been used as a self-report measure,[50] but does not adequately capture the DSM-IV criteria. With the support of the National Center for PTSD, Nader and colleagues recently developed the Clinician-Administered PTSD Scale–Child and Adolescent Version (CAPS-C).[51] Considerably easier to administer than the CAPS-C, the Child PTSD Symptom Scale (CPSS) is increasingly being used in research studies of pediatric PTSD.[52] Both the CAPS-C and the CPSS allow for reliable and valid current and lifetime diagnoses, and dimensional assessment of DSM-IV PTSD symptoms.

In addition to its use as a structured interview, the Pynoos version of the Reaction Index has been the most common scalar measure for assessing PTSD used as a self-report measure in epidemiological studies, including studies of hurricanes,[53] earthquake[54,55] and war zone exposure.[56] However, careful psychometric studies of the PTSD-RI have not been completed, and it also does not provide a stressor inventory or normative data. To address these problems, March and colleagues recently developed and normed a self-report measure of PTSD termed the Child and Adolescent Trauma Survey (CATS) (Table 10.1),[6] modeled on the Multidimensional

Table 10.1 Assessment requirements

Domain/subgroup	Population	Clinical	Treatment outcome
Criterion A	E	E	E
Core PTSD symptoms	E	E	E
Functioning	E	E	E
Loss/grief	R	R	R
Life events	R	R	O
Child intrinsic variables	E/R	E/R	E/R
Comorbidity	E/R	E/R	E/R
Social context	O	R	O
Parent psychopathology	O	E/R	O
Social cognition	O	E/R	O
Social skills	O	E/R	O
Biological	O	E/R	O
Outcome	NR	NR	E

E, essential; R, recommended; O, optional.

Anxiety Scale for Children (MASC)[57] and the DSM-IV PTSD criteria set.[31] In addition to a change-sensitive PTSD symptom scale,[58] the CATS is alone among self-report measures in including stable indices of non-PTSD life events and PTSD qualifying stressors.

With the caveat that parents in general are better at evaluating children's externalizing than internalizing symptoms,[59] a multi-method multi-trait evaluation of trauma-related symptoms is preferable, including information from multiple sources.[60] For example, parent/teacher measures, such as the Conners' Parent and Teacher Rating Scales,[61] are efficient adjuncts for assessing collateral externalizing symptoms. Self-report measures, such as the Children's Depression Inventory (CDI)[62] or the MASC,[56] can be used to assess internalizing comorbidities.

Lastly, very little is known about the role of moderating and mediating variables in either the development or treatment of PTSD in youth.[63,64] Demographic factors such as age,[65] gender,[20] race,[20] psychiatric comorbidity,[66] other life events,[66] negative cognitions,[20] and family functioning[65] have been suggested as potential predictor variables, but empirical studies of these predictors are mostly lacking in children.

Development

PTSD is a multiply determined disorder initiated by a high-magnitude stressor with symptoms maintained by a variety of cognitive and environmental processes that may serve as either risk or protective factors. Thus, the assessment of PTSD in children and adolescents necessarily must be embedded within the child's developmental and social matrices. Moreover, since post-traumatic sequelae vary with the nature of the stressor – witness the division in the field between abuse and sudden trauma research studies – and many children experience multiple events in both categories, the ability to map the event or events onto important domains of outcome within a developmental framework is critical to developing an intelligent treatment plan. To some extent, this renders the DSM-IV framework, which underemphasizes developmental differences and social contextual factors, less than adequate for evaluating childhood-onset PTSD. For example, some aspects of the PTSD symptom complex may be best reported by the affected child, others by parents, and still others by teachers or other observers, with some variation depending on the developmental stage of the child. Moreover, since the child's social matrix – neighborhood, family, peer, and school environments – may strongly influence the risk, characteristics, and course of PTSD and corollary symptoms, it is important to consider variables like loss, secondary adversities, family functioning and attachment-related symptoms, such as separation anxiety, when evaluating PTSD. Useful primarily for heuristic purposes, Figure 10.1 presents a much-simplified developmental model for the genesis and maintenance of PTSD in youth adapted from our previous work,[3,67,68] from Pynoos et al,[69] and by analogy from depression.[70]

Treatment

While it is beyond the scope of this chapter to review the extensive literature on the clinical treatment of pediatric PTSD, a wide variety of techniques have been asserted as effective in clinical practice.[3,71] Looked at

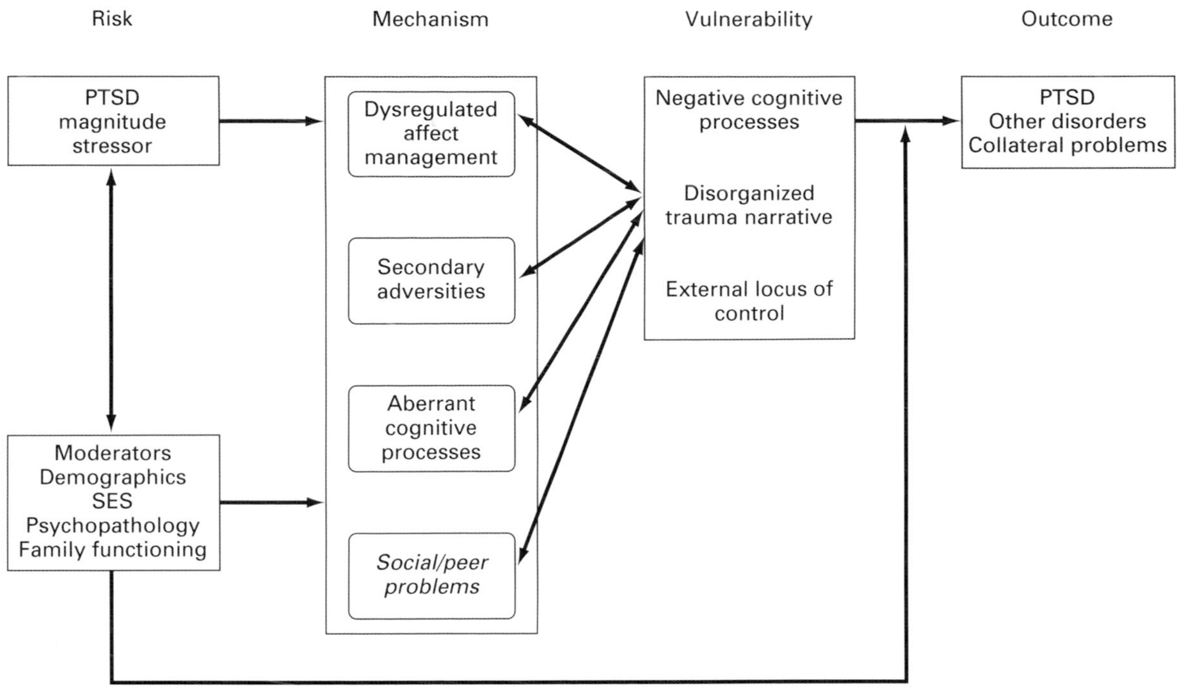

Figure 10.1. Developmental model.

from a broad vantage point, a 'prevention–intervention' model, which incorporates triage for children exposed to stressor events, supporting and strengthening coping skills for anticipated grief/trauma responses, treating other disorders that may develop or be exacerbated in the context of PTSD, and treatment for acute PTSD symptoms, is recommended.[72] While the horror of the trauma can never be erased and hence 'cure' may not be the appropriate treatment goal, victims can become well-functioning survivors if appropriate treatment is given and facilitation of healing takes place.

From the standpoint of evidence-based practice, recommendations for treatment are more narrowly defined. In a recent comprehensive review,[7] Cohen et al reached the following conclusions concerning the treatment of PTSD in youth:

Children and adolescents with PTSD would likely benefit from treatment focused on PTSD symptomatology. Of the available treatments, CBT has the most empirical support and is therefore the initial treatment of choice. The particular format of CBT should be dictated by the nature of the trauma, with specific protocols focused on either abuse or sudden trauma. Because of their favorable side effect profile and evidence supporting effectiveness in treating both depressive and anxiety disorders, SSRIs [selective serotonin reuptake inhibitors] often are the first psychotropic medication chosen for treating pediatric PTSD, especially when dictated by a SSRI-responsive comorbidity. Clonidine may be helpful for some children and adolescents with prominent hyperarousal symptoms, especially elevated startle responses.

Cognitive-behavioral psychotherapy

Although a wide variety of psychotherapeutic techniques have been employed,[3] empirical support for psychosocial treatments of PTSD in adults and children is strongest for cognitive-behavioral therapy.[7,73,74] Historically, behavior therapy (the BT in CBT) evolved within the theoretical framework of classical and operant conditioning. The cognitive interventions (the C in CBT) have assumed a more prominent role with the increasing recognition that cognitive processes powerfully mediate person–environment interactions. In the context of situational and/or cognitive processes, BT is sometimes referred to as nonmediational (emphasizing the direct influence of situations on behavior) and CT as mediational (emphasizing that thoughts and feelings underlie behavior). Behavioral therapists work with patients to change behaviors and thereby to reduce distressing thoughts and feelings. Cognitive therapists work to first change thoughts and feelings, with improvements in functional behavior following in turn. For the most part, these two main conceptual positions have been integrated within more recent approaches such as information processing.[74,75] Their clinical applications to treatment[76] have also been subsumed within the broad umbrella of social learning theory.[77]

March and colleagues recently completed a pilot study of group school-based CBT for PTSD after single-incident trauma, which draws significantly on earlier work in adults by Foa and colleagues.[74] As shown in Box 10.1, treatment took place over 18 weekly sessions. Each session includes a statement of goals, a careful review of the preceding week, introduction of new information, therapist-assisted 'nuts and bolts' practice, homework for the coming week, and monitoring procedures. Sessions 1 and 2 provide an overview of the treatment process, begin information-gathering, and introduce the concept of 'bossing back PTS' by giving PTSD a silly nickname. Session 1 also defines rules for group process, including confidentiality, turn-taking, rules for conflict resolution, and attendance procedures. Sessions 3–5 are devoted to anxiety management training.

Box 10.1. Typical treatment outline.

Session 1:	Getting started*
Session 2:	Naming and mapping
Session 3:	Anxiety management training 1
Session 4:	Anxiety management training 2
Session 5:	Grading feelings
Session 6:	Anger-coping 1
Session 7:	Anger-coping 2
Session 8:	Cognitive training 1
Session 9:	Cognitive training 2
Session 10a:	Introducing exposure and response prevention
Session 10b:	Pullout session
Session 11:	Trial exposure
Session 12:	Narrative exposure 1
Session 13:	Narrative exposure 2
Session 14:	Worst moment exposure 1
Session 15:	Worst moment exposure 2
Session 16:	Right beliefs
Session 17:	Relapse prevention/generalization
Session 18:	Graduation party*

*Sessions 1 and 18 are 90 minutes; all others are 50–60 minutes.

Session 3 introduces progressive, cue-controlled, differential muscle relaxation. Session 4 extends relaxation training by teaching diaphragmatic breathing to relieve 'suffocation' symptoms associated with panic states. Session 5 introduces fear thermometer scores in the form of an analog fear thermometer, using the fear thermometer to grade thoughts and feelings with respect to anxiety, anger, and PTS in response to traumatic reminders. Sessions 6 and 7 address anger/aggression by taking an interpersonal problem-solving approach to anger control.[78] Session 6 examines anger producing self-statements and, building on techniques learned in anxiety management training (AMT), introduces 'perspective-taking' as a cognitive strategy for managing angry cognitions and aggressive behaviors. Session 7 builds on session 6 by taking a role-playing approach to conflict resolution. Sessions 8 and 9 address cognitive training for 'bossing back PTS' by adapting the approach used for AMT and anger-coping more specifically to PTSD. Session 8 helps the child develop positive self-talk emphasizing personal efficacy, predictability and controllability of the environment, realistic risk appraisal, and positive statements countering PTS intrusions. Session 9 continues cognitive training, but more tightly couples CT to PTSD. Session 10a provides an overview of exposure and response prevention, and introduces the concept of the stimulus hierarchy. Session 10b is an individual session that has three goals:

1. Using a moment-by-moment trauma replay procedure, construction of a stimulus hierarchy based on identification of conditioned stimuli (traumatic reminders within fear structures) that are related to the child's trauma.
2. An introduction to narrative exposure.
3. Provision of corrective information regarding trauma-specific misattributions and distortions.

Sessions 5, 12 and 13 introduce the use of narrative exposure, where each child in turn tells his or her story to the group to encourage habituation. As indicated, the therapist/group members introduce corrective information regarding spatial/temporal distortions; global attributions reinforcing lack of personal efficacy; normalization; and positive coping. These sessions also involve practicing imaginal exposure and introduce in vivo exposure as homework. For example, the child who avoids going outside might spend time playing in the front yard, assuming that it is safe to do so. Homework involves selecting in vivo exposure targets. Sessions 14 and 15 extend the approach used in sessions 12 and 13 to the 'worst moment' for each child. Homework for these sessions involves practicing the techniques learned in the group for increasingly difficult in vivo exposure targets. In this context, the focus switches more to contrived exposure to traumatic reminders. Session 16 directly confronts PTSD-induced dysfunctional beliefs or schemes; homework is to practice substituting helpful beliefs for unskillful ones. Session 17 emphasizes that the children have learned how to 'boss back PTS' across many situations and into the future. The goal for this session is to summarize, review, reinforce, and promote generalization of the techniques of AMT, anger-coping, and exposure. Session 18 is a graduation party during which each child will receive a graduation certificate for 'becoming the boss of PTS'. Sessions 17 and 18 also fade therapist assistance.

Despite robust evidence favoring CBT as a treatment for PTSD across the age range, it is likely that most children do not receive state-of-the-art cognitive-behavioral interventions.[79] One reason is the lack of empirically supported manualized treatment protocols that can be exported to clinical settings.[80] Moreover, as Kendall Southam-Gerow point out,[79] controlled trials of protocol-driven treatments are clearly necessary before moving to effectiveness research protocols conducted in clinical populations. Thus, it is encouraging that protocols for treating PTSD stemming from both single-incident trauma[81] and sexual and physical abuse[82,83] are becoming more widely available.

Pharmacotherapy

Although PTSD has an exogenous origin and likely requires psychological treatment, the disorder is nevertheless, using Kardiner's term,[84] a true physioneurosis[39] and psychotropic medication may, in selected cases, prove helpful in relieving PTSD and collateral symptoms.[4] Ideally, medications should decrease intrusions, avoidance, and anxious arousal; minimize impulsivity and improve sleep; treat secondary disorders; and facilitate cognitive-behavioral interventions. On the other hand, while a variety of psychopharmacological agents have been advocated or used, including propranolol,[85] carbamezapine,[86] clonidine,[87] and various antidepressants,[88] relatively few data exist to guide the medicating of children and adolescents with these compounds.[88] Controlled trials in adults suggest that standard antidepressants may improve PTSD symptoms, with the SSRIs currently favored because of demonstrated efficacy and a more favorable side effect profile;[89] a similar response has been seen clinically in children and adolescents.[90] Clonidine has been shown to decrease startle responses in some children with PTSD[41] and Horrigan recently completed an open study in which a long-acting alpha-2 agonist, guanfacine, successfully reduced startle responses and nightmares in children with PTSD (Horrigan, personal communication), suggesting that the alpha-2 agonists may be helpful in some children with PTSD characterized by prominent hyperarousal symptoms.

Including families

Parental emotional reaction to the traumatic event and parental support of the child are potentially powerful influences on the child's PTSD symptoms. Hence, despite limited evidence to the contrary,[58] most experts assert that inclusion of parents and/or supportive others in treatment is important for resolution of PTSD symptoms for children.[3] At a minimum, including parents in treatment helps them monitor the child's symptomatology and learn appropriate behavioral management techniques, both in the intervals between treatment sessions and after therapy is terminated. In addition, helping parents resolve their emotional distress related to the trauma, to which the parent usually has had either direct or vicarious exposure, can help the parent be more perceptive of and responsive to the child's emotional needs.[91] Not surprisingly, parent interventions are considered imperative in the child abuse literature, where most authors recommend one or more parent-directed components.[7,82,92]

Combined treatment

It is widely recognized that assessment and treatment of PTSD must by necessity address a variety of symptoms or dysfunctions beyond those comprising or even attributable to PTSD per se.[3] However, there is little or no empirical evidence to support combining treatments within or across treatment modalities. In particular, there is no empirical evidence to support the common clinical belief that the combination of medication management and psychotherapy is superior to psychotherapy alone.

Duration of treatment

Clinically, most children and adolescents with uncomplicated PTSD will make substantial improvement with 12–20 sessions of PTSD-specific CBT. A smaller number of children require long-term treatment. Exposure to extensive violence, intrafamilial homicide or suicide, repetitive or prolonged abuse, or exposure to distressing events suggest that brief trauma work may not be enough. The presence of preexisting psychopathology in the child or a parent, prior history of abuse, or ongoing exposure to a disruptive living situation also suggest a need for intensive longer-term intervention. Long-term treatment can occur weekly or as 'pulsed intervention' based on the child's developmental phase, capacity for response, and clinical issues. Pulsed intervention assumes that brief therapy is suspended (rather than terminated) until further treatment becomes necessary – such as during developmental transitions, changes in living situation, formation of intimate relationships, marriage, etc. 'Pulsing' the treatment helps prevent ongoing helplessness by minimizing dependence on the therapist as 'the only one who really understands'. Unfortunately, severe PTSD requires arduous and critical dedication to treatment on the part of the patient and therapist. Longer-term therapy may also be necessary when issues related to character formation and capacity to form meaningful relationships are present.

Conclusion

There is incontrovertible evidence that PTSD occurs in children and adolescents in much the same form as in adults, though substantially colored by developmental and socioecological factors. Young persons with PTSD likely benefit from treatment focused on PTSD symptomatology. Of the available treatments, CBT has the most empirical support and is therefore the treatment of choice. The particular format of CBT should be dictated by the nature of the trauma, with specific protocols focused on either abuse or sudden trauma. Because of their favorable side effect profile and evidence supporting effectiveness in treating both depressive and anxiety disorders, SSRIs are often the first psychotropic medication chosen for treating pediatric PTSD, especially when dictated by an SSRI-responsive comorbidity. Given early recognition and adequate treatment, many if not most children can be helped to resume a normal developmental trajectory.

References

1. American Psychiatric Association, *Diagnostic and Statistical Manual of Mental Disorders* (DSM-III), 3rd edn (American Psychiatric Press: Washington, DC, 1980).
2. Terr LC, Psychic trauma in children: observations following the Chowchilla school bus kidnapping, *Annual Progress in Child Psychiatry and Child Development* (1982) 384–96.
3. March J, Amaya-Jackson J, Pynoos R, Pediatric post-traumatic stress disorder. In: Weiner J, ed, *Textbook of Child and Adolescent Psychiatry*, 2nd edn (American Psychiatric Press: Washington, DC, 1996).
4. Davidson J, March J, Traumatic stress disorders. In: Tasman A, Kay J, Lieberman J, eds, *Psychiatry* (WB Saunders: Philadelphia, 1996) 1085–98.

5. Pynoos RS, Traumatic stress and developmental psychopathology in children and adolescents. Sidran Press, Lutherville, MD, US 1994; 171:65–98.
6. March J, Assessment of pediatric post-traumatic stress disorder. In: Saigh P, Bremner D, eds, *Post-traumatic Stress Disorder* (American Psychological Press: Washington, DC, 1999) 199–218.
7. Cohen J, March J, Berliner L, Treatment guidelines for PTSD in children and adolescents. In: Foa E, ed, *ISTSS Treatment Guidelines for PTSD* (ISTSS: Chicago, in press).
8. Kessler RC, Sonnega A, Bromet E et al, Posttraumatic stress disorder in the National Comorbidity Survey, *Arch Gen Psychiatry* (1995) 52:1048–60.
9. Giaconia RM, Reinherz HZ, Silverman AB et al, Traumas and posttraumatic stress disorder in a community population of older adolescents, *J Am Acad Child Adolesc Psychiatry* (1995) **34**:1369–80.
10. Jenkins EJ, Bell CC, Violence among inner city high school students and post-traumatic stress disorder. Springer Publishing Co, Inc, New York, NY, US (1994) **246**:76–88.
11. Reiss D, Richters J, Radke-Yarrow M, Scharrf D, *Children and Violence* (Guilford: New York, 1993).
12. Pynoos RS, Nader K, Children who witness the sexual assaults of their mothers, *J Am Acad Child Adolesc Psychiatry* (1988) 27:567–72.
13. Schwarz ED, Kowalski JM, Posttraumatic stress disorder after a school shooting: effects of symptom threshold selection and diagnosis by DSM-III, DSM-III-R, or proposed DSM-IV, *Am J Psychiatry* (1991) **148**:592–7.
14. Clarke G, Sack WH, Goff B, Three forms of stress in Cambodian adolescent refugees, *J Abnorm Child Psychol* (1993) **21**:65–77.
15. Stuber ML, Nader K, Yasuda P et al, Stress responses after pediatric bone marrow transplantation: preliminary results of a prospective longitudinal study, *J Am Acad Child Adolesc Psychiatry* (1991) **30**:952–7.
16. Stoddard FJ, Norman DK, Murphy JM, A diagnostic outcome study of children and adolescents with severe burns, *J Trauma* (1989) **29**:471–7.
17. Brent DA, Risk factors for adolescent suicide and suicidal behavior: mental and substance abuse disorders, family environmental factors, and life stress, *Suicide Life Threat Behav* (1995) **25(Suppl)**:52–63.
18. Yule W, Udwin O, Murdoch K, The 'Jupiter' sinking: effects on children's fears, depression and anxiety, *J Child Psychol Psychiatry* (1990) **31**:1051–61.
19. Yule W, Williams RM, Post-traumatic stress reaction in children, *J Trauma Stress* (1990) **3**:279–95.
20. March J, Amaya-Jackson L, Terry R, Costanzo P, Post-traumatic stress in children and adolescents after an industrial fire, *J Am Acad Child Adolesc Psychiatry* (1997) **36**:1080–8.
21. Burke JD, Moccia P, Borus JF, Burns BJ, Emotional distress in fifth-grade children ten months after a natural disaster, *J Am Acad Child Psychiatry* (1986) **25**:536–41.
22. McFarlane A, Life events and psychiatric disorder: the role of a natural disaster, *Br J Psychiatry* (1987) **151**:362–7.
23. McNally RJ, Stressors that produce posttraumatic stress disorder in children. In: Davidson JRT, Foa EB, eds, *Posttraumatic Stress Disorder: DSM-IV and Beyond*, 1st edn (American Psychiatric Press: Washington, DC, 1993) 57–74.
24. Pynoos RS, Frederick CJ, Nader K et al, Life threat and posttraumatic stress in school-age children, *Arch Gen Psychiatry* (1987) **44**:1057–63.
25. Pynoos RS, Nader K, Children's memory and proximity to violence, *J Am Acad Child Adolesc Psychiatry* (1989) **28**:236–41.
26. Saigh PA, The development of posttraumatic stress disorder following four different types of traumatization, *Behav Res Ther* (1991) **29**:213–6.
27. Nader K, Stuber M, Pynoos RS, Posttraumatic stress reactions in preschool children with catastrophic illness: assessment needs, *Comprehensive Mental Health Care* (1991) **1**:223–39.
28. Kendall-Tackett KA, Williams LM, Finkelhor D, Impact of sexual abuse on children: a review and synthesis of recent empirical studies, *Psychol Bull* (1993) **113**:164–80.
29. Famularo R, Kinscherff R, Fenton T, Symptom differences in acute and chronic presentation of childhood post-traumatic stress disorder, *Child Abuse & Neglect* (1990) **14**:439–44.
30. Terr LC, Childhood traumas: an outline and overview, *Am J Psychiatry* (1991) **148**:10–20.
31. American Psychiatric Association, *Diagnostic and Statistical Manual of Mental Disorders* (DSM-IV), 4th edn (American Psychiatric Press: Washington, DC, 1994).
32. Eth S, Pynoos R, *Posttraumatic Stress Disorder in Children* (American Psychiatric Press: Washington, DC, 1985) .

33. Terr LC, *Too Scared to Cry: Psychic Trauma in Childhood*, 1st edn (Harper & Row: New York, 1990).
34. Pynoos RS, Nader K, Children's exposure to violence and traumatic death, *Psychiatric Annals* (1990) **20**:334–44.
35. Saylor CF, Swenson CC, Powell P, Hurricane Hugo blows down the broccoli: preschoolers' post-disaster play and adjustment, *Child Psychiatry Hum Dev* (1992) **22**:139–49.
36. Nader KO, Fairbanks LA, The suppression of reexperiencing: impulse control and somatic symptoms in children following traumatic exposure, *Anxiety, Stress & Coping: an International Journal* (1994) **7**:229–39.
37. Moradi AR, Doost HT, Taghavi MR et al, Everyday memory deficits in children and adolescents with PTSD: performance on the Rivermead Behavioural Memory Test, *J Child Psychol Psychiatry* (1999) **40**:357–61.
38. Putnam FW, Trickett PK, Child sexual abuse: a model of chronic trauma, *Psychiatry* (1993) **56**:82–95.
39. Perry BD, Neurobiological sequelae of childhood trauma: PTSD in children. American Psychiatric Press, Inc, Washington, DC, US (1994) **42**:233–55.
40. Perry BD, Pate JE, *Neurodevelopment and the Psychobiological Roots of Post-traumatic Stress Disorder* (Charles C Thomas: Springfield, IL, 1994) 326.
41. Ornitz E, Pynoos R, Startle modulation in children with post-traumatic stress disorder, *Am J Psychiatry* (1989) **146**:866–70.
42. Pynoos RS, Steinberg AM, Ornitz EM, Goenjian AK, Issues in the developmental neurobiology of traumatic stress, *Ann N Y Acad Sci* (1997) **821**:176–93.
43. Pitman R, Biological findings in posttraumatic stress disorder: implications for DSM-IV classification. In: Davidson J, Foa E, eds, *Posttraumatic Stress Disorder: DSM-IV and Beyond* (American Psychiatric Press: Washington, DC, 1992) 173–89.
44. Yule W, Canterbury R, The treatment of posttraumatic stress disorder in children and adolescents, *Int Rev Psychiatry* (1994) **6**:141–51.
45. Yule W, *Posttraumatic Stress Disorder* (Plenum: New York, 1994) **496**:223–40.
46. Brent DA, Perper JA, Moritz G et al, Posttraumatic stress disorder in peers of adolescent suicide victims: predisposing factors and phenomenology, *J Am Acad Child Adolesc Psychiatry* (1995) **34**:209–15.
47. Saigh PA, Mroueh M, Bremner JD, Scholastic impairments among traumatized adolescents, *Behav Res Ther* (1997) **35**:429–36.
48. Silverman W, Albano A, *The Anxiety Disorders Interview Schedule for DSM-IV, Child and Parent Versions* (The Psychological Corporation: San Antonio, TX, 1996).
49. Costello EJ, Angold A, March J, Fairbank J, Life events and post-traumatic stress: the development of a new measure for children and adolescents, *Psychol Med* (1998) **28**:1275–88.
50. Lonigan CJ, Shannon MP, Finch AJ et al, Children's reactions to a natural disaster: symptom severity and degree of exposure, *Adv Behav Res Ther* (1991) **13**:135–54.
51. Nader K, Blake D, Kriegler J, Pynoos R, Clinician Administered PTSD Scale for Children (CAPS-C), Current and Lifetime Diagnosis Version, and Instruction Manual. In.: UCLA Neuropsychiatric Institute and National Center for PTSD; 1994.
52. Foa EB, Johnson K, Feeny NC, Treadwell KT, The child PTSD symptom scale (CPSS): validation of a measure for children with PTSD, submitted.
53. Shaw JA, Applegate B, Tanner S et al, Psychological effects of Hurricane Andrew on an elementary school population, *J Am Acad Child Adolesc Psychiatry* (1995) **34**:1185–92.
54. Bradburn IS, After the earth shook: children's stress symptoms 6–8 months after a disaster, *Adv Behav Res Ther* (1991) **13**:173–9.
55. Goenjian AK, Pynoos RS, Steinberg AM et al, Psychiatric comorbidity in children after the 1988 earthquake in Armenia, *J Am Acad Child Adolesc Psychiatry* (1995) **34**:1174–84.
56. Nader KO, Pynoos RS, Fairbanks LA et al, A preliminary study of PTSD and grief among the children of Kuwait following the Gulf crisis, *Br J Clin Psychol* (1993) **32**:407–16.
57. March J, Parker J, Sullivan K et al, The Multidimensional Anxiety Scale for Children (MASC): factor structure, reliability and validity, *J Am Acad Child Adolesc Psychiatry* (1997) **36**:554–65.
58. March J, Amaya-Jackson L, Murry M, Schulte A, Cognitive-behavioral psychotherapy for children and adolescents with post-traumatic stress disorder following a single incident stressor, *J Am Acad Child Adolesc Psychiatry* (1998) **37**:585–93.
59. Costello E, Developments in child psychiatric epidemiology, *J Am Acad Child Adolesc Psychiatry* (1989) **28**:836–41.

60. Amaya-Jackson L, March J, Post-traumatic stress disorder in children and adolescents. In: Leonard HL, ed, *Child Psychiatric Clinics of North America: Anxiety Disorders* (WB Saunders: New York, 1993) 639–54.
61. Conners C, *Conners' Rating Scales* (Multi-Health Systems: Toronto, 1995).
62. Kovacs M, The Children's Depression Inventory (CDI), *Psychopharmacol Bull* (1985) 21:995–8.
63. Garbarino J, Kostelny K, Dubrow N, What children can tell us about living in danger, *Am Psychol* (1991) **46**:376–83.
64. March J, Amaya-Jackson L, Post-traumatic stress disorder in children and adolescents, *PTSD Research Quarterly* (1994) 4:1–7.
65. Green BL, Korol M, Grace MC et al, Children and disaster: age, gender, and parental effects on PTSD symptoms, *J Am Acad Child Adolesc Psychiatry* (1991) **30**:945–51.
66. Pynoos RS, Frederick C, Nader K, Arroyo W et al, Life threat and posttraumatic stress in school-age children, *Arch Gen Psychiatry* (1987) **44**:1057–63.
67. March J, *Anxiety Disorders in Children and Adolescents* (Guilford: New York, 1995).
68. Kendall P, Guiding theory for therapy with children and adolescents. In: Kendall P, ed, *Child and Adolescent Therapy* (Guilford: New York, 1993) 3–22.
69. Pynoos R, Steinberg A, Wraith R, A developmental model of childhood traumatic stress. In: Cicchetti D, Cohen D, eds, *Manual of Developmental Psychopathology: Risk Disorder, Adaptation* (John Wiley: New York, 1995) 72–95.
70. Goodman S, Gotlib I, Risk for psychopathology in the children of depressed mothers: a developmental model for understanding mechanisms of transmission, *Psychol Rev* in press.
71. Finkelhor D, Berliner L, Research on the treatment of sexually abused children: a review and recommendations, *J Am Acad Child Adolesc Psychiatry* (1995) **34**:1408–23.
72. American Academy of Child and Adolescent Psychiatry, Summary of the practice parameters for the assessment and treatment of children and adolescents with posttraumatic stress disorder, *J Am Acad Child Adolesc Psychiatry* (1998) **37**:997–1001.
73. Solomon SD, Gerrity ET, Muff AM, Efficacy of treatments for posttraumatic stress disorder: an empirical review, *JAMA* (1992) **268**:633–8.
74. Foa EB, Meadows EA, Psychosocial treatments for posttraumatic stress disorder: a critical review, *Ann Rev Psychol* (1997) **48**:449–80.
75. Foa E, Kozak M, Emotional processing and treatment of anxiety disorders: implications for psychopathology. In: Tuma A, Maser J, eds, *Anxiety and Anxiety Disorders* (Erlbaum: New Jersey, 1986).
76. Hibbs E, Jensen P, *Psychosocial Treatments for Child and Adolescent Disorders* (American Psychological Press: Washington, DC, 1996).
77. March J, Child psychiatry: cognitive and behavior therapies. In: Kaplan H, Saddock B, eds, *Comprehensive Textbook of Psychiatry*, vol 7 (Williams & Wilkins: New York, in press).
78. Lochman J, Lampron L, Gemmer T, Harris S, Anger coping intervention with aggressive children: a guide to implementation in school settings. In: Keller P, Heyman S, eds, *Innovations in Clinical Practice: A Source Book* (Professional Resource Exchange: Sarasota, FL, 1987) 339–56.
79. Kendall PC, Southam-Gerow MA, Issues in the transportability of treatment: the case of anxiety disorders in youths, *J Consult Clin Psychol* (1995) **63**:702–8.
80. Clarke GN, Improving the transition from basic efficacy research to effectiveness studies: methodological issues and procedures, *J Consult Clin Psychol* (1995) **63**:718–25.
81. March JS, Amaya-Jackson L, Murray MC, Schulte A, Cognitive-behavioral psychotherapy for children and adolescents with posttraumatic stress disorder after a single-incident stressor, *J Am Acad Child Adolesc Psychiatry* (1998) **37**:585–93.
82. Deblinger E, McLeer SV, Henry D, Cognitive behavioral treatment for sexually abused children suffering post-traumatic stress: preliminary findings, *J Am Acad Child Adolesc Psychiatry* (1990) **29**:747–52.
83. Cohen JA, Mannarino AP, A treatment outcome study for sexually abused preschool children: initial findings [published erratum appears in *J Am Acad Child Adolesc Psychiatry* (1996) **35**:835], *J Am Acad Child Adolesc Psychiatry* (1996) **35**:42–50.
84. Kardiner A, *The Traumatic Neurosis of War* (Paul B. Hoeber: New York, 1941).
85. Famularo R, Kinscherff R, Fenton T, Propranolol treatment for childhood posttraumatic stress disorder, acute type. A pilot study, *Am J Dis Child* (1988) 142:1244–7.

86. Looff D, Grimley P, Kuller F et al, Carbamazepine for PTSD [letter], *J Am Acad Child Adolesc Psychiatry* (1995) 34:703–4.
87. Newcorn JH, Schulz K, Harrison M et al, Alpha 2 adrenergic agonists. Neurochemistry, efficacy, and clinical guidelines for use in children, *Pediatr Clin North Am* (1998) 45:1099–22, viii.
88. Pfferbaum B, Posttraumatic stress disorder in children: a review of the last ten years, *J Am Acad Child Adolesc Psychiatry* (1997) 36:1503–11.
89. Davidson JR, Biological therapies for posttraumatic stress disorder: an overview, *J Clin Psychiatry* (1997) 58(Suppl 9):29–32.
90. Donnelly CL, Amaya-Jackson L, March JS, Psychopharmacology of pediatric posttraumatic stress disorder, *J Child Adolesc Psychopharmacol* (1999) 9:203–20.
91. Burman S, Allen-Meares P, Neglected victims of murder: children's witness to parental homicide, *Soc Work* (1994) 39:28–34.
92. Cohen JA, Mannarino AP, Factors that mediate treatment outcome of sexually abused preschool children, *J Am Acad Child Adolesc Psychiatry* (1996) 35:1402–10.

11

Grief and its relation to post-traumatic stress disorder

Holly G Prigerson, M Katherine Shear, Selby C Jacobs, Stanislav V Kasl, Paul K Maciejewski, Gabriel K Silverman, Meena Narayan and J Douglas Bremner

While the death of someone close is widely recognized as one of the most stressful events a person can experience,[1–5] bereavement has only recently been considered potentially 'traumatic'. New studies that permit bereavement to meet the first condition (Criterion A1) for post-traumatic stress disorder (PTSD) find that, particularly when the death is sudden and unexpected, recently bereaved persons can and do meet criteria for PTSD.[6–7] These results suggest that bereavement, especially under certain circumstances, can be traumatic and that the symptoms following from bereavement may qualify a person for a diagnosis of PTSD. What these findings do not indicate is the extent to which complicated bereavement reactions could be subsumed by a diagnosis of PTSD. By complicated bereavement, we mean the features that characterize extreme, debilitating reactions to loss that include symptoms of psychological trauma. For this reason, we call the syndrome 'traumatic grief', the features of which will be described below.

The aim of this chapter is to examine the extent of overlap between traumatic grief (TG) and PTSD. Determining the 'goodness of fit' between PTSD and TG has both conceptual and clinical implications. Aside from an academic interest in understanding the phenomenology of grief as a stress response syndrome, the distinctiveness of TG and PTSD diagnoses may signal to clinicians the need for different therapeutic approaches. If we find that the overlap between these two disorders is fairly complete, then the recommendation would be for clinicians to recognize the potential of bereavement to trigger the onset of PTSD, with little need for attention to a differential or comorbid diagnosis of TG. Alternatively, if we find the overlap between PTSD and TG to be only moderate, then the recommendation would be for clinicians to recognize the grief-specific nature of the bereaved person's emotional distress, to screen these patients separately for TG, and focus on the treatment of the symptoms associated with this distinct clinical entity.

In light of recent efforts to refine diagnostic criteria for TG, we are now in a better position than in the past to examine the relationship between TG and PTSD. In January of 1997, a panel of experts in the areas of bereavement, trauma, and psychiatric nosology[a] convened to discuss the need for diagnostic criteria for TG. The workshop began with a review of a series of studies of independent samples of bereaved people that demonstrated:

1. That symptoms of separation distress (for example, yearning, searching for the deceased, excessive loneliness resulting from the loss) form a single cluster with symptoms of traumatic distress (for example, intrusive thoughts about the deceased, feelings of numbness, disbelief, being stunned or dazed, fragmented sense of security and trust) and that this cluster was distinct from depressive and anxiety symptom clusters.[8–12]
2. That these symptoms lasted several years among a significant minority of bereaved subjects.[13–16]
3. That these symptoms, unlike depressive symptoms, did not respond to interpersonal psychotherapy either alone or in combination with a tricyclic antidepressant (nortriptyline).[17,18]
4. That these symptoms predicted substantial morbidity over and above depressive symptoms.[8–14]

The panel concluded that the evidence presented justified the development of diagnostic criteria for TG. Participants then discussed the symptoms that should be included in a diagnosis and, ultimately, proposed consensus criteria for TG (see Box 11.1). A recent study provided preliminary empirical support for most of the proposed symptoms,[19] and we are currently collecting field trial data to determine the optimal mix of symptoms and their severity, as well as the duration that provides the most accurate diagnosis for TG. In this chapter, we will review how much overlap exists between the proposed symptoms/criteria for TG and those that have been established for PTSD.

Before we discuss specific criteria, however, it is important to clarify what we mean by 'traumatic' grief. Contrary to the case with the 'traumatic bereavements' described by Raphael and Martinek[20] and Rynearson,[21] we do not wish to imply that the mode in which the death occurred was objectively traumatic (for example, natural or man-made disasters, murder). The trauma in the context of grief appears to be a 'separation trauma' that is rooted in a particularly strong attachment to the deceased, and feelings of extreme distress at the loss of this significant other. For a significant minority of bereaved individuals (roughly 20% by 6 months post-loss[8,9,19]), the impact of the loss leaves a deep and lasting impression on the survivor's identity and appears to overwhelm the survivor's coping capacity. Many of the symptoms associated with being devastated by another's death appear to resemble symptoms of PTSD (for

[a]The consensus panel included the following members: Holly G. Prigerson, PhD, conference organizer, Yale University, New Haven, CT; Charles F. Reynolds III, MD, conference co-organizer; David J. Kupfer, MD, conference co-organizer, University of Pittsburgh, Pittsburgh, PA; M. Katherine Shear, MD; conference co-organizer, University of Pittsburgh, Pittsburgh, PA; Selby C. Jacobs, MD, MPH, Yale University, New Haven, CT; Laurel C. Beery, B.S., University of Pittsburgh, Pittsburgh, PA; Jonathan Davidson, MD, Duke University, Durham, NC; Ellen Frank, PhD, University of Pittsburgh, Pittsburgh, PA; Paul K. Maciejewski, PhD, Yale University, New Haven, CT; Paul A. Pilkonis, PhD, University of Pittsburgh, Pittsburgh, PA; Thomas Widiger, PhD, University of Kentucky; Janet B.W. Williams, DSW, New York State Psychiatric Institute, New York, NY; Robert Weiss, PhD, University of Massachusetts, Boston, MA; Camille Wortman, PhD, Stony Brook, NY; Sidney Zisook, MD, University of California, San Diego, La Jolla, CA.

Box 11.1. Proposed criteria for traumatic grief.

Criterion A

1. The person has experienced the death of a significant other.
2. The response involves intrusive, distressing preoccupation with the deceased person (for example, yearning, longing, or searching).

Criterion B In response to the death, the following symptoms are marked and persistent:

1. Frequent efforts to avoid reminders of the deceased (for example, thoughts, feelings, activities, people, places).
2. Purposelessness or feelings of futility about the future.
3. Subjective sense of numbness, detachment, or absence of emotional responsiveness.
4. Feeling stunned, dazed, or shocked.
5. Difficulty acknowledging the death (for example, disbelief).
6. Feeling that life is empty or meaningless.
7. Difficulty imagining a fulfilling life without the deceased.
8. Feeling that part of oneself has died.
9. Shattered worldview (for example, lost sense of security, trust, or control).
10. Assumption of symptoms or harmful behaviors of, or related to, the deceased person.
11. Excessive irritability, bitterness, or anger related to the death.

Criterion C

Duration of disturbance (symptoms listed) is at least 2 months.

Criterion D

The disturbance causes clinically significant impairment in social, occupational, or other important areas of functioning.

example, reexperiencing phenomena and numbness). Consequently, our use of the word 'trauma' relates to the phenomenology of the symptoms rather than to the event involved in the etiology of the disorder.

Because TG is a reaction to a stressful life event and evokes several symptoms that appear similar to PTSD, we consider it to be a stress response syndrome. Yet, the question of how closely TG relates to PTSD needs to be carefully examined. Below we present available evidence on the degree to which the proposed symptoms of TG are redundant with DSM-IV[22] criteria for PTSD.

Traumatic grief and its fit with DSM-IV criteria for PTSD

In order to meet DSM-IV[22] criteria for a diagnosis of PTSD, a person must experience an event that has involved the actual or threatened death of or serious injury to the physical integrity of self or others. This event must also result in intense feelings of fear, helplessness, or horror. The second criterion requires that the event be reexperienced in at least one of several ways (for example, recurrent intrusive distressing thoughts, hallucinations), while the third criterion specifies that persistent avoidance of stimuli associated with the trauma and a general numbing of responsiveness be indicated in at least three ways (for instance, avoidance of reminders, diminished interest in significant activities, feelings of detachment from loved ones). The DSM-IV[22] stipulates that a person with PTSD must experience at least two symptoms of hyperarousal (for example, difficulties with sleeping or concentration, exaggerated startle response). All of these symptoms must be present for longer than 1 month, and persist for at least 3 months for a diagnosis of 'chronic' PTSD. The last requirement for a diagnosis of PTSD is that the aforementioned symptoms be associated with clinically significant distress or marked functional impairment. Below we apply these criteria to results we have obtained using our proposed criteria for TG.

Criterion A

In terms of diagnostic criteria for PTSD in the DSM-IV,[22] the first criterion ('A') refers to aspects of the event which purportedly make it 'traumatic' or 'catastrophic'. Thus, criterion 'A.1.' specifies that 'the person has to have experienced, witnessed, or was confronted with an event or events that involved actual or threatened death or serious injury, or a threat to the physical integrity of self or others' (p. 427). Individuals who have cared for a terminally ill loved one or who have mourned the death of a significant other would appear to satisfy this condition, thereby making bereavement an event that could trigger PTSD. Still, we should emphasize that for a diagnosis of TG, the trauma refers to the symptomatic response to the loss and not the traumatic nature of the event.

The second criterion for an event to be considered traumatic according to the DSM-IV[22] (PTSD criterion 'A.2.') is that the response to the experience must involve 'intense fear, helplessness, or horror. In children, this may be expressed instead by disorganized or agitated behavior' (p. 428). The proposed criteria for TG found in Box 11.1 include 'feelings of futility about the future' (TG criterion) and a 'shattered worldview' item (TG criterion B9) that has been operationalized in our clinical interview as symptoms reflecting a lost sense of 'security', 'control', and 'trust' (See Appendix 11.1, Traumatic Grief Evaluation of Response to Loss, TRGR2L, items B10–12). These symptoms suggest a general sense of helplessness, but helplessness itself is not explicitly included among the proposed criteria for TG.

While the impact of the loss on feelings of extreme fear, helplessness, and/or horror appears critical to determining the psychological trauma resulting from the loss, few data have been gathered to examine these reactions among the bereaved. Unpublished data from the Family Health Project (FHP: Investigators: Ostfeld, Kasl, Jacobs[23]) were used to explore this issue. The FHP collected data on spouses of patients found on critical care lists at the Hospital of St Raphael and Yale–New Haven Hospital in the United States state Connecticut. Subjects were interviewed soon after their spouses were identified on the critical care lists, and were interviewed again at 2 months, 6 months, 13 months, and 25 months post-intake. By the 6-month post-intake assessment, 150 spouses had been widowed and among these we found a significant association ($r=0.30$, $p<0.001$) between the Psychiatric Epidemiology Research Interview – Helplessness/Hopelessness Scale[24] and our proxy continuous measure of TG symptomatology. (The 11-items used in the TG proxy measure have been shown to be closely associated with the total scale score for the complete set of TG items [$r=0.94$, $p<0.001$] and to have a high degree of internal consistency [Cronbach's $\alpha=0.95$.[14]) Although these findings suggest that TG is associated with feelings of helplessness/ hopelessness, they are inconclusive for two primary reasons. First, the TG proxy measure did not contain the newly proposed 'shattered worldview' item. Second, the inclusion of 'hopelessness' is a particularly troublesome confounding measure because 'feelings of futility' and other items suggesting hopelessness are embedded among the TG criteria.

We suspect that 'fear' and 'horror' are not common or important features of TG associated with the most common form of bereavement – widowhood from natural causes – but await the collection of data that will allow for an empirical test of this hypothesis. Horror may be more likely to occur when the circumstances of loss are the result of savagery or the toll in terms of the number of lives lost is high as has recently been the case in genocide abroad (for example, Yugoslavia, Rwanda), or the result of random acts of violence as occur in United States inner cities. Still, in these circumstances it appears that it is the objectively traumatic nature of the loss that would be expected to result in feelings of being horrified and translate into a vulnerability to PTSD onset, and not TG specifically. In other words, bereavement often goes hand-in-hand with traumatic events such as earthquakes, natural and man-made accidents, but we would expect the horror of these experiences to result in a heightened risk of PTSD, and not necessarily TG. There is, however, reason to believe that TG would be highly comorbid with PTSD in such cases. Thus, although the reaction to the loss involves feelings of devastation evoked by the loss, at this point we are not convinced that individuals who meet our criteria for TG feel intensely horrified or frightened as a result of the death. More data are needed before firmer conclusions regarding the fit between TG and PTSD criterion A.2. can be drawn.

Criterion B

In addition to the above two components of criterion 'A', criterion 'B' for PTSD in the DSM-IV[22] requires that the event be reexperienced in one or more of the following ways: 'recurrent and intrusive distressing . . . images, thoughts, or perceptions . . . dreams . . . illusions, hallucinations, and dissociative flashback episodes . . . distress at exposure to internal and external cues that symbolize . . . an aspect of the event' (p. 428). In some sense, PTSD criterion B has the most extensive overlap with TG symptomatology. Unbidden, intrusive and distressing thoughts about the deceased, and assuming symptoms or harmful behaviors of the deceased, are included among the criteria proposed for TG.

But in contrast with PTSD, the reexperiencing phenomenon in TG has both positive and negative aspects to it. Unlike those who are traumatized by life-threatening accidents, rape, disasters, and other catastrophic events, individuals with TG are not always distressed by exposure to cues that remind them of the deceased. While the reexperiencing is affect-laden, it is not always upsetting. There is a yearning and searching for, and pining to be with, the person who died. In a group of grieving widowed persons, hallucinations of the deceased person have been found to be comforting.[25] 'Dissociative flashbacks' (which appears a strong term to describe this phenomenon), in which the survivor cognitively returns to times shared with the deceased person, appear to be common and we sometimes hear them described as providing solace. Still, while TG sufferers and people with normal bereavement reactions share a sense of comfort from memories of the deceased, those with TG also find the memories upsetting. In our experience, patients who suffer from TG appear to suffer conflict about the reexperiencing because it evokes both relief and distress. Reminders of the loss appear to evoke both pleasure and pain for the TG sufferer, while for the normally bereaved they may best be described as bittersweet, but not painful. The longing to reestablish a connection with the deceased is very strong, but the memories that reestablish the link to the deceased and their past also serve as painful reminders of the loss. Thus, unlike in the case of PTSD, for people who meet criteria for TG there appears to be a compulsion to ruminate about the deceased and the magnitude of their loss. The cost of the yearning to be reunited with the deceased appears to be the distress evoked by dwelling on the loss.

Obsessive thoughts about the deceased and the loss often lead to isolation and a loss of interest or engagement in meaningful activities. As benign as reexperiencing may seem in the case of normal bereavement, when we have examined the effects of a 'preoccupation with thoughts of the deceased' item on functional impairment we found it to be associated with an increased likelihood of adverse health behaviors (excessive consumption of alcohol, food, and tobacco), a heightened vulnerability to illness and increased severity of suicidal ideation.[26] Given that elderly White males, especially those who live alone, are lead candidates for completed suicide, a strong wish to be reunited with the deceased may translate into a death wish. If left to ruminate excessively about happier times prior to the loss, preoccupation with thoughts of the deceased may lead to passive or active suicidal intent. This is an idea that needs systematic testing. Despite the short-term emotional relief provided by thinking of happier times in the past, in the long term it appears that excessive reexperiencing can be harmful and should be targeted in the treatment of TG. In this way, while there is some comfort in the reexperiencing among TG sufferers, in both TG and PTSD, adverse consequences appear to result from a high degree of reexperiencing.

Criterion C

Next, the DSM-IV criterion 'C' specifies that persistent avoidance of stimuli associated with the trauma and numbing of general responsiveness must be demonstrated in three of the following ways: 'efforts to avoid thoughts or feelings . . . activities, places or people that arouse recollections of the trauma . . . inability to recall an important aspect of the trauma . . . markedly diminished interest or participation in significant activities, feeling of detachment . . . from others . . . restricted range of affect . . . sense of a foreshortened future'. While PTSD criterion C could be met for individuals who have a positive diagnosis of TG, important distinctions between the phenomenology of PTSD and TG with respect to avoidance and numbness need to be noted.

In a pilot study of 89 community-dwelling widows and widowers in Connecticut at an average of 5 months post-loss, we used item response theory (IRT) to test the performance of the consensus criteria proposed for TG. IRT techniques offer several advantages over classical test theory that are useful for the testing of unestablished diagnostic criteria. One important advantage is that IRT, unlike receiver operator characteristic (ROC) analyses, does not require a 'gold standard' diagnostic criterion against which to evaluate item performance. Rather, IRT allows for the performance of an individual item to be evaluated in relation to a commonly scaled, unidimensional TG 'attribute'. This commonly scaled attribute allows for the determination of the relative efficiency of items independent of any particular diagnostic algorithm. The item information functions (IIFs) produced by IRT analyses indicate the items, and the optimal frequency/severity for each item, that provide the greatest amount of information with reference to location on a common TG 'attribute' scale. IIFs provide estimates of which items, and what level of severity, serve as the best indicators of TG, assessed dimensionally rather than dichotomously (that is, no criterion for 'caseness' is required).

Severity scores obtained from a trained interviewer's assessment of TG using the Traumatic Grief Evaluation of Response to Loss (TRGR2L: see Appendix 11.1) were used in these IRT analyses. Although these results should be interpreted with caution given that they were not conducted on the recommended sample size of 300 subjects or more, they are suggestive of the marked differences in the performance of the avoidance and numbness items.

The IIFs displayed in Figure 11.1 indicate the amount of information provided for each symptom in reference to a standardized TG score (that is, the amount of 'traumatic griefness'). The results indicate that 'numbness' (TG

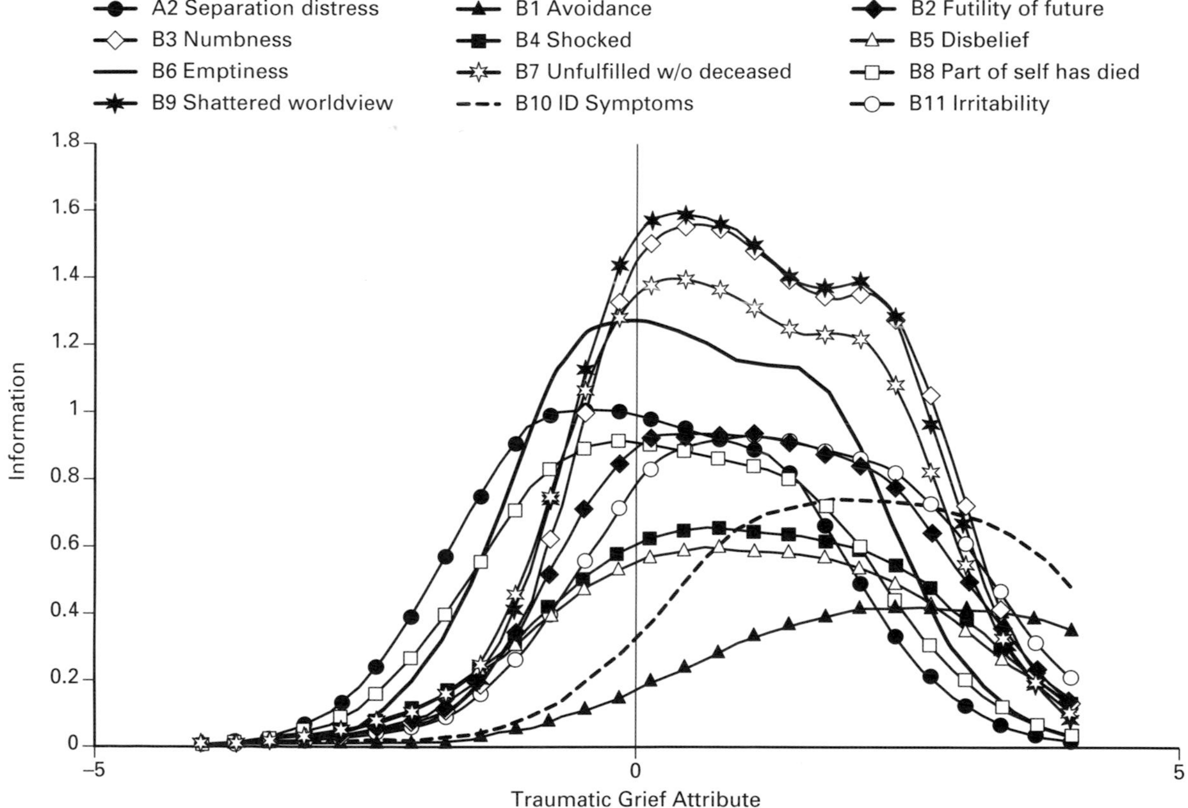

Figure 11.1. The amount of information provided by each of the proposed traumatic grief items with reference to a standardized score that assesses the severity of the traumatic grief attribute.

criterion B3), together with the 'shattered worldview' item (TG criterion B9), provided the most information about the TG attribute. This suggests that 'detachment' is one of the best performing indicators of TG. The 'shocked' item (TG criterion B4) refers to feeling 'stunned' or 'dazed' by the loss, which provided relatively little information about the TG attribute. If our sample had included individuals bereaved by sudden, unexpected deaths, these more shocking circumstances of the loss might have resulted in better performance of the 'stunned' and 'dazed' items. These results suggest that there may be less intense surprise about the death than is typical in PTSD resulting from objectively traumatic events such as assaults or accidents. Unlike in the case of frank PTSD, the numbness/detachment in TG may represent less of a tendency to dissociate from the *event* of the death than it represents a withdrawal from other *interpersonal relationships*, especially when they serve as reminders of the loss. This conclusion is supported by results obtained using the same sample of Connecticut widows and widowers. In a study of the quality of life impairments associated with TG, PTSD, and major depressive disorder (MDD), we found that subjects who met the proposed criteria for TG had significantly lower levels of social functioning than subjects who did not meet criteria for TG, while neither diagnoses of PTSD nor MDD entered in the same model were shown to influence significantly the widowed person's degree of social functioning.[27] TG appears more a consequence of interpersonal dysfunction than is the case with PTSD. A study by the authors is underway to examine the ways in which TG and PTSD are differentially affected by and a consequence of social support and social functioning.

The most notable distinction with PTSD concerns the 'avoidance' item (TG criterion B1). In Figure 11.1, 'avoidance' provided the least amount of information about the TG attribute and would not appear to efficiently distinguish individuals with TG from those without TG. Even Horowitz et al,[28] who propose 'avoidance' as one of their two core criteria for complicated grief, found the 'avoidant thoughts of deceased' item at the recommended 14 months post-loss diagnostic assessment had a sensitivity of only 0.26. In a study by Spooren et al[29] of Belgian parents who lost a child as a result of a traffic accident, the PTSD symptom of avoidance was notably rare. Thus, the available empirical evidence suggests that avoidance is neither a common feature of nor an efficient marker for TG. Further research is needed to confirm this hypothesis.

It should be noted, however, that in our treatment study when probed specifically for things they no longer do since the death, bereaved subjects do report avoidance of situations and activities that evoke loneliness and reminders of the loss. In our Inventory of Traumatic Grief, respondents are asked about their avoidance of thoughts of the deceased, and it may be that the avoidance relates more to reminders of the loss. It could be that the specific items used to assess avoidance have not been viewed as secondary to the loss, and a change in the wording of the item to refer to avoidance of the loss might yield greater endorsement of avoidance. We will be pilot testing this possibility in our field trial of the consensus criteria. Patients with TG report that they avoid doing things that they used to do with the deceased (for instance, going to movies, to the park, or even the hospital), not so much because they wish to avoid thinking about the deceased, but because they feel terribly alone when confronted with reminders of their loss. The avoidance is not of something dangerous, as would be the case in PTSD, but TG symptoms include a wish to avoid confronting the reality of the death, as is also indicated by a sustained sense of disbelief about the loss (TG criterion B5). In some sense, for TG sufferers there may be an avoidance of wanting to get on with their life, and this manifests itself as detachment and disengagement. This may explain why, in our initial experience, an exposure-based treatment produces markedly better results than those obtained for either interpersonal psychotherapy or antidepressant medication. TG therapy attempts to reduce, or desensitize TG sufferers to, the pain associated with reminders of the loss, thereby assisting in the processing of the loss and promoting a capacity for emotional reinvestment in people and activities in the post-loss environment.

Criterion D

For a person to meet criteria for the DSM-IV[22] diagnosis of PTSD, two or more symptoms of increased arousal must also be present (criterion 'D'). Examples of symptoms of heightened arousal in the DSM-IV[22] include: difficulty falling or staying asleep, irritability or outbursts of anger, difficulty concentrating, hypervigilance, or an exaggerated startle response. Criterion D for PTSD provides another set of symptoms of mixed relevance for TG.

Horowitz et al[28] also found that hypervigilance was only reported by 1.5% of his bereaved sample and that this item had a sensitivity of 0.03 at the recommended 14 months assessment of 'complicated grief'. As Raphael has noted, to the extent that there is hypervigilance in TG, it relates to scanning the environment for cues of the deceased, not fear that an unwanted horrible experience will reoccur.[20]

'Excessive irritability and anger' related to the loss are included among the proposed criteria for TG (criterion B11). The IRT analyses in Figure 11.1 indicate that the 'irritability' item provides a moderately high level of information about the TG attribute. Anecdotally, subjects who have met the proposed criteria for TG do complain about impaired concentration as a result of the loss.

While TG has been shown to predict poor subjective sleep,[14] in a study of late-life bereaved patients, McDermott et al[30] found that symptoms of TG were not significantly associated with the electroencephalographic (EEG) sleep abnormalities (for example, fragmentation of sleep and increase in rapid eye movement [REM] sleep intensity) proposed as core psychophysiological markers for PTSD.[31] A study underway that examines hypothalamic–pituitary–adrenal (HPA) axis function associated with TG versus normal bereavement (Narayan, Bremner, Prigerson, Charney, 'hypothalamic-pituitary–adrenal [HPA] function in traumatic grief and bereavement', sponsored by the National Center for PTSD) will shed additional light on neuroendocrine responses associated with TG. For example, supersuppression in response to a relatively small dose (0.5 mg) of dexamethasone would suggest a neurobiological similarity with PTSD.

Criterion E

The DSM-IV[22] specifies that the PTSD symptoms in criteria 'B', 'C', and 'D' must be present for longer than 1 month (criterion 'E'). Results from our studies and those of others have shown that the symptoms of TG may persist among a significant minority of bereaved individuals for several years.[13–18,32,33] While the results of analyses of the FHP data[14] revealed a significant time effect for the resolution of TG symptomatology in the first 2 years of bereavement ($F=111.87$, $df=3$, 288, $p<0.001$), the results of the orthogonal decomposition of the time effect indicated that the mean TG score declined quadratically – with a steep initial decline followed by a plateauing in the rate of resolution of TG grief symptoms (test for quadratic function: $F=43.41$, $df=1, 96$, $p<0.0001$). When we divided the sample between those in the upper 20% of the distribution of TG scores at baseline and those below that threshold, significant differences between the high and low group emerged for the rates of TG symptom resolution (group-by-time interaction: $F=10.69$, $df=3, 285$, $p<0.0001$). Post-hoc paired t-tests indicated that while subjects with low TG scores declined significantly on their severity of TG symptoms between the 2- and the 6-month assessments ($t=2.63$, $df=75$, $p<0.05$), those high on TG did not exhibit a significant decline in TG symptomatology during the same time period, nor between the 13- and the 25-month assessments. At the 25-month assessment, the mean level of TG symptoms among the high grief group most closely approximated the mean level of symptoms among the low grief group at their first, and most elevated, assessment (that is, mean TG levels of 26.6 and 30.8, respectively) and did not decline significantly thereafter. Thus, high levels of TG appeared to persist well beyond the 1-month stipulation and to correspond to a diagnosis of 'chronic' (duration of symptoms lasting 3 months or more) rather than 'acute' (less than 3 months) PTSD. This is consistent with results from the National Comorbidity Survey reported by Kessler et al,[34] in which more than one-third of subjects with an index episode of PTSD failed to recover even after many years. It is also consistent with Blank's[35] conclusion that 'most studies have found that PTSD often persists over time, or occurs long after the trauma' (p. 5).

Criterion F

The final criterion that needs to be met for the DSM-IV diagnosis of PTSD (criterion 'F') stipulates that the symptoms must cause 'clinically significant distress or impairment in social, occupational, or other important areas of functioning'. Over the past several years we have conducted several studies that indicate the wide variety of functional impairments associated with TG symptoms and a TG diagnosis.[8–16,26,27] We consistently find that TG (assessed either as a continuous symptom measure or as a dichotomous diagnosis) is associated with a heightened risk for such adverse outcomes as cardiac events, substance abuse, suicidality, impairments in social and physical functioning, decline in general health, increased bodily pain, and decreased energy. In these ways, TG symptomatology, like PTSD symptomatology, appears to be associated with clinically significant distress and functional impairment.

Overall diagnostic agreement

Although only limited data are available which contain concurrent diagnostic assessments of TG and PTSD, we are aware of two such data sets. The first was a study of friends of high school suicide victims who were assessed in a follow-up study 6 years following the friend's death. In this study, we found the rate of diagnostic agreement between a diagnosis of TG and that of PTSD to be low ($\phi = 0.34$), with only seven of the 15 who met criteria for TG also meeting criteria for PTSD.[13] In the pilot study of Connecticut widows and widowers, diagnoses for TG and PTSD were also shown to have a moderately high but far from complete overlap with each other (between TG and PTSD, $\phi = 0.47$). Of those diagnosed with TG (16/89), 63% did not meet criteria for PTSD (10/16), and 37.5% had *neither* a major depressive episode nor a PTSD diagnosis (6/16). These findings provide the strongest evidence to suggest that

TG and PTSD represent two distinct clinical entities given that nearly two-thirds of the subjects who met criteria for TG would have been missed by a PTSD diagnosis. They suggest that while there is overlap between these two disorders, the percentage of agreement is low enough to raise concerns about the appropriateness of a PTSD diagnosis for bereaved persons with TG.

Summary

If we review the necessary and sufficient conditions for a diagnosis of PTSD, it appears possible for people who meet criteria for TG also to meet these conditions. By definition, those who experience the death of someone close would satisfy the criterion A.1. 'stressor' condition. However, a necessary consequence of this traumatic exposure is that the bereaved person's response would involve intense fear, helplessness, or horror. Although more information about the horror resulting from a devastating loss is required before we can conclude that criterion A.2. does not apply to bereaved individuals with TG, we suspect the evidence will reveal fright to be a response of little significance for TG. To the extent these responses meet the threshold required for a diagnosis of PTSD, then the remaining PTSD criteria would be evaluated for their fit with TG.

With respect to the criterion B 'reexperiencing' phenomena, those with TG would easily meet the required single symptom of recurrent and intrusive distressing thoughts about the deceased. However, there are some very important differences in the quality of the intrusive thoughts. In TG, the intrusive thoughts relate to the deceased rather than to an event, and unlike in the case of PTSD from catastrophic events like fires and floods, the reexperiencing can be comforting as well as upsetting. A further important difference between the criteria for TG versus those for PTSD is that the element of 'separation distress', which evokes the intrusive thoughts in TG, is absent in PTSD. The core TG symptoms of yearning, pining, or searching for the deceased, or excessive emptiness or loneliness without the deceased, a sense that a part of the grieving person has died along with the deceased, lie at the heart of the bereaved person's emotional disturbance. Consequently, therapeutic aims for TG are to promote a transition from excessive, continued preoccupation with the deceased to new relationships and reengagement in the post-loss environment.

A person who met criteria for TG would likely meet the minimum of three of the criterion C avoidance and numbness symptoms. Detachment appears to be a hallmark of TG, and the sense of purposelessness, and diminished interest in people and things, are also symptoms of this disorder. Although the results we have found, together with the results of Horowitz et al[28] and Spooren et al,[29] raise a question about whether avoidance is a common behavior among the bereaved, and whether it is an efficient indicator of a pathological grief reaction, our clinical experience is different from this. However this question is resolved, avoidance in TG is not related to fear of the traumatic event, but to the intense sense of loneliness and despair evoked by the loss. It seems clear that when avoidance is present, it is an important focus of effective treatment, and that an exposure strategy serves to ameliorate the extreme sense of detachment and lack of enthusiasm, interest, and energy.

The PTSD criterion D, which stipulates that two of the five listed symptoms of hyperarousal must be present, could also be met by persons who meet criteria for TG who report irritability and difficulty concentrating. Still, the EEG sleep abnormalities associated with PTSD were not found among subjects who had syndromal level TG,[30] and Horowitz et al[28] found little evidence of hypervigilance. As Raphael and Martinek[20] have noted, the hypervigilance relates to a searching for cues of the deceased, rather than fears that the threatening event will reoccur. This suggests that while the hyperarousal criterion technically could be met, it would be misleading to conclude that bereaved people with TG suffer from excessive arousal.

Two remaining conditions are required for a PTSD diagnosis. PTSD criteria E and F, which relate to the duration of the disturbance and marked functional impairment, could easily be met by individuals with TG.

Taken together, all criteria for PTSD could be met by someone who received a diagnosis of TG. Nevertheless, as we have tried to illustrate, the phenomenology of the symptomatic response to a devastating loss appears to differ in many important ways from the symptomatic response to objectively traumatic events. TG does appear to be a stress response syndrome, but the distress is a function of the loss of someone whom the survivor believed was essential to his/her wellbeing, rather than evoked by exposure to a horrific event. The evidence presented in this chapter suggests that much of the emotional distress stemming from the loss, per se, might be missed if clinicians conceptualized the trauma strictly in terms of the criteria for PTSD outlined in the DSM-IV.[22]

As a further point of clarification, people who are exposed to an objectively traumatic event involving the death of someone close might develop *both* PTSD and TG. Our data sets have focused on conjugal bereavement from a spouse's naturally occurring death. Our discussion had been limited to the extent to which bereavement under these relatively normal circumstances could result in PTSD. There are numerous cases in which the death of a significant other is a result of a horrific event or disaster (such as earthquakes, fires, floods, gang violence), and we would expect a significant proportion of those exposed to traumatic events that involve the death of someone close to develop PTSD *and* TG. A study by Bremner et al[36] provides an example of how the response to an objective trauma may be influenced by interpersonal attachments. In this study of Vietnam veterans exposed to combat, those who went on to develop PTSD claimed that the most traumatic aspect of the Vietnam experience was seeing a friend get killed. The influence of attachment on the development of PTSD has also been noted by Ursano et al,[37] who found that disaster workers who identified with the deceased as a friend were more likely to have PTSD than those who did not. In this way, objectively traumatic events that involve the death of someone close would appear to put someone at risk for both PTSD and TG.

In conclusion, let us return to the question of the appropriateness of a PTSD diagnosis for those suffering from complicated bereavement reactions (defined by us as the criteria for TG). It seems that if the conceptualization of PTSD were modified to acknowledge that responses vary greatly depending on the nature of the traumatic exposure, then it might make more sense than it currently does to consider TG as one of many potential variants of a stress response syndrome. An emerging body of literature has brought a growing awareness that PTSD is not a monolithic disorder.[38–40] For example, a study by Peck et al[40] found that even among accident-induced psychological trauma, the PTSD symptoms associated with mountain climbing accidents were different from those secondary to automobile accidents. Finlay-Jones and Brown[41] have shown that events involving severe danger are causal agents in the onset of anxiety states, whereas events involving severe loss are causal agents for the onset of depressive disorders. As its name implies, traumatic grief appears to stem from severe losses that evoke a sense of extreme threat and, thereby, evoke symptoms of trauma. Bremner[39] has proposed a new category of trauma spectrum disorders in which the commonalities in stress symptoms would be recognized, while the distinctiveness of each outcome would also be appreciated. To the extent that losses, regardless of the circumstances in which the loss occurs, may be viewed as anxiety-provoking (as in the case of loss-induced adult separation anxiety), and this could be recognized under the umbrella of traumatic spectrum disorders, then TG might be appropriately classified among these other stress response syndromes.

Perhaps there exist two types of traumatic stress reactions, one that results primarily from the shock the event causes to the survivor's system and the fear that it engenders, and another that results primarily from the impact of the event on the survivor's identity and coping capacity. The latter would describe the TG response, as would a spectrum of loss or attachment disorders in which the survivor feels permanently disabled and powerfully changed by the loss of an important attachment object. Should a category of traumatic spectrum disorders be constructed, one which allows for the cohabitation of related yet not identical stress response syndromes, then it might be possible for TG to reside in a new and comfortable diagnostic home.

References

1. Holmes TH, Rahe RH, The social readjustment rating scale, *J Psychosom Res* (1967) 11:213–8.
2. Irwin M, Weiner H, Depressive symptoms and immune functions during bereavement. In: Zisook S, ed, *Biopsychosocial Aspects of Bereavement* (American Psychiatric Press: Washington, DC, 1987) 157–74.
3. Osterweis M, Solomon F, Green M, *Bereavement: Reactions, Consequences and Care* (National Academy Press: Washington, DC, 1984).
4. Shuchter SR, Zisook S, A multidimensional model of spousal bereavement. In: Zisook S, ed, *Biopsychosocial Aspects of Bereavement* (American Psychiatric Press: Washington, DC, 1987) 35–48.
5. Stroebe MS, Stroebe W, The mortality of bereavement. In: Stroebe MS, Stroebe W, Hansson RO, eds, *Handbook of Bereavement: Theory, Research, and Intervention* (Cambridge University Press: New York, 1993) 175–95.
6. Schut HAW, Keijser JD, Van Den Bout J, Dijkhuis JH, Post-traumatic stress symptoms in the first year of conjugal bereavement, *Anxiety Research*, (1991) 4:225-34.
7. Breslau N, Kessler RC, Chilcoat HD et al, Trauma and posttraumatic stress disorder in the community: the 1996 Detroit Area Survey of Trauma, *Arch Gen Psychiatry* (1998) 55:626-32.
8. Prigerson HG, Frank E, Kasl SV et al, Complicated grief and bereavement-related depression as distinct disorders: preliminary empirical validation in elderly bereaved spouses, *Am J Psychiatry* (1995) 152:22–30.
9. Prigerson HG, Maciejewski PK, Newsom J et al, The Inventory of Complicated Grief: a scale to measure maladaptive symptoms of loss, *Psychiatry Res* (1995) 59:65–79.
10. Chen JH, Bierhals AJ, Prigerson HG et al, Gender differences in health outcomes resulting from bereavement-related emotional distress, *Psychol Med* (1999) 29:367–80.
11. Prigerson HG, Shear MK, Newsom J et al, Anxiety among widowed elders: is it distinct from depression and grief? *Anxiety* (1996) 2:1–12.
12. Prigerson HG, Bierhals AJ, Kasl SV et al, Complicated grief as a distinct disorder from

bereavement-related depression and anxiety: a replication study, *Am J Psychiatry* (1996) **153**:1484–6.
13. Prigerson HG, Bridge J, Maciejewski P, Beery LC et al, Influence of traumatic grief on suicidal ideation among young adults, *Am J Psychiatry*, (1999) **156**:1994–5.
14. Prigerson HG, Bierhals AJ, Kasl SV et al, Traumatic grief as a risk factor for mental and physical morbidity, *Am J Psychiatry* (1997) **154**:616–23.
15. Prigerson HG, Shear MK, Frank E et al, Traumatic grief: a case of loss induced trauma, *Am J Psychiatry* (1997) **154**:1003–9.
16. Prigerson HG, Bierhals AJ, Wolfson L et al, Case histories of complicated grief, *Omega* (1997) **35**:9–24.
17. Pasternak RE, Reynolds CF, Schlernitzauer M et al, Acute open-trial nortriptyline therapy of bereavement-related depression in late life, *J Clin Psychiatry* (1991) **52**:307–10.
18. Reynolds CF, Miller MD, Pasternak RE et al, Treatment of bereavement-related major depressive episodes in later life: a controlled study of acute and continuation treatment with nortriptyline and interpersonal psychotherapy, *Am J Psychiatry* (1999) **152**:202–8.
19. Prigerson HG, Shear MK, Jacobs SC et al, Consensus criteria for traumatic grief: a preliminary empirical test, *Br J Psychiatry* (1999) **174**:67–73.
20. Raphael B, Martinek N, Assessing traumatic bereavement and posttraumatic stress disorder. In: Wilson JP, Keane TM, eds, *Assessing Psychological Trauma and PTSD* (Guilford Press: New York, 1997) 373–95.
21. Rynearson EK, Bereavement after homicide: a descriptive study. *Am J Psychiatry* (1984) **141**:1452–4.
22. American Psychiatric Association, *Diagnostic and Statistical Manual of Mental Disorders* (DSM-IV), 4th edn, (American Psychiatric Press: Washington, DC, 1994).
23. Jacobs SC, Kasl SV, Ostfield AM et al, The measurement of grief bereaved versus non-bereaved. *Hosp J* (1986) **2**:21–36.
24. Dohrenwend BP, Levav I, Shrout PE, Screening scales from Psychiatric Epidemiology Research Interview (PERI). In: Weissman MM, Myers JK, Ross CE, eds, *Community Surveys of Psychiatric Disorders* (Rutgers University Press: New Brunswick, NJ, 1986) 349–75.
25. Rees WD, The hallucinations of widowhood, *BMJ* (1971) **4**:37–41.
26. Prigerson HG, Hall M, Reynolds CF III, The relation between complicated grief symptoms and long-term functioning. Presented at the American Psychological Association Meeting Symposium on Intrusive Thoughts and Health, Toronto, 9 August 1995.
27. Silverman GK, Jacobs SC, Kasl SV et al, The association between a diagnosis of traumatic grief and quality of life impairments, *Psychol Med* in press.
28. Horowitz MJ, Siegel B, Holen A et al, Criteria for complicated grief, *Am J Psychiatry* (1997) **154**:905–10.
29. Spooren DJ, Henderick H, Jannes C, A retrospective study of parents bereaved from a child in a traffic accident. Service satisfaction, available support and psychiatric sequelae, *Omega*, in press.
30. McDermott O, Prigerson HG, Reynolds CF et al, Sleep in the wake of complicated grief: a preliminary report, *Biol Psychiatry* (1997) **41**:710–16.
31. Ross RJ, Ball WA, Sullivan KA, Caroff SN, Sleep disturbance as the hallmark of Posttraumatic Stress Disorder, *Am J Psychiatry* (1989) **146**:697–707.
32. Jacobs S, *Pathologic Grief: Maladaptation to Loss* (American Psychiatric Press: Washington, DC, 1993).
33. Zisook S, DeVaul RA, Unresolved grief, *Am J Psychoanal* (1985) **45**:370–9.
34. Kessler RC, Sonnega A, Bromet E et al, Posttraumatic stress disorder in the National Comorbidity Survey, *Arch Gen Psychiatry* (1995) **52**:1048–60.
35. Blank AS, The longitudinal course of posttraumatic stress disorder. In: Davidson JRT, Foa B, eds, *Posttraumatic Stress Disorder: DSM IV and Beyond* (American Psychiatric Press: Washington, DC, 1993) 3–22.
36. Bremner JD, Southwick SM, Charney DS, Etiologic factors in the development of posttraumatic stress disorder. In: Mazure CM, ed, *Stress and Psychiatric Disorders* (American Psychiatric Press: Washington, DC, 1994) 149–86.
37. Ursano RJ, Fullerton C, Kao TC, Posttraumatic stress disorder and identification in disaster workers, *Am J Psychiatry* (1999) **156**:353–9.
38. Prigerson HG, Narayan M, Slimack M et al, Pathways to traumatic stress syndromes, *Curr Opin Psychiatry* (1998) **11**:149–52.
39. Bremner JD, Acute and chronic responses to psychological trauma: where do we go from here? *Am J Psychiatry* (1999) **156**:349–51.

40. Peck DF, Robertson A, Zeffert S, Psychological sequelae of mountain accidents: a preliminary study, *J Psychosom Res* (1996) 41:55–63.

41. Finlay-Jones R, Brown GW, Types of stressful life event and the onset of anxiety and depressive disorders, *Psychol Med* (1981) 11:803–15.

Appendix 11.1. Traumatic grief evaluation of response to loss (TRGR2L)

Holly G Prigerson, Paul K Maciejewski, Stanislav V Kasl, M Katherine Shear, Selby C Jacobs

Patient Name:____

ID Number: ____

Evaluation Date: (Mo) ______________(Day) ______________(Year) ________

Rater Name: ____

Instructions:

This instrument is to be used to provide an objective measure of the frequency and intensity of the symptoms that a patient with Traumatic Grief disorder has experienced during the past month.

Variable names appear in (CAPS)

CRITERION A: SEPARATION DISTRESS

A1. Have you recently experienced the loss of a significant other?
- 0 = No
- 1 = Yes

Criterion Met: If response is '1' for A1. Y/N (A1)

A2.1. Do you yearn or long for the deceased?
Frequency: (PREOC FREQ)
A2.1a. How often have you felt this way?
- 0 = Never (less than once a month)
- 1 = Rarely (once a month or more, less than once a week)
- 2 = Sometimes (once a week or more, less than once a day)
- 3 = Often (once every day)
- 4 = Always (several times every day)

Intensity: (PREOC INTEN)
A2.1b. How strong was this feeling?
- 0 = Not present
- 1 = Mild
- 2 = Moderate
- 3 = Severe
- 4 = Extreme

A2.2. Do you find yourself searching for the deceased?
Frequency: (PREOC FREQ)
A2.2a. How often have you felt this way?
0 = Never (less than once a month)
1 = Rarely (once a month or more, less than once a week)
2 = Sometimes (once a week or more, less than once a day)
3 = Often (once every day)
4 = Always (several times every day)

Intensity: (PREOC INTEN)
A2.2b. How strong was this feeling?
0 = Not present
1 = Mild
2 = Moderate
3 = Severe
4 = Extreme

A2.3. Do you feel lonely as a result of the death?
Frequency: (PREOC FREQ)
A2.3a. How often have you felt this way?
0 = Never (less than once a month)
1 = Rarely (once a month or more, less than once a week)
2 = Sometimes (once a week or more, less than once a day)
3 = Often (once every day)
4 = Always (several times every day)

Intensity: (PREOC INTEN)
A2.3b. How strong was this feeling?
0 = Not present
1 = Mild
2 = Moderate
3 = Severe
4 = Extreme

Criterion Met: If frequency and intensity is at least '3' for 2 of the 3 A2 Criteria

Then A2 is met: Y/N (A2)

Criterion A: If Criteria A1 and A2 are met, then Criterion A has been met. Y/N (CRITA)

CRITERION B: TRAUMATIC DISTRESS

First, determine if the respondent has met the threshold level to endorse each item. If the respondent endorses at least 6 of the Criterion B items, then s/he has met the Criterion B requirement for a diagnosis of Traumatic Grief.

B1. Was the loss traumatic for you?

0 = loss, but not traumatic
1 = loss moderately traumatizing
2 = loss severely traumatizing

Criterion Met: If Criterion B1 is '1' or more then it is met. Y/N (B1)

B2. Do you feel numb or detached from people?

Frequency: (NUMB FREQ)
How often have you felt this way?

0 = Never (less than once a month)
1 = Rarely (once a month or more, less than once a week)
2 = Sometimes (once a week or more, less than once a day)
3 = Often (once every day)
4 = Always (several times every day)

Intensity: (NUMB INTEN)
How strong was this feeling?

0= Not present
1 = Mild
2 = Moderate
3 = Severe
4 = Extreme

Criterion Met: If frequency and intensity are at least '2'. Y/N (B2)

B3. Do you feel stunned, dazed or shocked about the death?

Frequency: (STUNNED FREQ)
How often have you felt this way?

0 = Never (less than once a month)
1 = Rarely (once a month or more, less than once a week)
2 = Sometimes (once a week or more, less than once a day)
3 = Often (once every day)
4 = Always (several times every day)

Intensity: (STUNNED INTEN)
How strong was this feeling?

0 = Not present
1 = Mild
2 = Moderate

3 = Severe
4 = Extreme

Criterion Met: If frequency and intensity are at least '3'. Y/N (B3)

B4. Do you feel disbelief over the death?
Frequency: (DISB FREQ)
How often have you felt this way?
0 = Never (less than once a month)
1 = Rarely (once a month or more, less than once a week)
2 = Sometimes (once a week or more, less than once a day)
3 = Often (once every day)
4 = Always (several times every day)

Intensity: (DISB INTEN)
How difficult was it for you to believe that your loved one had died?
0 = Not present
1 = Mild
2 = Moderate
3 = Severe
4 = Overwhelming

Criterion Met: If frequency and intensity are at least '3'. Y/N (B4)

B5. Do you actively avoid reminders of the deceased (for example, thoughts, feelings, activities, people, places)?
Frequency (AVOID FREQ)
How often do you find yourself avoiding reminders of the deceased?
0 = Never (less than once a month)
1 = Rarely (once a month or more, less than once a week)
2 = Sometimes (once a week or more, less than once a day)
3 = Often (once every day)
4 = Always (several times every day)

Intensity: (AVOID INTEN)
How strong was this feeling?
0 = Not present
1 = Mild
2 = Moderate
3 = Severe
4 = Overwhelming

Criterion Met: If frequency and intensity are at least '3'. Y/N (B5)

B6. Do you feel a sense of futility about the future?
Frequency: (FUTIL FREQ)
How often have you felt this way?

0 = Never (less than once a month)
1 = Rarely (once a month or more, less than once a week)
2 = Sometimes (once a week or more, less than once a day)
3 = Often (once every day)
4 = Always (several times every day)

Intensity: (FUTIL INTEN)
How strong were these feelings?

0 = Not present
1 = Mild
2 = Moderate
3 = Severe
4 = Overwhelming

Criterion Met: If frequency and intensity are at least '3'. Y/N (B6)

B7. Do you feel that life is empty or meaningless?
Frequency: (EMPTY FREQ)
How often have you felt this way?

0 = Never (less than once a month)
1 = Rarely (once a month or more, less than once a week)
2 = Sometimes (once a week or more, less than once a day)
3 = Often (once every day)
4 = Always (several times every day)

Intensity: (EMPTY INTEN)
How strong was the sense of emptiness as a result of the death?

0 = Not present
1 = Mild
2 = Moderate
3 = Severe
4 = Overwhelming

Criterion Met: If frequency and intensity are at least '3'. Y/N (B7)

B8. Do you have difficulty imagining a fulfilling life without the deceased?
Frequency: (FULFILL FREQ)
How often have you felt this way?

0 = Never (less than once a month)
1 = Rarely (once a month or more, less than once a week)
2 = Sometimes (once a week or more, less than once a day)

3 = Often (once every day)
4 = Always (several times every day

Intensity: (FULFILL INTEN)
How strong was this feeling?
0 = Not present
1 = Mild
2 = Moderate
3 = Severe
4 = Overwhelming

Criterion Met: If frequency and intensity are at least '3'. Y/N (B8)

B9. Do you feel that a part of yourself has died?
Frequency: (SELF DIED FREQ)
How often have you felt this way?
0 = Never (less than once a month)
1 = Rarely (once a month or more, less than once a week)
2 = Sometimes (once a week or more, less than once a day)
3 = Often (once every day)
4 = Always (several times every day)

Intensity: (SELF DIED INTEN)
How strong was this feeling?
0 = Not present
1 = Mild
2 = Moderate
3 = Severe
4 = Overwhelming

Criterion Met: If frequency and intensity are at least '3'. Y/N (B9)

B10. Have you experienced symptoms or recognized harmful behaviors in yourself that are similar to those of the deceased?
Frequency: (SYMPT FREQ)
How often have you felt this way?
0 = Never (less than once a month)
1 = Rarely (once a month or more, less than once a week)
2 = Sometimes (once a week or more, less than once a day)
3 = Often (once every day)
4 = Always (several times every day)

Intensity: (SYMPT INTEN)
How strong was this feeling?

0 = Not present
1 = Mild
2 = Moderate
3 = Severe
4 = Overwhelming

Criterion Met: If frequency and intensity are at least '3'. Y/N (B10)

B11. Do you feel a lost sense of security as a result of the loss?
Frequency: (SECURE FREQ)
How often have you felt this way?

0 = Never (less than once a month)
1 = Rarely (once a month or more, less than once a week)
2 = Sometimes (once a week or more, less than once a day)
3 = Often (once every day)
4 = Always (several times every day)

Intensity: (SECURE INTEN)
How strong was this feeling?

0 = Not present
1 = Mild
2 = Moderate
3 = Severe
4 = Overwhelming

Criterion Met: If frequency and intensity are at least '3'. Y/N (B11)

B12. Do you feel a lost sense of control as a result of the loss?
Frequency: (CONTROL FREQ)
How often have you felt this way?

0 = Never (less than once a month)
1 = Rarely (once a month or more, less than once a week)
2 = Sometimes (once a week or more, less than once a day)
3 = Often (once every day)
4 = Always (several times every day)

Intensity: (CONTROL INTEN)
How strong was this feeling?

0 = Not present
1 = Mild
2 = Moderate
3 = Severe
4 = Overwhelming

Criterion Met: If frequency and intensity are at least '3'. Y/N (B12)

B13. Do you feel mistrustful of others as a result of the loss?
Frequency: (TRUST FREQ)
How often have you felt this way?

0 = Never (less than once a month)
1 = Rarely (once a month or more, less than once a week)
2 = Sometimes (once a week or more, less than once a day)
3 = Often (once every day)
4 = Always (several times every day)

Intensity: (TRUST INTEN)
How strong was this feeling?

0 = Not present
1 = Mild
2 = Moderate
3 = Severe
4 = Overwhelming

Criterion Met: If frequency and intensity are at least '3'. Y/N (B13)

B14. Do you feel angry or bitter as a result of the loss?
Frequency: (ANGER FREQ)
How often have you felt this way?

0 = Never (less than once a month)
1 = Rarely (once a month or more, less than once a week)
2 = Sometimes (once a week or more, less than once a day)
3 = Often (once every day)
4 = Always (several times every day)

Intensity: (ANGER INTEN)
How strong was this feeling?

0 = Not present
1 = Mild
2 = Moderate
3 = Severe
4 = Overwhelming

Criterion Met: If frequency and intensity are at least '3'. Y/N (B14)

B15. Do you feel on edge or anxious?
Frequency: (ANXIOUS FREQ)
How often have you felt this way?

0 = Never (less than once a month)
1 = Rarely (once a month or more, less than once a week)
2 = Sometimes (once a week or more, less than once a day)
3 = Often (once every day)
4 = Always (several times every day)

Intensity: (ANXIOUS INTEN)
How strong was this feeling?

0 = Not present
1 = Mild
2 = Moderate
3 = Severe
4 = Overwhelming

Criterion Met: If frequency and intensity are at least '3'. Y/N (B15)

CRITERION B: If respondent endorsed at least 8 of the 15 items above, then s/he met requirements for Criterion B. Y/N (CRITB)

CRITERION C: DURATION Duration of disturbance (symptoms listed for Criteria A and B) is at least two months. Y/N (CRITC)

How many months has it been since your spouse died? __________ (MONTHS FROM LOSS)

How many months ago would you say your feelings of grief began? __________ (ONSET)

How long would you say that you have been grieving? __________ (DURATION)

Have there been times when you did not have pangs of grief and then these feelings began to bother you again? 1 = Yes 2 = No (EPISODIC)

Can you describe how your feelings of grief have changed over time?

____

____

____

CRITERION D: IMPAIRMENT Disturbance causes marked and persistent dysfunction in social, occupational, or other important domains. Y/N (CRITD)

____

Has the subject met each of the above criteria needed for a diagnosis of traumatic grief? Y/N (TOTCRIT)

AFTER ADMINISTERING THIS INTERVIEW, IN YOUR JUDGMENT DO YOU BELIEVE THIS PERSON TO BE SUFFERING FROM A CLINICALLY SIGNIFICANT/DIAGNOSABLE LEVEL OF TRAUMATIC GRIEF?

YES **NO** (RTASS)

12

Ethnocultural issues

Alexander C McFarlane

> There is an objective truth – which she might call historical fact as opposed to historical interpretation. And you have to reach for it . . . the most important thing any human being can do is to be as objective as possible about the past, that is the only thing on which a secure identity – individual or society – can be based. And linked to this is the feeling that doing it is a virtual impossibility. Because the moment you try, all the forces of delusion, self-aggrandisement, guilt, brain-washing by public perceptions, conspire to distort the past almost as soon as it has happened.[1]

Introduction

Post-traumatic stress disorder (PTSD) is a unique disorder because it conveys how the environment and the process of adjustment to severe traumatic stress can be extremely detrimental to an individual's adaptation. The process of interaction between internal and social resources brings into focus how individuals' experience and the meaning which they assign to an event play a critical role in psychological outcome. The attribution of meaning involves looking at the individual's personal relationships in the context of society and culture. This embeddedness of experience implies that PTSD is not an illness implicit to the individual alone, as it also involves an interaction with the sociocultural environment over time.[2] The belief that individuals can control their own destiny is only a relatively recent notion and it is one of the dimensions in which cultural expectations define the impact of experience on psychological wellbeing. Religion and the prevailing cultural norms about restitution and dealing with grief are cultural domains where resources can mitigate the impact of trauma.[3]

This chapter will discuss these issues whilst accepting the importance of the role of the neurobiology and the universality of the psychological stress response.[4] These form the stage on which ethnic and cultural factors are played out. Perhaps most important to this process is the dimension of intrusion and avoidance in the traumatic stress response.[5] These axes of reaction are manifest in both individuals' cognitive and affective domains and the way that society at large contains and relives trauma. The critical aspect of this process is the subtle manner in which the past often comes to be played out in the future and moulds the shape and effect of current reactions and attitudes without the roots being recognized.

The role of culture is easy to lose in the world of objectivity and statistically based research with the current ascendancy of biological observations. The stated importance of an ethnocultural perspective can be dismissed as platitudinous in the world of reductionism because of few facts and many assertions. The contributions which it makes do not have the same focused objective dimensions as does research into changes in specific domains of neurotransmitter systems, for example. However, there is a great need to look at the relevance of more empirically based observations about trauma to the lives of traumatized people and the meanings they ascribe to their suffering.[6]

Definition of culture

Culture is a phenomenon which has several dimensions: it is the distinctive practices and beliefs as well as a development or improvement of the intellect or behaviour due to education, training or experience. The idea that it is a process which involves active development and change is implicit in the use of the word to describe the act or processing of cultivated land, animals, etc.[7] The definitions of culture are as many and varied as cultures which exist. One of the primary characteristics of a culture is that it provides a context for survival. Rappaport[8] has described a complex set of relationships between quite divergent variables in a society, comparing it to an ecosystem where the culture is defined as the system which is evolved to ensure the survival of the population in the context of the resources available. Thus culture has a regulatory function which is experienced as an ideology by the population, whereas its contribution to survival is latent and unconscious among the members of the culture.[9]

Culture contributes divergent tensions, not the least of which comes from the human need for dependence, and therefore its loss becomes traumatic.[3] Individuals who are strongly identified with a culture and its values are protected and buffered by the support and sense of identity which it provides, particularly at times of trauma. The power of culture lies in the fact that it is a protector, integrator and security system.[10] This protection is at a cost because it limits individuality and freedom of expression and the loss leaves a deep sense of disorientation.

Culture provides a frame of belief which assists in dealing with illness and traumatic events as well as their causes. This function has a dimension which persists and does not disappear with treatment or the reconstruction of the damage after a disaster. Traumatic events do have predictable consequences which are unavoidable, although they can be minimized through preparation, training and risk appraisal. Distress, loss and sickness must therefore be managed and adapted to by both individuals and groups. Culture is the vehicle which embodies the values enriching these processes and the rituals contributing to healing. Suffering and illness are profound personal experiences as well as communications to the group.[3]

The traumatic stress field is one which is especially influenced by these forces. The nature of a traumatic experience is partly defined by cultural expectations about risk. Fatalistic cultures are accepting of the existence of traumatic events because they have external and unmodifiable risks and these must be constantly faced. However, this belief system can undermine the potential for successful mitigation of risk, although it provides a useful set of beliefs and constructs for dealing with tragedy when it arises. The social system also provides valuable models for how to adapt once the trauma has arisen. The models of intervention which we propose in the face of disaster, such as debriefing, are in part social movements which mobilize belief systems and support networks and give cultural permission to emote and seek help.[11] These belief systems help overcome the natural resistance to asking for help and the cultural tradition of not showing pain or distress. The advocacy for particular treatment approaches also comes from subcultural beliefs about the benefits and superiority of one treatment over another in the context of competing tribes of therapist. This internecine battle is often disguised with the language of science, which emphasizes the differences between approaches rather than the non-specific aspects of treatment and the common origins of many competing approaches.

There are also often major cultural gulfs between clinicians and their patients. This divide is summarized in this quote about the inability of the welfare professions to document and intervene in child abuse until recent times.

> In England, a different factor was at work during those years, and that a mind-set prevailed which allowed damage and abuse to go unrecognised. They were the years of scrupulous professional regard for what was thought of as 'working class culture'. In their numbing desire to be 'non-judgemental', educated people in the welfare trade did not 'talk down' to the economically disadvantaged nor teach them how to live their lives. So the dysfunctional became a model, and their expectations for their clients – of stability and routine in child care, for example – were low. They had every bit of jargon at their fingertips, and liberal clichés bubbled on their lips; it was just in practical observation that they were deficient.[12]

Most discussion of culture and trauma focus on the comparison between different societies and the way that they adapt and create meaning in response to particular types of experience or the phenomenology of the stress response in culturally distinct groups. Victims' status itself creates a distinct cultural group and behavioural expectations. This latter dimension of the forces and influence of culture is possibly of most significance to clinicians.

The cultural determination of meaning

The personal meaning of traumatic experience of the individual is influenced by the social context in which it occurs. Victims and the significant people in their surroundings may have different and fluctuating assessments both of the reality of what has happened and of the extent of their suffering.[13] As a result, victims and witnesses may have strongly conflicting agendas in the need for repair: heal, forget or take revenge. At the individual level, this dynamic can be seen as one of the forces which is played out in the repressed memory debate, where the accused have used scientific argument to alienate and deny the traumatic reality of the victims. These conflicts between a trauma's meaning to victims and witnesses create an environment for the trauma to be perpetuated. When it comes to the conflict of nations, soon not the trauma itself but the allocation of blame and responsibility may become the central issue.

Many personal testimonies of trauma survivors describe the absence of support by the people on whom they counted, and being blamed for bringing horrendous experiences upon themselves, which left deeper scars than the actual traumatic events themselves.[13a] Similarly victims often feel ashamed and disgusted by their own failure to prevent what has happened. Thus, for many victims a violation of their self and social ideals becomes part of the traumatic experience. This is also true for nations who have been beaten in war. This sense of self-betrayal is particularly acute if a nation was unprepared and did not anticipate the intentions or strength of their enemy. Members of that nation may find it difficult to respect those who fought or the leaders who played a part in the loss of national pride. The liberators and the resistance fighters can become powerful reminders of this shame.

Once the period of a trauma is over there can be a dramatic shift in attitudes. Ironically, both a victim of PTSD, and the larger society that may be expected to respond with compassion, forbearance or financial sacrifices, have a stake in believing that the trauma is not really the cause of the individual's suffering. Society becomes resentful about having its illusions of safety and predictability disturbed by people who remind them of how fragile security can be. One of the reasons for this failure of empathy is the gulf between the experience of the victim and their ability to express it in language which provokes empathy in those who do not know the experience.

The conflict between the individual and social need

External validation of the reality of a traumatic experience in a safe and supportive context is a vital aspect of preventing and treating post-traumatic stress. However, the creation of such a context for recovery can become very complicated when the psychological needs of victims are in conflict with their social network. When victims' helplessness persists, as in chronic PTSD, or when the meaning of the trauma is secret, forbidden or unacceptable, such as occurs in intrafamilial abuse, or state violence, the trauma fails to elicit donation of resources, restitution or the metering out of justice. In the restoration of government at the end of a war there may be a conflict between the resistance leadership and the established holders of power who went into the safety of exile. Validation of bravery of the resistance fighters may threaten a non-democratic government which was installed at liberation because this enhances their legitimate political profile. Lack of validation and support is likely to perpetuate the haunting traumatic memories which evoke a sense of victimization and social alienation.

One of the paradoxes about the predicament of survivors (whether they be soldiers or civilian victims) is that the larger social group often lacks any realistic understanding of their predicament. Primo Levi, who was an Italian chemist who survived the death camps of Nazi Germany, wrote passionately about the changed perception of the victims of this terrible incarceration. In the years immediately following the war he described how:

> I encountered people who didn't want to know anything, because the Italians, too, had suffered, after all, even those who didn't go to the camps! They used to say, 'For heaven's sakes, it's all over,' and so I remained quiet for a long time.[14]

In 1955 Levi noted that it had become 'indelicate' to speak of the camps – 'One risks being accused of setting up as a victim, or of indecent exposure'. Thus was confirmed the terrible, anticipatory dream of the victims, during and after the camps: that no one would listen, and if they listened they wouldn't believe. . . . Once people did start to listen, and believe, the other obsession of the survivor began to eat away at Levi – the shame, and guilt, of survival itself, made worse in his case by the embarrassment of fame. Why should he, Levi, have survived? Had he made compromises that others had refused? Had others died in his place? . . . His only resource to ward off the enemies of memory was words. But 'the trade of clothing facts in words', he wrote, 'is bound by its very nature to fail'.

The importance of language – that we can communicate and we must communicate, that language is vital to humanity and the deprivation of language is the first step of destruction of a man – was enforced within the camp (words were replaced by blows – 'that was how we knew we were no longer men').[15]

For the victims of individual and hidden traumas such as child abuse and domestic violence, the recurrence of the victimization and denial by the immediate social network is far more insidious and hence harder to identify.[16] Due to the social stigma attached to these forms of trauma, their occurrence is kept hidden, which means that there is very little chance of any realistic social awareness emerging. This was also the lot of the 'comfort women' enslaved by the Japanese army.[17] The women's movement has been the voice for these concerns and has greatly contributed to the breaking down of the social dismissal of sexual violence. This collective advocacy has challenged the minimization of the black and silent world of familial abuse which shatters the advocated social ideals of modern conservative politicians.

Victims of trauma often become objects of passionate concern from those around them, concern that may have no direct reflection on their actual wellbeing. Often voiceless about their innermost fears, and becoming accustomed to passive acquiescence, victims of trauma are vulnerable to use for a variety of political and social ends, both for good and ill; they can be nurtured or idealized, and just as easily spurned, stigmatized and rejected. Between 1947 and 1982, Israeli society moved from the latter to the former position with respect to its attitude toward Holocaust survivors, without ever resting in the middle of the pendulum by treating them as fellow human beings who had been exposed to the unspeakable.[18] Bloom[19] has described how the field of traumatic stress emerged out of a political process advocating compassion for the Vietnam veterans. They were seen as the victims of government policy and the resultant terror of collective violence.

The problem and the nature of traumatic memory

The most dramatic achievement of human culture is language. It has no innate or independent existence, yet it has driven an enormous amount of human evolution.[20] Language also defines and binds cultures. It is challenging to consider that before the existence of the gramophone, language could only be understood as a collective social memory. It is a phenomenon that can only exist between individuals. As the sophistication of societies increases it becomes the pervasive glue which creates the ties between groups and defines the boundaries which are more or less permeable between cultures.

The limitation of language becomes apparent when experiences occur so infrequently between individuals that there is no collective way of expressing the nature and consequences of that event.[21] By definition these experiences have the capacity to fall outside the world of the spoken culture. Hence the expression of traumatic experience is a much more complex task than appears at first hand. War is the greatest collective human trauma and the need to write history and develop military tactics has necessitated its exploration. There is a variety of data which suggest there is an immense difficulty in constructing a true representation of war.

Janet[22] highlighted that another of the critical dimensions of traumatic experience is the difficulty of creating a representation of it in narrative memory. The event becomes trapped in the primary sensory memories rather than developing a transformed and more symbolic structure which has a linguistic base. Hence the very nature of traumatic experience is its propensity to bypass linguistic representation.[23] Perhaps one way of conceptualizing this phenomenon is to consider that traumatic experiences are defined by their capacity to disrupt the use of language. Creative expression does not naturally emerge to convey these events. One of the most boring jobs for the officers in World War II was censoring the letters of the men, who seemed to have enormous difficulty capturing the nature of terror and the chaos of combat.[24] Siegfried Sassoon reflected the social consequences of this problem, conveying their experience in his peace statement which was published in *The Times* and read out in the House of Commons.[25]

> I have seen and endured the sufferings of the troops, and I can no longer be a party to prolong these sufferings for ends which I believe to be evil and unjust. I am not protesting against the conduct of the War, but against the political errors and insincerities for which the fighting men are being sacrificed. On behalf of those who are suffering now I make this protest against the deception which is being practised on them; also I believe that I may help to destroy the callous complacency with which the majority of those at home regard the continuance of agonies which they do not share, and which they have not sufficient imagination to realise. (p. 218)[26]

Grasping the nature of the trauma therefore requires a great deal of imagination and empathy if the truth is not to be avoided. The listener or interpreter which may be the broader culture has to compensate for the fact that most victims have impaired capacity to translate the intense emotions and perceptions related to the trauma into communicable language. Not being able to give a coherent account of the trauma to others, or even to oneself, without feeling traumatized all over again, makes it difficult for a culture to create representations of these experiences. The combination of the wish of the bystander not to be disturbed by the raw emotions of injured people and the problems of victims articulating what they feel and need makes it extremely difficult to stay focused on working through the impact of the trauma. Instead of clear-cut statements that convey the reality of what has happened, traumatic memories start leading a life of their own as disturbing symptoms.[26]

When the memories of the trauma remain unprocessed, traumatized individuals tend to become like Pavlov's dogs: subtle reminders become conditional stimuli to re-experience frightening feelings and perceptions belonging to the past. Hence social and cultural rituals which do not process the experience have the capacity to sustain the trauma and inflict pain by touching the wound which has not healed. This emphasizes that cultures should ideally provide some symbolic transformation of an experience. To facilitate social healing they should provide hope in the recall of horror. They must tell the story of suffering whilst not wounding the bereaved by adding the dread of their memories of the dead. They must encourage reconciliation rather than driving retribution and motivating a further cycle of violence by creating a universal image of suffering where no one is spared the agony of violence. The message is to heal but not through the romanticization of victors or the humiliation of those who were routed.

The awareness in a society of the memories which drive its values and the roots of its culture are critical to healthy identifications and preventing an acting out of old wounds in social prejudices and victimizations. Grossman[27] has highlighted how the increasing distance we have from birth and death in developed societies means that we have lost the experiences that teach respect for life and death. Increasingly, Western cultural ideas are subject to distortions through the media, which feast on trauma and suffering, and the aggression depicted in the cinema and video games. This portrays a far more aggressive and ruthless world than reality demonstrates historically, since there have been tremendous prohibitions to killing even in war. The identification of youth with this Hollywood culture and its implicit messages may explain the spate of violent crime being committed by youth across the Western world. Previously, the importance of submission as a strategy and an understanding that much aggression was a threatening posture rather than a desire to kill was implicit cultural knowledge. The danger of living in a media-driven culture is that it both misrepresents long-standing inhibitions against violence and also destroys the cultural diversity which has been the core of the survival of social groups.

Cross-cultural studies

There are a variety of case reports which have examined the trauma response in particular minority groups.[9] These reports often convey unique and stark cultural comparisons but the perspective of the heightened sensitivity to difference in the outside observer is what drives these comparisons. When these perceived distinctions are subjected to scientific observation, what is striking is the relative lack of data suggesting cultural specificity in the trauma response, although the healing rituals vary greatly.[28] A sensitivity to this variance is an important issue for the development of humanitarian aid to Third World disasters and civil wars. The problems of ethnic conflict and the refugee crisis which often follows are going to be a growing international problem emphasizing the importance of this body of knowledge.[29] The other groups who have been of particular interest are refugees who have been resettled in new host countries and victims of torture and gross human rights violations.[30]

The large epidemiological studies of Vietnam veterans provide a particular insight into outcome of minorities in response to one category of event. The National Vietnam Veterans Readjustment Study (NVVRS)[31] oversampled several minorities and found that in contrast to the White rate of PTSD of 13.7%, Blacks had a rate of 20.6% and Hispanics 27.6%. There was also a suggestion that when they became ill there was also a greater degree of disability and social maladjustment. However, the increased rate of disorder in the Blacks was accounted for by increased combat exposure. These were analogous findings to those of Laufer et al,[32] who similarly found greater impact of combat on Blacks. Similar observations were made about Maori soldiers in the New Zealand army who served in Vietnam where combat exposure level, rank and combat role accounted for the greater morbidity.[33] These findings are not representative of the general population. In the National Comorbidity Study, Kesseler et al[34] found that Whites had the higher rates of traumatization and PTSD. The most important cultural finding in this study was that for the same trauma, women had double the rate of PTSD of men. The embeddedness of women in their culture and attachments is one explanation for this vulnerability.[3] Trauma involves the carrying of the pain of those around one, which is particularly costly if individuals have strong attachments.

Case studies have exemplified some of the dimensions of war which can have specific effects on minorities.[35,36] For example, Asian Americans fighting in the Vietnam War were more closely identified with the Viet Cong, which created many points of confusion in separating the self from the victim.[37] This is the reverse of the phenomenon observed in Southeast Asian refugees in the USA,[38,39] where the lack of social integration was an important stressor. Studies of refugee populations which make prevalence estimates are difficult to interpret because the representativeness of the sample is often hard to determine, but they do demonstrate the extreme traumatization of these people and the need for humanitarian concerns not to be lost within the walls of cultural and geographical isolation.

Natural disasters create by far the greatest devastation in Third World countries[40] because of the lack of risk management and the poor quality of building materials and construction standards (97.5% of disaster victims are in developing countries[41]). Yet these events have been given little attention in epidemiological research because of the imperatives of survival in these economies. The prevalence studies which have been conducted are generally difficult to interpret because of the non-representative samples studied (for example, the 1989 Mexico earthquake,[42] the Amero mudslide[41]). Some important exceptions exist, including the study of the Armenian earthquake and the Puerto Rico floods and mudslides which had been previously sampled in the Epidemiological Catchment Area (ECA) study.[43] There are also a series of more recent events which have been studied but few of the data have found their way into the Western literature. The Kobe earthquake in Japan which killed thousands of people has been extensively examined and demonstrated some of the methodological issues about underreporting symptoms due to the cultural tradition of *bushido*, where there is great shame associated with inappropriate displays of emotion.[9] The Iraqi occupation of Kuwait has also been studied using a strict epidemiological approach and demonstrated the similarities of response in a Moslem and Western culture and that gender stereotyping seemed to have little impact.[44]

The similarities of the trauma response across cultures present significant support for the integrity of PTSD as a distinct diagnosis. A study of Khmer adolescent refugees suggested that PTSD as a result of war trauma surmounted the barriers of culture and language.[45] Implicit in PTSD is the notion that relatively independent of the nature of the traumatic stressor, the context and the culture, there is a similar phenomenology and epidemiology. This observation supports the idea of trauma as a unifying concept in contrast to the imperative of focusing on individual groups of victims. What cross-cultural studies have identified is the impact of culture on the road to care and the nature of treatment which is acceptable to the patient. For example, treatment-seeking Iranian torture victims living in Germany had poorer knowledge of German.[46] A useful strategy is to work in collaboration with traditional healers who address the health beliefs of the victims.[47] It appears that racial origin does not influence the response to treatment in a Veterans Affairs system.[48] This is an example which should also be followed in the context of Western society, where there is often a significant divide between the health beliefs of the patient and the professional.[48a] Studies of the mental health literacy of populations demonstrates major divergences in the beliefs within a culture about the effectiveness and appropriateness of different treatments.[49]

The way culture influences the presentation of symptoms

Studies of refugee populations have highlighted the propensity to somatization of PTSD in non-Western groups.[50,51] The irony is that the majority of patients in First World settings also present with these concerns but the doctor's apostolic role persuades the patient to avoid this method of complaint and focus on the cognitive and affective symptoms.[52] The history of trauma-related syndromes has focused on the role of somatization.[53] In the 1890s there was a major focus on the investigation of hysteria and its multiple manifestations. During World Wars I and II there were epidemics of conversion disorders, especially in battle situations where the soldiers were given little opportunity for the expression of their fear through action. The description of the phenomenology of these reactions did not unravel the importance of the expression of the trauma in the symptoms. Latterly, following the Vietnam War, there was the belief that the multiple ailments of the servicemen were due to their exposure to the herbicide Agent Orange.[54] Predictably, following the 1990 war against Iraq, the Gulf War syndrome rather than PTSD has emerged as the critical health issue where the somatic distress of the servicemen is the critical concern.

The other force at work in these situations is the role of compensation and the impact that litigation has on symptoms and their presentation. The suspicion of exaggeration and malingered distress is one of the cultural stigmas which haunt the trauma victim. There are two competing narratives in the legal arena which demonstrate how distress can be modified by the context and the listener. The counsel for the defence has little compunction in voicing suspicion and derision about the victim's complaints in contrast to the plaintiff's counsel, who will subtly encourage and seek out real and imagined complaints. The impact of the culture of the law on the definition of the field and the public debate surrounding victims is a major social force. The critic Robert Hughes in *Culture of Complaint*[55] discussed the issue that how society conceptualizes personal responsibility is dramatically influenced by the adversarial tradition. In its extremes these tensions become manifest in the false memory debate and concerns about alien abduction and satanic ritual abuse. The multiple opinions which can be expressed about victims demonstrate the depth of divergence within a dominant culture.

The impact of trauma on culture

The twentieth century was marked by major international conflicts and unprecedented loss of life in war. World War I was a cataclysm that partly occurred because of the failure of military tactics to deal with the consequences of the new weapons and their destructive power. This conflict challenged conventional forms of expression and the abstract art movement was strongly influenced by a recognition that realism had failed to prepare people for what transpired.[56] The uncertainty and the emergence of new forms of disaster such as the atomic bomb, AIDS and environmental degradation have left a pall of uncertainty and threat hanging over the world. The world of art and philosophy has tried to grapple with this new reality of chance. In this way the threat of loss and the awareness of the brutality of the world have come to change art and culture in dramatic ways. Perhaps the most dramatic shifts occurred in the social dislocation and rebellion against authority at the time of the Vietnam War. Trauma is an abiding theme of the twentieth century and has dominated our attempts to find cultural and political identity. Trauma is the constant concern of the media and as a major social preoccupation becomes a powerful organizing force. The need remains to develop a cultural narrative for traumatic situations which allows more effective organization to prevent the cycles of violence which we see being played out in places such as Yugoslavia. The misrepresentation of conflict and its consequences in romanticism and nationalism are major threats to peace and survival.

This indicates that the effect of trauma on culture is a bidirectional phenomenon. Just as culture provides a social vehicle for healing, cultures are changed and subcultures arise in an attempt to accommodate the effects of disasters, perceived social threats and wars. Culture represents the need which people have for stories to heal suffering. Scientifically proved treatments are insufficient. There is a need for rituals to assist in healing. The rituals of bereavement and the narratives which are used to contend with death take on many different forms which all serve the same purpose: to integrate a person's experience into the stream of social adaptation.

Thus there are a series of ways in which culture can assist in the understanding of suffering and the healing of these wounds.[9]

1. The comparison of different cultures can assist in understanding the nature of trauma and the ways of dealing with and resolving these traumas.
2. Studying groups who belong to minority cultures embedded in a larger social group can assist in understanding the impact of belonging to one culture while being embedded in a different host culture.
3. The impact of a minority culture being overrun by an exogenous group can be a specific type of trauma in its own right which can disrupt the normal healing rituals of the minority culture and leave the entire group highly vulnerable to trauma.

References

1. Barker P, 1998, cited in Annan G, Ghosts, *New York Review*, 20 May 1999.
2. Bronfenbrenner U, Nature–nurture reconceptualized in developmental perspective: a bioecological model, *Psychol Rev* (1994) **10**:568–86.
3. de Vries MW, Trauma in cultural perspective. In: van der Kolk BA, McFarlane AC, Wesiaeth L, eds, *Traumatic Stress: The Effects of Overwhelming Experience on Mind, Body and Society* (Guilford: New York, 1996) 398–413.
4. Yehuda R, McFarlane AC, Conflict between current knowledge about PTSD and its conceptual basis, *Am J Psychiatry* (1995) **152**:1705–13.
5. American Psychiatric Association, *Diagnostic and Statistical Manual of Mental Disorders*, 4th edn (American Psychiatric Association: Washington, DC, 1994).
6. Wilson EO, *Consilience: The Unity of Knowledge* (Little, Brown: Boston, 1998).
7. *Heinemann Australian Dictionary*, 4th edn (Heinemann Educational Australia: Richmond, Victoria, 1992).
8. Rappaport, RA, *Ritual Ecology and Systems* (Yale University Press: New Haven, CT, 1984) 1–7.
9. Chemtob CM, Posttraumatic stress disorder, trauma and culture. In: Mak FL, Nadelson CC, eds, *International Review of Psychiatry*, vol 2 (American Psychiatric Press: Washington, DC, 1996) 257–92.
10. Brown GW, Prudo R, Psychiatric disorders in a rural and an urban population: vol 1. Aetiology of depression, *Psychol Med* (1981) 11:581–99.
11. Raphael B, Meldrum L, McFarlane AC, Does debriefing after psychological trauma work? *BMJ* (1995) **310**:1479–80.
12. Mantel H, Killer children, *New York Review of Books*, 20 May 1999, 4–5.
13. Winter J, *Sites of Memory, Sites of Mourning. The Great War in European Cultural History* (Cambridge University Press: Cambridge, 1995).

13a. Lifton RJ, *Home from the War* (Basic Books: New York, 1973).

14. Tedeschi G, 1995, cited in Caracciolo N, *Uncertain Refuge: Italy and the Jews During the Holocaust* (University of Illinois Press: Illinois, 1995).
15. Judt T, The courage of the elementary, *New York Review of Books*, 20 May 1999, 31–8.
16. Herman J, *Trauma and Recovery* (Basic Books: New York, 1992).
17. Buruma I, *The Wages of Guilt: Memories of War in Germany and Japan* (Meridian Press: New York, 1995).
18. Solomon Z, From denial to recognition: attitudes toward Holocaust survivors from World War II to the present, *J Trauma Stress* (1995) **8**:215–28.
19. Bloom SL, Our hearts and our hopes are turned to peace: Origins of the International Society for Traumatic Stress Studies. In: Shalev AY, Yehuda R, McFarlane AC, eds, *International Handbook of Human Response to Trauma* (Kluwer/Plenum: New York, 2000) 27–50.
20. Deacon TW, *The Symbolic Species. The Co-evolution of Language and the Brain* (WW Norton: New York, 1997).
21. American Psychiatric Association, *Diagnostic and Statistical Manual of Mental Disorders*, 3rd edn (American Psychiatric Association: Washington, DC, 1980).
22. Janet P, *Les Médications Psychologiques* (Felix Alcan: Paris, 1919).
23. van der Kolk BA, The psychobiology of traumatic memory: clinical implications of neuroimaging studies, *Ann N Y Acad Sci* (1997) **821**:99–113.
24. Fussell P, *The Great War and Modern Memory* (Oxford University Press: London, 1975).
25. Sassoon S, *Memoirs of an Infantry Officer* (Faber and Faber: London, 1930).
26. Langer LL, *Holocaust Testimonies: The Ruins of Memory* (Yale University Press: New Haven, CT, 1991).
27. Grossman D, *On Killing: the Psychological Cost of Learning to Kill in War and Society* (Little, Brown: Boston, 1997).
28. Frueh BC, Brady KL, de Arellano MA, Racial differences in combat-related PTSD: empirical findings and conceptual issues, *Clin Psychol Rev* (1998) **18**:287–305.
29. de Girolamo G, McFarlane AC, Epidemiology of victims of intentional violence: a review of the literature. In: Mak FL, Nadelson CC, eds, *Int Rev Psychiatry*, vol 2 (American Psychiatric Press: Washington, DC, 1996) 93–119.
30. Silove D, Torture and refugee trauma; implications for nosology and treatment of posttraumatic syndromes. In: Mak FL, Nadelson CC, eds, *International Review of Psychiatry* (American Psychiatric Press: Washington, DC, 1996) 211–32.
31. Kulka RA, Schlenger WE, Fairbank JA et al, *Trauma and the Vietnam War Generation: Report of Findings from the National Vietnam Veterans Readjustment Study* (Brunner/Mazel: New York, 1990).

32. Laufer KS, Yager T, Frey-Wouters E et al, *Comparative Adjustment of Veterans and their Peers*, vol 3. *Post-war Trauma: Social and Psychological Problems of Vietnam Veterans in the Aftermath of the Vietnam War* (Center for Policy Research: New York, 1981).
33. MacDonald C, Chamberlain K, Long N, Race, combat and PTSD in a community sample of New Zealand Vietnam war veterans, *J Trauma Stress* (1997) **10**:117–24.
34. Kessler RC, Bromet E, Hughes M, Nelson CB, Posttraumatic stress disorder in the National Comorbidity Survey, *Arch Gen Psychiatry* (1995) **52**:1048–60.
35. Loo LM, An integrative-sequential treatment model for posttraumatic stress disorder: a case study of the Japanese-American internment and redress, *Clin Psychol Rev* (1993) **13**:89–117.
36. Hamada R, Chemtob CM, Sautner B et al, Ethnic identity and Vietnam: a Japanese-American Vietnam veteran with PTSD, *Hawaii Med J* (1988) **47**:100–09.
37. Loo CM, Singh K, Scurfield R, Kilauano B, Race-related stress among Asian American veterans: a model to enhance diagnosis and treatment, *Cultural Diversity in Mental Health* (1998) **4**:75–90.
38. Kinzie DJ, Boehnlein JK, Leung PK et al, The prevalence of posttraumatic stress disorder and its clinical significance among southeast Asian refugees, *Am J Psychiatry* (1990) **147**:913–17.
39. Mattson S, Mental health of southeast Asian refugee women: an overview, *Health Care Women Int* (1993) **14**:155–65.
40. Green BL, Cross-national and ethnocultural issues in disaster research. In: Marsella AJ, Friedman MJ, Gerrity ET, Scurfield RM, eds, *Ethnocultural Aspects of Posttraumatic Stress Disorder: Issues, Research and Clinical Applications* (American Psychological Association: Washington, DC, 1996) 341–61.
41. Lima BR, Pai S, Santacruz H et al, Psychiatric disorders in primary health care clinics one year after a major Latin American disaster, *Stress Medicine* (1991) **7**:25–32.
42. de la Puente R, The mental health consequences of the 1985 earthquakes in Mexico, *Int J Ment Health* (1990) **19**:21–9.
43. Soloman SD, Canino GJ, Appropriateness of DSM-III-R criteria for posttraumatic stress disorder, *Compr Psych* (1990) **31**: 227–37.
44. McFarlane AC, van der Kolk BA, The long-term effect of psychological trauma: a public health issue in Kuwait, *Med Principles Pract* (1996) **5**:59–75.
45. Sack WH, Seeley JR, Clarke GN, Does PTSD transcend cultural barriers? A study from the Khmer Adolescent Refugee Project, *J Am Acad Child Adolesc Psychiatry* (1997) **36**:49–54.
46. Priebe S, Esmaili S, Long-term mental sequelae of torture in Iran – who seeks treatment? *J Nerv Ment Dis* (1997) **185**:74–7.
47. Scurfield RM, Healing the warrior: admission of two American Indian war-veteran cohort groups to a specialised inpatient PTSD unit, *Am Indian Alsk Native Ment Health Res* (1995) **6**:1–22.
48. Rosenheck R, Fontana A, Race and outcome of treatment for veterans suffering from PTSD, *J Trauma Stress* (1996) **9**:343–51.
48a. Schreiber S, Migration, traumatic bereavement and transcultural aspects of psychological healing: loss and grief of a refugee woman from Begameder county in Ethiopia, *Br J Med Psychol* (1995) **68**:135–42.
49. Jorm AF, Korten AE, Jacomb PA et al, 'Mental health literacy': a survey of the public's ability to recognise mental disorder and their beliefs about the effectiveness of treatment, *Med J Aust* (1997) **166**: 182–6.
50. Cheung P, Somatisation as a presentation in depression and post-traumatic stress disorder among Cambodian refugees, *Aust N Z J Psychiatry* (1993) **27**:422–8.
51. Kirmayer LJ, Confusion of the senses: implications of ethnocultural variations in somatoform and dissociative disorders for PTSD. In: Marsella AJ, Friedman MJ, Gerrity ET, Scurfield RM, eds, *Ethnocultural Aspects of Posttraumatic Stress Disorder: Issues, Research and Clinical Applications* (American Psychological Association: Washington, DC, 1996) 131–63.
52. Balint M, *The Doctor, his Patient and the Illness* (Pitman: London, 1957).
53. Showalter E, *Hystories. Hysterical Epidemics and Modern Culture* (Picador: London, 1997).
54. Hall W, The Agent Orange controversy after the Evatt Royal Commission, *Med J Aust* (1986) **145**:219–25.
55. Hughes R, *Culture of Complaint: The Fraying of America* (Oxford University Press: New York, 1993).
56. Conrad P, *Modern Times: Modern Places. Life and Art in the 20th Century* (Thames and Hudson: London, 1998).

13

Post-traumatic stress disorder – future prospects and needs

David Nutt, Jonathan Davidson and Joseph Zohar

As will be evident from the preceding chapters in this book, post-traumatic stress disorder (PTSD) is undoubtedly one of the most important of the anxiety disorders, both in terms of human and societal costs. Moreover, with the possible exception of GAD, it is also the least well understood and managed. To some extent these failures of understanding and management are understandable. The diagnostic concept is a recent one which has undergone some evolution and which in some quarters is only now becoming accepted. The fact that there have been relatively few good controlled trials that have demonstrated efficacy of either drug or psychological treatments has meant that doctors and other health care providers have shied away from making the diagnosis as they were unsure of what to do next.

One important aspect of this problem is that PTSD patients suffer from 'double stigma': the well known, and not so easy to shake, stigma of mental disorder, and the somewhat unusual 'internal stigma'. Many psychiatrists do not actually believe that PTSD is a 'real' disorder, but rather tend to see it as a 'compensation neurosis', a way to 'milk' financial payback. It would therefore be important to convey to our colleagues that although a minority of patients try to abuse the syndrome, the vast majority of PTSD patients do suffer from a real (and disabling) disorder that needs to be better studied and understood.

We hope this volume has helped in rectifying some of the misunderstandings and ignorance in this field. The scale of the problem is clear, as are the ways to diagnose and treat. The relationship to other disorders and to grief has been explored and possible brain mechanisms explained. Still, there is a great deal to be answered and the purpose of this chapter is to highlight some of these issues as well as pointing possible ways forward.

Diagnosis

Perhaps the biggest challenge in this field is the disentangling of PTSD from depression.

The issue here is not about symptoms, which can generally be delineated, but causality, both biological and psychological. The literature on depression is well aware of the impact that early life trauma can have in predisposing to later mood disorder, but this area has not really attempted to address key questions such as whether early trauma resulting in PTSD produces a different form or prognosis of later depression. One particularly important issue is that of steroid hormone dysregulation. Chapter 5 explains the important conceptual difference between PTSD (low cortisol levels probably from hypersensitive feedback) and depression (high levels due to deficient feedback). The dexamethasone suppression test has fallen somewhat into disuse following a promising beginning. Perhaps the lack of specificity in the test reflects the presence of two groups of depressed people – those with primary high cortisol depression and those with secondary post-PTSD depression with low cortisol and a different dexamethasone response? Conversely, could a diagnostic test based on hypersensitive feedback be developed for PTSD? Perhaps, but account would have to be taken of the consequences of secondary major depression.

Rating scales

Two important psychometric tasks that confront PTSD are to develop (a) a simple screening test and (b) a scale by which response to treatment can be monitored. These may or not be one and the same insofar as scale content is concerned.

Instruments can be grouped into those completed by an observer (interview-based) and those filled out by the patient (self-rated). Interview-based scales in common use include the CAPS (Clinician Administered PTSD Scale), the SIP (Structured Interview for PTSD) and the eight-item derivative of the SIP (TOP-8). A brief global scale, the SPRINT (Short PTSD Rating Instrument) is under development. Self-rating scales include the Impact of Event Scale Revised (IES-R), the Mississippi Combat and Non-combat Scales, the Penn Inventory, the Foa PTSD Symptom Scale (PSS), the Davidson Trauma Scale (DTS) and its four-item screening derivative, the SPAN.

While the CAPS and SIP are widely used, well-established and valid for DSM-IV criteria, they are somewhat lengthy, and therefore not ideal for routine clinical or research use, especially if repeated use is foreseen. Time equates with cost in the practice setting and briefer scales may have greater utility. The TOP-8 represents a start and has been shown to reflect treatment change sensitively, as well to detect differences between SSRI and placebo. It shows good psychometric properties,[1,2] and takes only about 10 minutes to complete at most. Its contents incorporate symptoms from all four PTSD clusters.

Currently lacking is a global measure of PTSD which includes all core symptoms, other important associated symptoms (such as somatization) as well as disability relating to the disorder. We have developed such a scale, the Short PTSD Rating Instrument (SPRINT) and are currently in the process of developing and testing this scale. Preliminary data look promising (Connor et al, unpublished).

Among the self-ratings, a promising new scale has been developed for the purpose of serving as a diagnostic screen. This scale, which consists of the following four symptoms taken from the DTS, startle, physiological arousal, anger, numbing, is referred to as the SPAN.[3] It performed at greater than 80% level of diagnostic accuracy. Further development of this scale is now under way in a broader section of the population. We believe it to be an important task to develop a brief self-rated screener for PTSD to be used in primary care and other settings where the disorder may be seen. One important provision to keep in mind is that trauma must always be identified and related to the intrusive and avoidant symptoms. However, it is of interest that the two screeners which have recently been developed through psychometric methods, one an interview[4] and the other self-rated,[3] both found lowest utility for 'classical' intrusive symptoms of re-experiencing and found greater diagnostic utility for avoidance, numbing and hyperarousal.

Mechanisms

The idea that PTSD is associated with supersensitive glucocorticoid receptors has already been mentioned, but there is a lot we do not understand about this process. Is the sensitivity genetically determined or acquired? And at what level does it occur? Secondary questions relate to the action of steroids in PTSD – if the subsensitivity is contributing to the persistence of the disorder then would a course of cortisol or prednisolone sufficient to induce a normal end organ response be of benefit?

The neuroimaging studies present another perplexing picture as both depression and PTSD are associated with smaller hippocampi and this is presumed to be due to cortisol-related damage. It is understandable how high levels of cortisol as in depression could cause neuronal death, but how could low levels? Presumably if the steroid receptors are supersensitive then they could mediate intracellular processes of equivalent magnitude to those produced by higher cortisol levels in people with normal feedback responses. But then when hippocampal neurons are lost one would expect decreased inhibitory output from the hippocampus to the hypothalamus. This in turn would lead to an increased output of either CRF or vasopressin (or both) so that cortisol levels would then begin to rise. Thus the endocrine aspects of PTSD would be self-limiting. Obviously, good-quality longitudinal studies are critical if this complex question is to be resolved, and a combination of serial imaging plus neuroendocrine challenges would be necessary.

It would also be helpful if an animal model of steroid receptor supersensitivity could be developed, although the mice overexpressing corticosteroid receptors are an interesting move in this direction.

When to treat?

PTSD is by definition a disorder that is related to specific external event(s). It can therefore provide us with a unique and unparalleled opportunity to test different types of intervention, either as prevention, or as an attempt to modify its course. Very little is known so far on the impact of early pharmacological intervention as the majority of controlled studies that have been performed took place months and years after the trauma. In medicine, if we are faced with a situation in which there is a 20% or more chance of developing a chronic and disabling disorder, an intense effort for prevention is carried out, and these are indeed roughly the figures for severe trauma.

It is surprising, therefore, that the major efforts so far in PTSD have been directed at treatment rather than at prevention. It is even more striking since the effect size of the available treatments studied up until now is modest. In this regard there are several areas in need of future exploration. One that is poorly researched is the value of, and best process for, early intervention. It is strange that the psychiatric condition with the clearest onset (at least in adulthood) has not yet had a proper evaluation of early drug treatment. In contrast there have been many examples of natural and man-made disasters being the subject of a range of psychological interventions. It is undoubtedly important for us to know whether early intervention with drugs that have proven utility later on would help prevent the onset of the illness. In this category one could consider the range of antidepressants, anticonvulsants and perhaps even benzodiazepines. Admittedly the relatively low conversion rate from acute stress to full PTSD means that such studies would need a large number of subjects. However, PTSD is common and once established can be quite hard to treat, so prevention could well be economically as well as medically viable.

One suggestion to make early intervention trials more practicable is to determine if biological markers such as heart rate and cortisol levels at the time of the incident do usefully predict illness development. If they did reliably then they could be used to define and enrich groups that were of high risk of developing PTSD and in whom it would be viable to explore the effects of early treatment. One could envisage that some of the newer antidepressants, such as nefazodone and mirtazapine, which are free from the sleep disrupting effects of the SSRIs and can actually improve sleep, might be particularly suitable for this sort of approach. We would actively encourage that such trials be carried out. It may be that, in view of the adverse affects of the alpha-2 antagonist yohimbine in PTSD, mirtazapine, which is also an alpha-2 blocker, might cause some symptom worsening.

Currently available therapies

The first point to make is that the field is in its infancy and despite the multitude of minor trials there is relatively little strong evidence to support clear endorsement of any particular drug, although the SSRIs appear to have the best portfolio so far. Indeed, one, sertraline, has obtained an indication for PTSD in the United States. What is clear is that different classes of drug work on different symptom clusters. Thus the SSRIs seem to do best for numbing whereas the alpha-2 agonist drugs are good against autonomic hyperactivity and the benzodiazepines have good sleep-promoting properties.

In clinical practice one often resorts to selecting combinations of drugs based on a knowledge of effects and side effects. It would be helpful to have well-controlled trials of combinations in order to develop clear guidelines on their optimal interactions. More speculatively it may then be possible to synthesize new compounds tailored to have the combination pharmacology in a single molecule.

New approaches to drug treatment

The exciting discoveries in the peptide field in recent years have given as new perspective to the future therapy of both depression and anxiety. We now have clinical experience with the use of peptide antagonists for CRF, CCK and substance P (neurokinin NK1). CRF antagonists are under evaluation for the treatment of depression and would be fascinating to explore in PTSD, in both the acute and the chronic phase of the illness. Presumably by reducing CRF drive cortisol levels would fall, so reducing the extent of the supersensitive feedback. This might then be predicted to allow other brain processes the opportunity to reset.

CCK, especially when acting via the CCK-B receptor, is a peptide intimately involved in anxiety and panic attacks.[5] Antagonists to CCK-B receptors have been made and tried in humans as potential therapies for panic disorder. Although these results have been disappointing it may be that these compounds would be of more value in other anxiety disorders, possibly in a preventative role. Such ideas could presumably be relatively easily studied in animal models where it could be established whether these drugs were able to prevent stress-induced behavioural changes.

Although originally discovered through their role in pain pathways, the neurokinin family of peptides and receptors have more recently been shown to be also involved in emotional behaviour. This field has developed rapidly in the past couple of years following the discovery of selective high-affinity antagonists for these receptors and the promising clinical results in depression.[6] A number of competing compounds are now under investigation by a variety of companies. Again the evidence that depression should be the main target for these compounds is not well established. NK1 receptor antagonists have been shown to be effective in animal stress models, which was part of the rationale for their being tried in depression. It would seem equally plausible that they could be effective in PTSD, especially if used in the early phases of the illness. The side-effect profile of these compounds is very favourable in comparison with that of other classes of antidepressants and there is no reason to expect any particular problems in the PTSD population. Indeed some of these NK1 receptor antagonists have been tried in some anxiety disorders without apparent problems and in the depression trial MK-869 was also shown to reduce anxiety.[6]

The role of the benzodiazepines in PTSD is currently unclear, with the best study, of alprazolam, showing some evidence of a worse outcome over 6 months. This may reflect complications due to sedation and memory impairment that prevent the sufferer developing other cognitive or behavioural strategies to deal with the trauma. However it may be that the drug was not given near enough to the time of the trauma to be effective. We have argued elsewhere[7] that benzodiazepines would only be active if taken within a short period, ideally hours or less, after the incident in order to limit the embedding of the traumatic memories.

Another approach is to use benzodiazepines with somewhat different profiles of action, and lower potency, such as partial or subtype selective agonists. In recent years a number of benzodiazepine partial agonists have been developed and several have been studied in humans. The best studied is pagoclone which has been shown to have some utility in panic disorder.[8] The advantage of these drugs is that they have much less effect on cognitive function than full agonists. They can therefore be used at high doses to saturate benzodiazepine receptors,which means that if endogenous inverse agonists are being produced in patients with PTSD, their actions will be completely blocked.

Other approaches to blocking the onset of PTSD can also be considered. These include the use of glutamate antagonists as the main glutamate receptors (AMPA and NMDA) which have critical involvement in the laying down of memories. Antagonists of both receptor type now exist and some have been tested in humans for other purposes. Whilst this is a difficult strategy to pursue due to the intimate involvement of the glutamate system in all memory formation as well as consciousness, there may be examples of where it could be valuable, for example after severe trauma that has a high likelihood of progressing to PTSD, such as violent rape, torture, etc.

How do currently effective treatments work at the molecular level?

This is an important issue if we are to begin to develop new specific therapies. One way to address this question is to adapt techniques from other branches of psychiatry such as the study of antidepressant action in depression. Techniques which allow the acute lowering of brain levels and function of 5-hydroxytryptamine (5HT) and noradrenaline using the tryptophan depletion paradigm and alpha-methylparatyrosine, respectively, have radically revised our theories of how antidepressant drugs work to lift mood. We now know that in patients who are well on a serotonergic antidepressant, removing or reducing precursor availability by tryptophan depletion will cause the re-emergence of symptoms in up to 70% of subjects but is without effect in those patients whose depression has been lifted by noradrenergic agents.[9] Conversely, depleting noradrenaline by using the tyrosine hydroxylase inhibitor alpha-methylparatyrosine (alphaMPT) will cause relapse in a similar proportion of people who are well on noradrenergic drugs (but not in those well on SSRIs). These findings have had a major impact on the field, turning on its head prevailing theories that antidepressants work through down-regulation of postsynaptic receptors or second messenger processes. They clearly suggest the mode of therapeutic action of antidepressants the increasing of transmitter concentrations in the synaptic cleft.

This experimental and conceptual approach is beginning to be used in other conditions with interesting results (Table 13.1). For instance in OCD patients who had made some recovery on SSRIs tryptophan depletion was without effect on OCD symptoms; i.e. it did not cause even a partial relapse.[10] In contrast, in panic disorder it has recently been shown to reverse the therapeutic benefit of the SSRI paroxetine.[11] What might one predict in PTSD? As no depletion experiments appear to have been carried out in untreated PTSD patients the position is quite uncertain but of great theoretical interest.

Noradrenaline depletion studies appear not yet to have been tried in the anxiety disorders. One could argue that PTSD, especially the autonomic and intrusive elements, might respond to depletion in a therapeutic way. Strangely alphaMPT, which is occasionally used in patients with phaeochromocytomas,

Table 13.1 Tryptophan depletion studies and the mode of action of antidepressants in psychiatric disorder

Disorder	Treatment	Effect
Depression	SSRI/MAOI	Majority relapse
	Noradrenergic agent	No effect
Obsessive compulsive disorder (OCD)	SRI (SSRI/clomipramine)	No effect
Panic disorder	SSRI (paroxetine)	Relapse on provocation

SSRI, selective serotonin reuptake inhibitors; MAOI, monoamine oxidase inhibitors.

can cause anxiety, so this may be less likely. Nevertheless, the experiment would be worth doing and certainly it would be of great conceptual importance to find out if the anti-PTSD actions of noradrenergic agents would be offset by depletion.

One issue that will have to be taken on board is that of symptom provocation. In the depression and panic disorder studies depressive mood changes were seen to occur spontaneously during the period of depletion. However, the anxiety response in panic was only revealed by challenge with a panicogen, in this case flumazenil.[11] We would suggest that if similar experiments are conducted in PTSD, the paradigm should include a stimulus that will lead to provocation of symptoms in untreated patients, such as a video presentation of trauma.

Imaging: receptors and endogenous transmitters

A number of current theories of PTSD are amenable, or soon will be, to testing using neuroimaging techniques. Table 13.2 shows a current list of validated positron emission tomography (PET) and single photon emission computed tomography (SPECT) probes that can be used to estimate receptor number in human brain, and so allow testing theories that these receptors change in PTSD.

The growing availability of receptor and enzyme targeted probes for neuroimaging means that the possibility of measuring endogenous transmitter release is now very real. Current tracers allow the estimation of synaptic levels of dopamine (by ^{11}C-raclopride competition) and endogenous opioids (by ^{11}C-diprenorphine competition). Similarly the possibility of an endogenous benzodiazepine being released can be tested by observing displacement of ^{11}C-flumazenil. Probes that may be useful for assessing 5HT receptors are now available and one, ^{11}C-WAY100635 has already been used to study the brain mechanisms of depression[12] and panic.[13] Probes for noradrenaline and NK1 receptors are in the pipeline. One very exciting recent development is the identification of a new probe for

Table 13.2 Currently available validated probes for human receptor imaging

Receptor	PET	SPECT
Dopamine D2	^{11}C-raclopride; ^{11}C-spiperone	^{123}I-IBZM
Dopamine turnover	^{18}F-DOPA	
Dopamine uptake site	^{11}C-bCIT	^{123}I-bCIT
GABA-A/BDZ	^{11}C-flumazenil	^{123}I-iomazenil
	^{11}C-Ro 15-4513	^{123}I-NNC
$5HT_{1A}$ receptor	^{11}C-WAY100635	
$5HT_2$ receptor	^{11}C-altanserin, ^{11}C-spiperone	
5HT uptake	^{11}C-McN-5652	^{123}I-bCIT
Opiate (all)	^{11}C-diprenorphine	
Opiate -Mu receptor	^{11}C-carfentanyl	

PET, positron emission tomography; SPECT, single photon emission computed tomography.

the GABA-A/benzodiazepine receptor ^{11}C-Ro 15-4513. This appears to have selectivity for limbic receptors and may also give a measure of endogenous GABA-A activity.[14,15] Some theories of stress/trauma encoding and reliving implicate limbic GABA-A processes[16,17] and others have noted that some patients with PTSD seem to show altered sensitivity of the GABA-A receptor.[18] It may now be possible to directly test these theories using this probe.

Perhaps the most immediately relevant issue relating to endogenous ligands is the question of the possible role of endogenous opioids in PTSD. Many animal studies have shown that stress will release endogenous opioids and it has been possible to demonstrate this using in vivo binding. It has been suggested on the basis of blocking experiments with the antagonist naloxone that numbing and other symptoms of PTSD could reflect endogenous opioid release.[19] If this is true then the release of such substances could in theory be demonstrated by displacement of diprenorphine or carfentanyl tracer using an experimental paradigm similar to that which has been developed for the study of epilepsy.[20] Moreover this approach could help address the ongoing question of alterations in opioid receptors in PTSD. The issue of a possible endogenous inverse agonist benzodiazepines has been touched on and needs to be properly evaluated by assessment of ^{11}C-flumazenil or ^{11}C-Ro 15-4513 displacement during re-experiencing.

Conclusions

PTSD is a major psychiatric disorder with all the personal and social costs that go with such illnesses. There is growing recognition of the scale of the problem that it presents and the need to treat the condition seriously. The emerging literature suggests that the SSRIs may be the first-line drug treatment although other agents with different modes of action have been shown to be effective in smaller-scale studies. Nevertheless, there is a great need for more and better treatments and for a better understanding of how drug treatments work. Psychological treatments are also effective when conducted in centres of excellence and ways of extending this approach into the general psychiatric and primary care arena need to be explored. Theories of the neurobiology of PTSD are growing in credibility and new human imaging techniques may allow some of these to be directly tested in the not too distant future. Taken together these developments offer considerable hope to the many (long) sufferers from PTSD.

References

1. Davidson JRT, Colket JT, The eight-item treatment-outcome post-traumatic stress disorder scale: a brief measure to assess treatment outcome in post-traumatic stress disorder, *Int Clin Psychopharmacol* (1997) 12:41–5.
2. Connor KM, Davidson JRT, Further psychometric assessment of the TOP-8: a brief interview-based measure of PTSD, *Depression and Anxiety* (1999) 9:135–7.
3. Meltzer-Brody S, Churchill E, Davidson JRT, Derivation of the SPAN: a brief diagnostic screening test for PTSD, *Psychiatry Res* (1999) 88:63–70.
4. Breslau N, Peterson EL, Kesler RC, Schultz LR, Short Screening Scale for SDM-IV posttraumatic stress disorder, *Am J Psychiatry* (1999) 156: 908–11.
5. Van Megen HJGM, Westenberg HGM, den Boer JA, Kahn RS, Cholecystokinin in anxiety, *Eur Neuropsychopharmacol* (1996) 6:263–80.

6. Kramer MS, Cutler NR, Feighner J et al, Distinct mechanism for antidepressant activity by blockade of central substance P receptors, *Science* (1998) **281**:1640–5.
7. O'Brien M, Nutt DJ, Loss of consciousness and PTSD: a clue to aetiology and treatment? *Br J Psychiatry* (1998) **173**:102–4.
8. Sandford JJ, D'Orlando KJ, Gamman RE, Nutt DJ, Pilot crossover trial of pagoclone and placebo in patients with DSM-IV panic disorder. Proceedings of the Twenty-first CINP Congress, Glasgow, 12–16 July 1998, Abstract PW14045.
9. Delgado PL, Charney DS, Price LH et al, Serotonin function and the mechanism of antidepressant action: reversal of antidepressant-induced remission by rapid depletion of plasma tryptophan, *Arch Gen Psychiatry* (1990) **47**:411–18.
10. Barr LC, Goodman WK, McDougle CJ et al, Tryptophan depletion in patients with obsessive-compulsive disorder who respond to serotonin reuptake inhibitors, *Arch Gen Psychiatry* (1994) **51**:309–17.
11. Nutt DJ, Forshall S, Bell C et al, Mechanisms of action of selective serotonin reuptake inhibitors in the treatment of psychiatric disorders, *Eur Neuropsychopharmacol* (1999) **9(Suppl 3)**:S81–S86.
12. Sargent PA, Kjaer KH, Bench CJ et al, Brain serotonin-1A receptor binding measured by positron emission tomography with [11C]Way-100635: effects of depression and antidepressant treatment, *Arch Gen Psychiatry* (2000) **57**:174–80.
13. Sargent PA, Nash J, Hood S et al, 5HT1A receptor binding in panic disorder; comparison with depressive disorders and healthy volunteers using PET and [11C]Way-100635. Abstract presented at Human Brain Mapping Conference, San Antonio, Texas, June 2000.
14. Onoe H, Tsukada H, Nishiyama S et al, A subclass of GABAA/benzodiazepine receptor exclusively localised in the limbic system, *Neuroreport* (1996) **8**:117–22.
15. Feeney A, Lingford-Hughes A, Hume S et al, The characterisation of 11C-Ro 15-4513 as a PET ligand. Abstract presented at the BAP Conference, Cambridge, 16–19 July 2000. *J Psychopharmacol* (in press).
16. Adamec RE, Evidence that NMDA-dependent limbic neural plasticity in the right hemisphere mediates pharmacological stressor (FG-7142)-induced lasting increases in anxiety-like behavior. Study 1 – Role of NMDA receptors in efferent transmission for the cat amygdala, *J Psychopharmacology* (1998) **12**:122–8.
17. Nutt DJ, The psychobiology of post-traumatic stress disorder, *J Clin Psychiatry* (2000) **61(Suppl. 5)**: 24–9.
18. Coupland NJ, Lillywhite A, Bell CE et al, A pilot controlled study of the effects of flumazenil in post traumatic stress disorder, *Biol Psychiatry* (1997) **41**:988–90.
19. Pitman PK, Overview of biological themes in PTSD, *Ann N Y Acad Science* (1997) **821**:1–9.
20. Koepp MJ, Richardson MP, Brooks DJ, Duncan JS, Focal cortical release of endogenous opioids during reading-induced seizures, *Lancet* (1998) **352**:952–5.

Appendix

Post-traumatic stress disorder assessment

Two important psychometric tasks that confront the physician in post-traumatic stress disorder (PTSD) are to develop (a) a simple screening test and (b) a scale by which response to treatment can be monitored. These may or not be one and the same insofar as scale content is concerned.

Instruments can be grouped into those completed by an observer (interview-based) and those filled out by the patient (self-rated). Interview-based scales in common use include the CAPS (Clinician Administered PTSD Scale), the SIP (Structured Interview for PTSD) and the eight-item derivative of the SIP (TOP-8). A brief global scale, the SPRINT (Short PTSD Rating Instrument) is under development. Self-rating scales include the Impact of Event Scale – Revised (IES-R), the Mississippi Combat and Non-combat Scales, the PENN Inventory, the Foa PTSD Symptom Scale (PSS), the Davidson Trauma Scale (DTS) and its four-item screening derivative, the SPAN.

While the CAPS and SIP are widely used, well established and valid for DSM-IV criteria, they are somewhat lengthy, and therefore not ideal for routine clinical or research use, especially if repeated use is foreseen. Time equates with cost in the practice setting and briefer scales may have greater utility. The TOP-8 represents a start and has been shown sensitively to affect treatment change, as well as to detect differences between selective serotonin reuptake inhibitors (SSRI) and placebo. It shows good psychometric properties,[1,2] and takes only about 10 minutes to complete at most. Its contents incorporate symptoms from all four PTSD chapters.

Currently lacking is a global measure of PTSD which includes all core symptoms, other important associated symptoms (such as somatization), as well as disability relating to the disorder. We have developed such a scale, the Short PTSD Rating Instrument (SPRINT), and are currently in the process of developing and testing this scale. Preliminary data look promising.[3]

Among the self-ratings, a promising new scale has been developed for the purpose of serving as a diagnostic screen. This scale, which consists of the following four symptoms taken from the DTS, startle, physiological arousal, anger, and numbing, is referred to as the SPAN.[4] It performed at greater than 80% level of diagnostic accuracy. Further development of this scale is now under way in a broader section of the population. We believe it to be an important task to develop a brief self-rated screener for PTSD to be used in primary care and other settings where the disorder may be seen. One important provision to keep in mind is that trauma must always be identified and related to the intrusive and avoidant symptoms. However, it is of interest that the two screeners which have recently been developed through psychometric methods, one an interview[5] and the other self-rated,[4] both found lowest utility for 'classical' intrusive symptoms of re-experiencing and found greater diagnostic utility for avoidance, numbing and hyperarousal.

References

1. Davidson JRT, Colket JT, The eight-item treatment-outcome post-traumatic stress disorder scale: a brief measure to assess treatment outcome in post-traumatic stress disorder, *Int Clin Psychopharmacol* (1997) 12:41–5.
2. Connor KM, Davidson JRT, Further psychometric assessment of the TOP-8: a brief interview-based measure of PTSD, *Depression and Anxiety* (1999) 9:135–7.
3. Connor KM et al, unpublished data 2000.
4. Meltzer-Brody S, Churchill E, Davidson JRT, Derivation of the SPAN: a brief diagnostic screening test for PTSD, *Psychiatry Res* (1999) **88**:63–70.
5. Breslau N, Peterson EL, Kersler RC, Schultz LR, Short screening scale for DSM-IV posttraumatic stress disorder, *Am J Psychiatry* (1999) 156:908–11.

Clinician-Administered PTSD Scale for DSM-IV

Criterion A. The person has been exposed to a traumatic event in which both of the following were present:

(1) the person experienced, witnessed, or was confronted with an event or events that involved actual or threatened death or serious injury, or a threat to the physical integrity of self or others
(2) the person's response involved intense fear, helplessness, or horror. Note: In children, this may be expressed instead by disorganized or agitated behavior

I'm going to be asking you about some difficult or stressful things that sometimes happen to people. Some examples of this are being in some type of serious accident; being in a fire, a hurricane, or an earthquake; being mugged or beaten up or attacked with a weapon; or being forced to have sex when you didn't want to. I'll start by asking you to look over a list of experiences like this and check any that apply to you. Then, if any of them do apply to you, I'll ask you to briefly describe what happened and how you felt at the time.

Some of these experiences may be hard to remember or may bring back uncomfortable memories or feelings. People often find that talking about them can be helpful, but it's up to you to decide how much you want to tell me. As we go along, if you find yourself becoming upset, let me know and we can slow down and talk about it. Also, if you have any questions or you don't understand something, please let me know. Do you have any questions before we start?

ADMINISTER CHECKLIST, THEN REVIEW AND INQUIRE UP TO THREE EVENTS. IF MORE THAN THREE EVENTS ENDORSED, DETERMINE WHICH THREE EVENTS TO INQUIRE (E.G., FIRST, WORST, AND MOST RECENT EVENTS; THREE WORST EVENTS; TRAUMA OF INTEREST PLUS TWO OTHER WORST EVENTS, ETC.)

IF NO EVENTS ENDORSED ON CHECKLIST: *(Has there ever been a time when your life was in danger or you were seriously injured or harmed?)*

IF NO: *(What about a time when you were threatened with death or serious injury, even if you weren't actually injured or harmed?)*

IF NO: *(What about witnessing something like this happen to someone else or finding out that it happened to someone close to you?)*

IF NO: *(What would you say are some of the most stressful experiences you have had over your life?)*

EVENT #1

What happened? *(How old were you? Who else was involved? How many times did this happen? Life threat? Serious injury?)* **How did you respond emotionally?** *(Were you very anxious or frightened? Horrified? Helpless? How so? Were you stunned or in shock so that you didn't feel anything at all? What was that like? What did other people notice about your emotional response? What about after the event – how did you respond emotionally?)*	*Describe (e.g., event type, victim, perpetrator, age, frequency):* *A. (1)* *Life threat? NO YES {self ____ other ____}* *Serious injury? NO YES {self ____ other ____}* *Threat to physical integrity? NO YES {self ____ other ____}* *A. (2)* *Intense fear/help/horror? NO YES {during ____ after ____}* *Criterion A met? NO PROBABLE YES*

EVENT #2

What happened? *(How old were you? Who else was involved? How many times did this happen? Life threat? Serious injury?)* **How did you respond emotionally?** *(Were you very anxious or frightened? Horrified? Helpless? How so? Were you stunned or in shock so that you didn't feel anything at all? What was that like? What did other people notice about your emotional response? What about after the event – how did you respond emotionally?)*	*Describe (e.g., event type, victim, perpetrator, age, frequency):* *A. (1)* *Life threat? NO YES {self ___ other ___}* *Serious injury? NO YES {self ___ other ___}* *Threat to physical integrity? NO YES {self ___ other ___}* *A. (2)* *Intense fear/help/horror? NO YES {during ___ after ___}* *Criterion A met? NO PROBABLE YES*

EVENT #3

What happened? *(How old were you? Who else was involved? How many times did this happen? Life threat? Serious injury?)* **How did you respond emotionally?** *(Were you very anxious or frightened? Horrified? Helpless? How so? Were you stunned or in shock so that you didn't feel anything at all? What was that like? What did other people notice about your emotional response? What about after the event – how did you respond emotionally?)*	*Describe (e.g., event type, victim, perpetrator, age, frequency):* *A. (1)* *Life threat? NO YES {self ___ other ___}* *Serious injury? NO YES {self ___ other ___}* *Threat to physical integrity? NO YES {self ___ other ___}* *A. (2)* *Intense fear/help/horror? NO YES {during ___ after ___}* *Criterion A met? NO PROBABLE YES*

For the rest of the interview, I want you to keep (EVENTS) in mind as I ask you some questions about how they may have affected you.

I'm going to ask you about twenty-five questions altogether. Most of them have two parts. First, I'll ask if you've ever had a particular problem, and if so, about how often in the past month *(week)*. Then I'll ask you how much distress or discomfort that problem may have caused you.

Criterion B. The traumatic event is persistently reexperienced in one (or more) of the following ways:

1. **(B-1)** recurrent and intrusive distressing recollections of the event, including images, thoughts, or perceptions. **Note:** In young children, repetitive play may occur in which themes or aspects of the trauma are expressed.

Frequency	*Intensity*	***Past week***
Have you ever had unwanted memories of (EVENT)? What were they like? *(What did you remember?)* [IF NOT CLEAR:] *(Did they ever occur while you were awake, or only in dreams?)* [EXCLUDE IF MEMORIES OCCURRED ONLY DURING DREAMS] **How often have you had these memories in the past month *(week)*?** 0 Never 1 Once or twice 2 Once or twice a week 3 Several times a week 4 Daily or almost every day ***Description/Examples***	**How much distress or discomfort did these memories cause you? Were you able to put them out of your mind and think about something else?** *(How hard did you have to try?)* **How much did they interfere with your life?** 0 None 1 Mild, minimal distress or disruption of activities 2 Moderate, distress clearly present but still manageable, some disruption of activities 3 Severe, considerable distress, difficulty dismissing memories, marked disruption of activities 4 Extreme, incapacitating distress, cannot dismiss memories, unable to continue activities *QV (specify)* ________________	***F*** ____ ***I*** ____ ***Past month*** ***F*** ____ ***I*** ____ ***Sx: Y N*** ***Lifetime*** ***F*** ____ ***I*** ____ ***Sx: Y N***

2. (B-2) recurrent distressing dreams of the event. **Note:** In children, there may be frightening dreams without recognizable content.

Frequency	Intensity	Past week
Have you ever had unpleasant dreams about (EVENT)? Describe a typical dream. *(What happens in them?)* **How often have you had these dreams in the past month *(week)*?** 0 Never 1 Once or twice 2 Once or twice a week 3 Several times a week 4 Daily or almost every day ***<u>Description/Examples</u>***	**How much distress or discomfort did these dreams cause you? Did they ever wake you up?** [IF YES:] *(What happened when you woke up? How long did it take you to get back to sleep?)* [LISTEN FOR REPORT OF ANXIOUS AROUSAL, YELLING, ACTING OUT THE NIGHTMARE] *(Did your dreams ever affect anyone else? How so?)* 0 None 1 Mild, minimal distress, may not have awoken 2 Moderate, awoke in distress but readily returned to sleep 3 Severe, considerable distress, difficulty returning to sleep 4 Extreme, incapacitating distress, did not return to sleep *QV (specify)* ___________________	*F* _____ *I* _____ ***<u>Past month</u>*** *F* _____ *I* _____ *Sx:* *Y N* ***<u>Lifetime</u>*** *F* _____ *I* _____ *Sx:* *Y N*

3. (B-3) acting or feeling as if the traumatic event were recurring (includes a sense of reliving the experience, illusions, hallucinations, and dissociative flashback episodes, including those that occur on awakening or when intoxicated). **Note:** In young children, trauma-specific reenactment may occur.

Frequency	*Intensity*	*Past week*
Have you ever suddenly acted or felt as if (EVENT) were happening again? *(Have you ever had flashbacks about {EVENT}?)* [IF NOT CLEAR:] *(Did this ever occur while you were awake, or only in dreams?)* {EXCLUDE IF OCCURRED ONLY DURING DREAMS} **Tell me more about that. How often has that happened in the past month** ***(week)?***	**How much did it seem as if (EVENT) were happening again?** *(Were you confused about where you actually were or what you were doing at the time?)* **How long did it last? What did you do while this was happening?** *(Did other people notice your behavior? What did they say?)*	*F* _____ *I* _____ *Past month* *F* _____
0 Never 1 Once or twice 2 Once or twice a week 3 Several times a week 4 Daily or almost every day *Description/Examples*	0 No reliving 1 Mild, somewhat more realistic than just thinking about event 2 Moderate, definite but transient dissociative quality, still very aware of surroundings, daydreaming quality 3 Severe, strongly dissociative (reports images, sounds, or smells) but retained some awareness of surroundings 4 Extreme, complete dissociation (flashback), no awareness of surroundings, may be unresponsive, possible amnesia for the episode (blackout) *QV (specify)* ____________________	*I* _____ *Sx: Y N* *Lifetime* *F* _____ *I* _____ *Sx: Y N*

4. (B-4) intense psychological distress at exposure to internal or external cues that symbolize or resemble an aspect of the traumatic event

Frequency	Intensity	Past week
Have you ever gotten emotionally upset when something reminded you of (EVENT)? *(Has anything ever triggered bad feelings related to (EVENT)?)* **What kinds of reminders made you upset? How often in the past month *(week)*?** 0 Never 1 Once or twice 2 Once or twice a week 3 Several times a week 4 Daily or almost every day *Description/Examples*	**How much distress or discomfort did (REMINDERS) cause you? How long did it last? How much did it interfere with your life?** 0 None 1 Mild, minimal distress or disruption of activities 2 Moderate, distress clearly present but still manageable, some disruption of activities 3 Severe, considerable distress, marked disruption of activities 4 Extreme, incapacitating distress, unable to continue activities *QV (specify)* ____________	*F* ____ *I* ____ ***Past month*** *F* ____ *I* ____ *Sx: Y N* ***Lifetime*** *F* ____ *I* ____ *Sx: Y N*

5. **(B-5)** physiological reactivity on exposure to internal or external cues that symbolize or resemble an aspect of the traumatic event

Frequency	***Intensity***	***Past week***
Have you ever had any physical reactions when something reminded you of (EVENT)? *(Did your body ever react in some way when something reminded you of (EVENT)?)* **Can you give me some examples?** *(Did your heart race or did your breathing change? What about sweating or feeling really tense or shaky?)* **What kinds of reminders triggered these reactions? How often in the past month *(week)*?** 0 Never 1 Once or twice 2 Once or twice a week 3 Several times a week 4 Daily or almost every day ***Description/Examples***	**How strong were (PHYSICAL REACTIONS)? How long did they last?** *(Did they last even after you were out of the situation?)* 0 No physical reactivity 1 Mild, minimal reactivity 2 Moderate, physical reactivity clearly present, may be sustained if exposure continues 3 Severe, marked physical reactivity, sustained throughout exposure 4 Extreme, dramatic physical reactivity, sustained arousal even after exposure has ended *QV (specify)* ________________	*F* ____ *I* ____ ***Past month*** *F* ____ *I* ____ *Sx: Y N* ***Lifetime*** *F* ____ *I* ____ *Sx: Y N*

Criterion C. Persistent avoidance of stimuli associated with the trauma and numbing of general responsiveness (not present before the trauma), as indicated by three (or more) of the following:

6. (C-1) efforts to avoid thoughts, feelings, or conversations associated with the trauma

Frequency	Intensity	Past week
Have you ever tried to avoid thoughts or feelings about (EVENT)? *(What kinds of thoughts or feelings did you try to avoid?)* **What about trying to avoid talking with other people about it?** *(Why is that?)* **How often in the past month (*week*)?** 0 Never 1 Once or twice 2 Once or twice a week 3 Several times a week 4 Daily or almost every day *Description/Examples*	**How much effort did you make to avoid (THOUGHTS/FEELINGS/ CONVERSATIONS)?** *(What kinds of things did you do? What about drinking or using medication or street drugs?)* [CONSIDER ALL ATTEMPTS AT AVOIDANCE, INCLUDING DISTRACTION, SUPPRESSION, AND USE OF ALCOHOL/DRUGS] **How much did that interfere with your life?** 0 None 1 Mild, minimal effort, little or no disruption of activities 2 Moderate, some effort, avoidance definitely present, some disruption of activities 3 Severe, considerable effort, marked avoidance, marked disruption of activities, or involvement in certain activities as avoidant strategy 4 Extreme, drastic attempts at avoidance, unable to continue activities, or excessive involvement in certain activities as avoidant strategy *QV (specify)* ________________	*F* _____ *I* _____ ***Past month*** *F* _____ *I* _____ *Sx: Y N* ***Lifetime*** *F* _____ *I* _____ *Sx: Y N*

7. (C-2) efforts to avoid activities, places, or people that arouse recollections of the trauma

Frequency	*Intensity*	*Past week*
Have you ever tried to avoid certain activities, places, or people that reminded you of (EVENT)? *(What kinds of things did you avoid? Why is that?)* **How often in the past month** ***(week)*****?** 0 Never 1 Once or twice 2 Once or twice a week 3 Several times a week 4 Daily or almost every day *Description/Examples*	**How much effort did you make to avoid (ACTIVITIES/PLACES/ PEOPLE)?** *(What did you do instead?)* **How much did that interfere with your life?** 0 None 1 Mild, minimal effort, little or no disruption of activities 2 Moderate, some effort, avoidance definitely present, some disruption of activities 3 Severe, considerable effort, marked avoidance, marked disruption of activities or involvement in certain activities as avoidant strategy 4 Extreme, drastic attempts at avoidance, unable to continue activities, or excessive involvement in certain activities as avoidant strategy *QV (specify)* ________	*F* ____ *I* ____ *Past month* *F* ____ *I* ____ *Sx: Y N* *Lifetime* *F* ____ *I* ____ *Sx: Y N*

8. (C-3) inability to recall an important aspect of the trauma

Frequency	***Intensity***	***Past week***
Have you had difficulty remembering some important parts of (EVENT)? Tell me more about that. *(Do you feel you should be able to remember these things? Why do you think you can't?)* **In the past month *(week)*, how much of the important parts of (EVENT) have you had difficulty remembering?** *(What parts do you still remember?)* 0 None, clear memory 1 Few aspects not remembered (less than 10%) 2 Some aspects not remembered (approx 20-30%) 3 Many aspects not remembered (approx 50-60%) 4 Most or all aspects not remembered (more than 80%) ***Description/Examples***	**How much difficulty did you have recalling important parts of (EVENT)?** *(Were you able to recall more if you tried?)* 0 None 1 Mild, minimal difficulty 2 Moderate, some difficulty, could recall with effort 3 Severe, considerable difficulty, even with effort 4 Extreme, completely unable to recall important aspects of event *QV (specify)* ________________	***F*** _____ ***I*** _____ ***Past month*** ***F*** _____ ***I*** _____ ***Sx: Y N*** ***Lifetime*** ***F*** _____ ***I*** _____ ***Sx: Y N***

9. (C-4) markedly diminished interest or participation in significant activities

Frequency	Intensity	Past week
Frequency **Have you been less interested in activities that you used to enjoy?** *(What kinds of things have you lost interest in? Are there some things you don't do at all anymore? Why is that?)* [EXCLUDE IF NO OPPORTUNITY, IF PHYSICALLY UNABLE, OR IF DEVELOPMENTALLY APPROPRIATE CHANGE IN PREFERRED ACTIVITIES] **In the past month *(week)*, how many activities have you been less interested in?** *(What kinds of things do you still enjoy doing?)* **When did you first start to feel that way?** *(After the {EVENT}?)* 0 None 1 Few activities (less than 10%) 2 Some activities (approx 20-30%) 3 Many activities (approx 50-60%) 4 Most or all activities (more than 80%) ***Description/Examples***	***Intensity*** **How strong was your loss of interest?** *(Would you enjoy {ACTIVITIES} once you got started?)* 0 No loss of interest 1 Mild, slight loss of interest, probably would enjoy after starting activities 2 Moderate, definite loss of interest, but still has some enjoyment of activities 3 Severe, marked loss of interest in activities 4 Extreme, complete loss of interest, no longer participates in any activities ***QV (specify)*** ______________ ***Trauma-related?*** *1 definite 2 probable 3 unlikely* *Current* _____ *Lifetime* _____	***Past week*** ***F*** _____ ***I*** _____ ***Past month*** ***F*** _____ ***I*** _____ ***Sx:* Y N** ***Lifetime*** ***F*** _____ ***I*** _____ ***Sx:* Y N**

10. (C-5) feeling of detachment or estrangement from others

Frequency	***Intensity***	***Past week***
Have you felt distant or cut off from other people? What was that like? How much of the time in the past month *(week)* have you felt that way? When did you first start to feel that way? *(After the {EVENT}?)* 0 None of the time 1 Very little of the time (less than 10%) 2 Some of the time (approx 20-30%) 3 Much of the time (approx 50-60%) 4 Most or all of the time (more than 80%) ***Description/Examples***	**How strong were your feelings of being distant or cut off from others?** *(Who do you feel closest to? How many people do you feel comfortable talking with about personal things?)* 0 No feelings of detachment or estrangement 1 Mild, may feel "out of synch" with others 2 Moderate, feelings of detachment clearly present, but still feels some interpersonal connection 3 Severe, marked feelings of detachment or estrangement from most people, may feel close to only one or two people 4 Extreme, feels completely detached or estranged from others, not close with anyone ***QV (specify)*** ____________ ***Trauma-related?*** *1 definite 2 probable 3 unlikely* *Current* _____ *Lifetime* _____	***F*** _____ ***I*** _____ ***Past month*** ***F*** _____ ***I*** _____ ***Sx: Y N*** ***Lifetime*** ***F*** _____ ***I*** _____ ***Sx: Y N***

11. (C-6) restricted range of affect (e.g., unable to have loving feelings)

Frequency	Intensity	Past week
Have there been times when you felt emotionally numb or had trouble experiencing feelings like love or happiness? What was that like? *(What feelings did you have trouble experiencing?)* **How much of the time in the past month *(week)* have you felt that way? When did you first start having trouble experiencing (EMOTIONS)?** *(After the {EVENT}?)* 0 None of the time 1 Very little of the time (less than 10%) 2 Some of the time (approx 20-30%) 3 Much of the time (approx 50-60%) 4 Most or all of the time (more than 80%) *Description/Examples*	**How much trouble did you have experiencing (EMOTIONS)?** *(What kinds of feelings were you still able to experience?)* [INCLUDE OBSERVATIONS OF RANGE OF AFFECT DURING INTERVIEW] 0 No reduction of emotional experience 1 Mild, slight reduction of emotional experience 2 Moderate, definite reduction of emotional experience, but still able to experience most emotions 3 Severe, marked reduction of experience of at least two primary emotions (e.g., love, happiness) 4 Extreme, completely lacking emotional experience ***QV (specify)*** ______ ***Trauma-related?*** *1 definite 2 probable 3 unlikely* *Current* _____ *Lifetime* _____	***F*** _____ ***I*** _____ ***Past month*** ***F*** _____ ***I*** _____ ***Sx: Y N*** ***Lifetime*** ***F*** _____ ***I*** _____ ***Sx: Y N***

12. (C-7) sense of a foreshortened future (e.g., does not expect to have a career, marriage, children, or a normal life span)

Frequency	*Intensity*	*Past week*
Have there been times when you felt there is no need to plan for the future, that somehow your future will be cut short? Why is that? [RULE OUT REALISTIC RISKS SUCH AS LIFE-THREATENING MEDICAL CONDITIONS] **How much of the time in the past month *(week)* have you felt that way? When did you first start to feel that way?** *(After the {EVENT}?)* 0 None of the time 1 Very little of the time (less than 10%) 2 Some of the time (approx 20-30%) 3 Much of the time (approx 50-60%) 4 Most or all of the time (more than 80%) *Description/Examples*	**How strong was this feeling that your future will be cut short?** *(How long do you think you will live? How convinced are you that you will die prematurely?)* 0 No sense of a foreshortened future 1 Mild, slight sense of a foreshortened future 2 Moderate, sense of a foreshortened future definitely present, but no specific prediction about longevity 3 Severe, marked sense of a foreshortened future, may make specific prediction about longevity 4 Extreme, overwhelming sense of a foreshortened future, completely convinced of premature death *QV (specify)* ________________ *Trauma-related?* *1 definite 2 probable 3 unlikely* *Current* _____ *Lifetime* _____	*F* _____ *I* _____ ***Past month*** *F* _____ *I* _____ *Sx: Y N* ***Lifetime*** *F* _____ *I* _____ *Sx: Y N*

Criterion D. Persistent symptoms of increased arousal (not present before the trauma), as indicated by two (or more) of the following:

13. (D-1) difficulty falling or staying asleep

Frequency	***Intensity***	***Past week***
Have you had any problems falling or staying asleep? How often in the past month *(week)*? When did you first start having problems sleeping? *(After the {EVENT}?)* 0 Never 1 Once or twice 2 Once or twice a week 3 Several times a week 4 Daily or almost every day Sleep onset problems? Y N Mid-sleep awakening? Y N Early a.m. awakening? Y N Total # hrs sleep/night ____ Desired # hrs sleep/night ____	**How much of a problem did you have with your sleep?** *(How long did it take you to fall asleep? How often did you wake up in the night? Did you often wake up earlier than you wanted to? How many total hours did you sleep each night?)* 0 No sleep problems 1 Mild, slightly longer latency, or minimal difficulty staying asleep (up to 30 minutes loss of sleep) 2 Moderate, definite sleep disturbance, clearly longer latency, or clear difficulty staying asleep (30-90 minutes loss of sleep) 3 Severe, much longer latency, or marked difficulty staying asleep (90 min to 3 hrs loss of sleep) 4 Extreme, very long latency, or profound difficulty staying asleep (> 3 hrs loss of sleep) ***QV (specify)*** __________ ***Trauma-related?*** *1 definite 2 probable 3 unlikely* *Current* ____ *Lifetime* ____	***F*** ____ ***I*** ____ ***Past month*** ***F*** ____ ***I*** ____ ***Sx: Y N*** ***Lifetime*** ***F*** ____ ***I*** ____ ***Sx: Y N***

14. **(D-2)** irritability or outbursts of anger

Frequency	***Intensity***	***Past week***
Have there been times when you felt especially irritable or showed strong feelings of anger? Can you give me some examples? How often in the past month ***(week)*****? When did you first start feeling that way?** *(After the {EVENT}?)* 0 Never 1 Once or twice 2 Once or twice a week 3 Several times a week 4 Daily or almost every day ***Description/Examples***	**How strong was your anger?** *(How did you show it?)* [IF REPORTS SUPPRESSION:] *(How hard was it for you to keep from showing your anger?)* **How long did it take you to calm down? Did your anger cause you any problems?** 0 No irritability or anger 1 Mild, minimal irritability, may raise voice when angry 2 Moderate, definite irritability or attempts to suppress anger, but can recover quickly 3 Severe, marked irritability or marked attempts to suppress anger, may become verbally or physically aggressive when angry 4 Extreme, pervasive anger or drastic attempts to suppress anger, may have episodes of physical violence *QV (specify)* __________________ ***Trauma-related?*** *1 definite 2 probable 3 unlikely* *Current* _____ *Lifetime* _____	***F*** _____ ***I*** _____ ***Past month*** ***F*** _____ ***I*** _____ ***Sx: Y N*** ***Lifetime*** ***F*** _____ ***I*** _____ ***Sx: Y N***

15. (D-3) difficulty concentrating

Frequency	Intensity	
<u>*Frequency*</u> **Have you found it difficult to concentrate on what you were doing or on things going on around you? What was that like? How much of the time in the past month *(week)*? When did you first start having trouble concentrating?** *(After the {EVENT}?)* 0 None of the time 1 Very little of the time (less than 10%) 2 Some of the time (approx 20-30%) 3 Much of the time (approx 50-60%) 4 Most or all of the time (more than 80%) <u>*Description/Examples*</u>	<u>*Intensity*</u> **How difficult was it for you to concentrate?** [INCLUDE OBSERVATIONS OF CONCENTRATION AND ATTENTION IN INTERVIEW] **How much did that interfere with your life?** 0 No difficulty with concentration 1 Mild, only slight effort needed to concentrate, little or no disruption of activities 2 Moderate, definite loss of concentration but could concentrate with effort, some disruption of activities 3 Severe, marked loss of concentration even with effort, marked disruption of activities 4 Extreme, complete inability to concentrate, unable to engage in activities *QV (specify)* ____________ ***Trauma-related?*** *1 definite 2 probable 3 unlikely* *Current* _____ *Lifetime* _____	<u>***Past week***</u> ***F*** _____ ***I*** _____ <u>***Past month***</u> ***F*** _____ ***I*** _____ *Sx:* ***Y N*** <u>***Lifetime***</u> ***F*** _____ ***I*** _____ *Sx:* ***Y N***

16. (D-4) hypervigilance

Frequency **Have you been especially alert or watchful, even when there was no real need to be?** *(Have you felt as if you were constantly on guard?)* **Why is that? How much of the time in the past month** ***(week)*****? When did you first start acting that way?** *(After the {EVENT}?)* 0 None of the time 1 Very little of the time (less than 10%) 2 Some of the time (approx 20-30%) 3 Much of the time (approx 50-60%) 4 Most or all of the time (more than 80%) *Description/Examples*	*Intensity* **How hard did you try to be watchful of things going on around you?** [INCLUDE OBSERVATIONS OF HYPERVIGILANCE IN INTERVIEW] **Did your (HYPERVIGILANCE) cause you any problems?** 0 No hypervigilance 1 Mild, minimal hypervigilance, slight heightening of awareness 2 Moderate, hypervigilance clearly present, watchful in public (e.g., chooses safe place to sit in a restaurant or movie theater) 3 Severe, marked hypervigilance, very alert, scans environment for danger, exaggerated concern for safety of self/family/home 4 Extreme, excessive hypervigilance, efforts to ensure safety consume significant time and energy and may involve extensive safety/checking behaviors, marked watchfulness during interview *QV (specify)* ________________ *Trauma-related?* *1 definite 2 probable 3 unlikely* *Current* _____ *Lifetime* _____	*Past week* *F* _____ *I* _____ *Past month* *F* _____ *I* _____ *Sx: Y N* *Lifetime* *F* _____ *I* _____ *Sx: Y N*

17. (D-5) exaggerated startle response

Frequency	***Intensity***	***Past week***
Have you had any strong startle reactions? When did that happen? *(What kinds of things made you startle?)* **How often in the past month *(week)*? When did you first have these reactions?** *(After the {EVENT}?)* 0 Never 1 Once or twice 2 Once or twice a week 3 Several times a week 4 Daily or almost every day ***Description/Examples***	**How strong were these startle reactions?** *(How strong were they compared to how most people would respond?)* **How long did they last?** 0 No startle reaction 1 Mild, minimal reaction 2 Moderate, definite startle reaction, feels "jumpy" 3 Severe, marked startle reaction, sustained arousal following initial reaction 4 Extreme, excessive startle reaction, overt coping behavior (e.g., combat veteran who "hits the dirt") ***QV (specify)*** ________________ ***Trauma-related?*** *1 definite 2 probable 3 unlikely* *Current* _____ *Lifetime* _____	***F*** _____ ***I*** _____ ***Past month*** ***F*** _____ ***I*** _____ ***Sx: Y N*** ***Lifetime*** ***F*** _____ ***I*** _____ ***Sx: Y N***

Criterion E. Duration of the disturbance (symptoms in Criteria B, C, and D) is more than 1 month.

18. onset of symptoms

[IF NOT ALREADY CLEAR:] **When did you first start having (PTSD SYMPTOMS) you've told me about?** *(How long after the trauma did they start? More than six months?)*	________ ***total # months delay in onset*** ***With delayed onset (≥ 6 months)?*** ***NO YES***

19. duration of symptoms

[CURRENT] **How long have these (PTSD SYMPTOMS) lasted altogether?** [LIFETIME] **How long did these (PTSD SYMPTOMS) last altogether?**	*Duration more than 1 month?* *Total # months duration* *Acute (< 3 months) or chronic (≥ 3 months)?*	***Current*** ***NO YES*** ________ ***acute chronic***	***Lifetime*** ***NO YES*** ________ ***acute chronic***

Criterion F. The disturbance causes clinically significant distress or impairment in social, occupational, or other important areas of functioning.

20. subjective distress

[CURRENT] **Overall, how much have you been bothered by these (PTSD SYMPTOMS) you've told me about?** [CONSIDER DISTRESS REPORTED ON EARLIER ITEMS] [LIFETIME] **Overall, how much were you bothered by these (PTSD SYMPTOMS) you've told me about?** [CONSIDER DISTRESS REPORTED ON EARLIER ITEMS]	0 None 1 Mild, minimal distress 2 Moderate, distress clearly present but still manageable 3 Severe, considerable distress 4 Extreme, incapacitating distress	***Past week*** _____ ***Past month*** _____ ***Lifetime*** _____

21. impairment in social functioning

[CURRENT] **Have these (PTSD SYMPTOMS) affected your relationships with other people? How so?** [CONSIDER IMPAIRMENT IN SOCIAL FUNCTIONING REPORTED ON EARLIER ITEMS] [LIFETIME] **Did these (PTSD SYMPTOMS) affect your social life? How so?** [CONSIDER IMPAIRMENT IN SOCIAL FUNCTIONING REPORTED ON EARLIER ITEMS]	0 No adverse impact 1 Mild impact, minimal impairment in social functioning 2 Moderate impact, definite impairment, but many aspects of social functioning still intact 3 Severe impact, marked impairment, few aspects of social functioning still intact 4 Extreme impact, little or no social functioning	***Past week*** _____ ***Past month*** _____ ***Lifetime*** _____

22. impairment in occupational or other important area of functioning

[CURRENT – IF NOT ALREADY CLEAR] **Are you working now?** IF YES: **Have these (PTSD SYMPTOMS) affected your work or your ability to work? How so?** [CONSIDER REPORTED WORK HISTORY, INCLUDING NUMBER AND DURATION OF JOBS, AS WELL AS THE QUALITY OF WORK RELATIONSHIPS. IF PREMORBID FUNCTIONING IS UNCLEAR, INQUIRE ABOUT WORK EXPERIENCES BEFORE THE TRAUMA. FOR CHILD/ ADOLESCENT TRAUMAS, ASSESS PRE-TRAUMA SCHOOL PERFORMANCE AND POSSIBLE PRESENCE OF BEHAVIOR PROBLEMS] IF NO: **Have these (PTSD SYMPTOMS) affected any other important part of your life?** [AS APPROPRIATE, SUGGEST EXAMPLES SUCH AS PARENTING, HOUSEWORK, SCHOOLWORK, VOLUNTEER WORK, ETC.] **How so?** [LIFETIME – IF NOT ALREADY CLEAR] **Were you working then?** IF YES: **Did these (PTSD SYMPTOMS) affect your work or your ability to work? How so?** [CONSIDER REPORTED WORK HISTORY, INCLUDING NUMBER AND DURATION OF JOBS, AS WELL AS THE	0 No adverse impact 1 Mild impact, minimal impairment in occupational/other important functioning 2 Moderate impact, definite impairment, but many aspects of occupational/other important functioning still intact 3 Severe impact, marked impairment, few aspects of occupational/other important functioning still intact 4 Extreme impact, little or no occupational/other important functioning	***Past week*** _____ ***Past month*** _____ ***Lifetime*** _____

▶

QUALITY OF WORK RELATIONSHIPS. IF PREMORBID FUNCTIONING IS UNCLEAR, INQUIRE ABOUT WORK EXPERIENCES BEFORE THE TRAUMA. FOR CHILD/ ADOLESCENT TRAUMAS, ASSESS PRE-TRAUMA SCHOOL PERFORMANCE AND POSSIBLE PRESENCE OF BEHAVIOR PROBLEMS] IF NO: **Did these (PTSD SYMPTOMS) affect any other important part of your life?** [AS APPROPRIATE, SUGGEST EXAMPLES SUCH AS PARENTING, HOUSEWORK, SCHOOLWORK, VOLUNTEER WORK, ETC.] **How so?**		

Global Ratings

23. global validity

ESTIMATE THE OVERALL VALIDITY OF RESPONSES. CONSIDER FACTORS SUCH AS COMPLIANCE WITH THE INTERVIEW, MENTAL STATUS (E.G., PROBLEMS WITH CONCENTRATION, COMPREHENSION OF ITEMS, DISSOCIATION), AND EVIDENCE OF EFFORTS TO EXAGGERATE OR MINIMIZE SYMPTOMS.	0 Excellent, no reason to suspect invalid responses 1 Good, factors present that may adversely affect validity 2 Fair, factors present that definitely reduce validity 3 Poor, substantially reduced validity 4 Invalid responses, severely impaired mental status or possible deliberate "faking bad" or "faking good"

24. global severity

ESTIMATE THE OVERALL SEVERITY OF PTSD SYMPTOMS. CONSIDER DEGREE OF SUBJECTIVE DISTRESS, DEGREE OF FUNCTIONAL IMPAIRMENT, OBSERVATIONS OF BEHAVIORS IN INTERVIEW, AND JUDGMENT REGARDING REPORTING STYLE.	0 No clinically significant symptoms, no distress and no functional impairment 1 Mild, minimal distress or functional impairment 2 Moderate, definite distress or functional impairment but functions satisfactorily with effort 3 Severe, considerable distress or functional impairment, limited functioning even with effort 4 Extreme, marked distress or marked impairment in two or more major areas of functioning	***Past week*** _____ ***Past month*** ***Lifetime*** _____

25. global improvement

RATE TOTAL OVERALL IMPROVEMENT PRESENT SINCE THE INITIAL RATING. IF NO EARLIER RATING, ASK HOW THE SYMPTOMS ENDORSED HAVE CHANGED OVER THE PAST 6 MONTHS. RATE THE DEGREE OF CHANGE, WHETHER OR NOT, IN YOUR JUDGMENT, IT IS DUE TO TREATMENT.	0 Asymptomatic 1 Considerable improvement 2 Moderate improvement 3 Slight improvement 4 No improvement 5 Insufficient information

Current PTSD Symptoms

Criterion A met (traumatic event)?	*NO*	*YES*
_____ *# Criterion B sx (≥ 1)?*	*NO*	*YES*
_____ *# Criterion C sx (≥ 3)?*	*NO*	*YES*
_____ *# Criterion D sx (≥ 2)?*	*NO*	*YES*
Criterion E met (duration ≥ 1 month)?	*NO*	*YES*
Criterion F met (distress/impairment)?	*NO*	*YES*

CURRENT PTSD (Criteria A-F met)?	*NO*	*YES*

IF CURRENT PTSD CRITERIA ARE MET, SKIP TO ASSOCIATED FEATURES.

IF CURRENT CRITERIA ARE NOT MET, ASSESS FOR LIFETIME PTSD. IDENTIFY A PERIOD OF AT LEAST A MONTH SINCE THE TRAUMATIC EVENT IN WHICH SYMPTOMS WERE WORSE.

Since the (EVENT), has there been a time when these (PTSD SYMPTOMS) were a lot worse than they have been in the past month? When was that? How long did it last? *(At least a month?)*

IF MULTIPLE PERIODS IN THE PAST: **When were you bothered the most by these (PTSD SYMPTOMS)?**

IF AT LEAST ONE PERIOD, INQUIRE ITEMS 1-17, CHANGING FREQUENCY PROMPTS TO REFER TO WORST PERIOD: **During that time, did you (EXPERIENCE SYMPTOM)? How often?**

Lifetime PTSD Symptoms

Criterion A met (traumatic event)? *NO* *YES*

_____ *# Criterion B sx (≥ 1)?* *NO* *YES*

_____ *# Criterion C sx (≥ 3)?* *NO* *YES*

_____ *# Criterion D sx (≥ 2)?* *NO* *YES*

Criterion E met (duration ≥ 1 month)? *NO* *YES*

Criterion F met (distress/impairment)? *NO* *YES*

LIFETIME PTSD (Criteria A-F met)? *NO* *YES*

Associated Features

26. guilt over acts of commission or omission

Frequency	***Intensity***	***Past week***
Have you felt guilty about anything you did or didn't do during (EVENT)? Tell me more about that. *(What do you feel guilty about?)* **How much of the time have you felt that way in the past month *(week)*?** 0 None of the time 1 Very little of the time (less than 10%) 2 Some of the time (approx 20-30%) 3 Much of the time (approx 50-60%) 4 Most or all of the time (more than 80%) ***Description/Examples***	**How strong were these feelings of guilt? How much distress or discomfort did they cause?** 0 No feelings of guilt 1 Mild, slight feelings of guilt 2 Moderate, guilt feelings definitely present, some distress but still manageable 3 Severe, marked feelings of guilt, considerable distress 4 Extreme, pervasive feelings of guilt, self-condemnation regarding behavior, incapacitating distress ***QV (specify)*** _______________	***F*** _____ ***I*** _____ ***Past month*** ***F*** _____ ***I*** _____ ***Sx: Y N*** ***Lifetime*** ***F*** _____ ***I*** _____ ***Sx: Y N***

27. survivor guilt [APPLICABLE ONLY IF MULTIPLE VICTIMS]

Frequency	*Intensity*	*Past week*
Have you felt guilty about surviving (EVENT) when others did not? Tell me more about that. *(What do you feel guilty about?)* **How much of the time have you felt that way in the past month** ***(week)*****?** 0 None of the time 1 Very little of the time (less than 10%) 2 Some of the time (approx 20-30%) 3 Much of the time (approx 50-60%) 4 Most or all of the time (more than 80%) 8 N/A *Description/Examples*	**How strong were these feelings of guilt? How much distress or discomfort did they cause?** 0 No feelings of guilt 1 Mild, slight feelings of guilt 2 Moderate, guilt feelings definitely present, some distress but still manageable 3 Severe, marked feelings of guilt, considerable distress 4 Extreme, pervasive feelings of guilt, self-condemnation regarding survival, incapacitating distress *QV (specify)* ________________	*F* _____ *I* _____ *Past month* *F* _____ *I* _____ *Sx: Y N* *Lifetime* *F* _____ *I* _____ *Sx: Y N*

28. a reduction in awareness of his or her surroundings (e.g., "being in a daze")

Frequency	***Intensity***	***Past week***
Have there been times when you felt out of touch with things going on around you, like you were in a daze? What was that like? [DISTINGUISH FROM FLASHBACK EPISODES] **How often has that happened in the past month *(week)*?** [IF NOT CLEAR:] *(Was it due to an illness or the effects of drugs or alcohol?)* **When did you first start feeling that way?** *(After the {EVENT}?)* 0 Never 1 Once or twice 2 Once or twice a week 3 Several times a week 4 Daily or almost every day ***Description/Examples***	**How strong was this feeling of being out of touch or in a daze?** *(Were you confused about where you actually were or what you were doing at the time?)* **How long did it last? What did you do while this was happening?** *(Did other people notice your behavior? What did they say?)* 0 No reduction in awareness 1 Mild, slight reduction in awareness 2 Moderate, definite but transient reduction in awareness, may report feeling "spacy" 3 Severe, marked reduction in awareness, may persist for several hours 4 Extreme, complete loss of awareness of surroundings, may be unresponsive, possible amnesia for the episode (blackout) ***QV (specify)*** ____________ ***Trauma-related?*** *1 definite 2 probable 3 unlikely* *Current* _____ *Lifetime* _____	***F*** _____ ***I*** _____ ***Past month*** ***F*** _____ ***I*** _____ ***Sx: Y N*** ***Lifetime*** ***F*** _____ ***I*** _____ ***Sx: Y N***

29. derealization

Frequency	***Intensity***	***Past week***
Have there been times when things going on around you seemed unreal or very strange and unfamiliar? [IF NO:] *(What about times when people you knew suddenly seemed unfamiliar?)* **What was that like? How often has that happened in the past month (*week*)?** [IF NOT CLEAR:] *(Was it due to an illness or the effects of drugs or alcohol?)* **When did you first start feeling that way?** *(After the {EVENT}?)* 0 Never 1 Once or twice 2 Once or twice a week 3 Several times a week 4 Daily or almost every day ***Description/Examples***	**How strong was (DEREALIZATION)? How long did it last? What did you do while this was happening?** *(Did other people notice your behavior? What did they say?)* 0 No derealization 1 Mild, slight derealization 2 Moderate, definite but transient derealization 3 Severe, considerable derealization, marked confusion about what is real, may persist for several hours 4 Extreme, profound derealization, dramatic loss of sense of reality or familiarity *QV (specify)* ________________ *Trauma-related?* *1 definite 2 probable 3 unlikely* *Current* _____ *Lifetime* _____	***F*** _____ ***I*** _____ ***Past month*** ***F*** _____ ***I*** _____ ***Sx: Y N*** ***Lifetime*** ***F*** _____ ***I*** _____ ***Sx: Y N***

30. depersonalization

Frequency	*Intensity*	*Past week*
Have there been times when you felt as if you were outside of your body, watching yourself as if you were another person? [IF NO:] *(What about times when your body felt strange or unfamiliar to you, as if it had changed in some way?)* **What was that like? How often has that happened in the past month *(week)*? [IF NOT CLEAR:]** *(Was it due to an illness or the effects of drugs or alcohol?)* **When did you first start feeling that way?** *(After the {EVENT}?)* 0 Never 1 Once or twice 2 Once or twice a week 3 Several times a week 4 Daily or almost every day *Description/Examples*	**How strong was (DEPERSONALIZATION)? How long did it last? What did you do while this was happening?** *(Did other people notice your behavior? What did they say?)* 0 No depersonalization 1 Mild, slight depersonalization 2 Moderate, definite but transient depersonalization 3 Severe, considerable depersonalization, marked sense of detachment from self, may persist for several hours 4 Extreme, profound depersonalization, dramatic sense of detachment from self *QV (specify)* ________________ *Trauma-related?* *1 definite 2 probable 3 unlikely* *Current* _____ *Lifetime* _____	***F*** _____ ***I*** _____ ***Past month*** ***F*** _____ ***I*** _____ ***Sx: Y N*** ***Lifetime*** ***F*** _____ ***I*** _____ ***Sx: Y N***

CAPS SUMMARY SHEET

Name:________________________ ID#:________ Interviewer:________________________

Study:____________ Date:________

A. Traumatic event:

B. Reexperiencing symptoms	*PAST WEEK*			*PAST MONTH*			*LIFETIME*		
	Freq	*Int*	*F+I*	*Freq*	*Int*	*F+I*	*Freq*	*Int*	*F+I*
(1) intrusive recollections									
(2) distressing dreams									
(3) acting or feeling as if event were recurring									
(4) psychological distress at exposure to cues									
(5) physiological reactivity on exposure to cues									
B subtotals									
Number of Criterion B symptoms (need 1)									

C. Avoidance and numbing symptoms	*PAST WEEK*			*PAST MONTH*			*LIFETIME*		
	Freq	*Int*	*F+I*	*Freq*	*Int*	*F+I*	*Freq*	*Int*	*F+I*
(6) avoidance of thoughts or feelings									
(7) avoidance of activities, places, or people									
(8) inability to recall important aspect of trauma									
(9) diminished interest in activities									
(10) detachment or estrangement									
(11) restricted range of affect									
(12) sense of a foreshortened future									
C subtotals									
Number of Criterion C symptoms (need 3)									

D. Hyperarousal symptoms	*PAST WEEK*			*PAST MONTH*			*LIFETIME*		
	Freq	*Int*	*F+I*	*Freq*	*Int*	*F+I*	*Freq*	*Int*	*F+I*
(13) difficulty falling or staying asleep									
(14) irritability or outbursts of anger									
(15) difficulty concentrating									
(16) hypervigilance									
(17) exaggerated startle response									
D subtotals									
Number of Criterion D symptoms (need 2)									

Total Freq, Int, and Severity (F+I)	*PAST WEEK*			*PAST MONTH*			*LIFETIME*		
	Freq	*Int*	*F+I*	*Freq*	*Int*	*F+I*	*Freq*	*Int*	*F+I*
Sum of subtotals (B+C+D)									

E. Duration of disturbance	*CURRENT*	*LIFETIME*
(19) duration of disturbance at least one month	*NO YES*	*NO YES*

F. Significant distress or impairment in functioning	*PAST WEEK*	*PAST MONTH*	*LIFETIME*
(20) subjective distress			
(21) impairment in social functioning			
(22) impairment in occupational functioning			
AT LEAST ONE ≥ 2?	*NO YES*	*NO YES*	*NO YES*

PTSD diagnosis	*CURRENT*	*LIFETIME*
PTSD PRESENT – ALL CRITERIA (A-F) MET?	*NO YES*	*NO YES*
Specify: (18) with delayed onset (≥ 6 months delay)	*NO YES*	*NO YES*
(19) acute (< 3 months) or chronic (≥ 3 months)	*acute chronic*	*acute chronic*

Global ratings	*PAST WEEK*	*PAST MONTH*	*LIFETIME*
(23) global validity			
(24) global severity			
(25) global improvement			

Associated features	*PAST WEEK*			*PAST MONTH*			*LIFETIME*		
	Freq	*Int*	*F+I*	*Freq*	*Int*	*F+I*	*Freq*	*Int*	*F+I*
(26) guilt over acts of commission or omission									
(27) survivor guilt									
(28) reduction in awareness of surroundings									
(29) derealization									
(30) depersonalization									

Treatment Outcome PTSD Scale (TOP-8) (Selected items)

Initials ______ ID # ______ Date ______ Visit # ______

The interviewer should identify which traumatic event is the most bothersome and then rate how much each symptom has troubled the subject during the past week. Event: ____________________________

Have you experienced painful images, thoughts or memories of the trauma which you couldn't get out of your mind even though you may have wanted to? Have these been recurrent?

0 = not at all
1 = mild: rarely and not bothersome
2 = moderate: at least once a week and/or produces some distress
3 = severe: at least 4 times per week or moderately distressing
4 = extremely severe: daily or produces so much distress that patient cannot work or function socially

____

Have you experienced less interest (pleasure) in things that you used to enjoy?

0 = no loss of interest
1 = one or two activities less pleasurable
2 = several activities less pleasurable
3 = most activities less pleasurable
4 = almost all activities less pleasurable

____

Do you have less to do with other people than you used to? Do you feel estranged from other people?
0 = no problem
1 = feels detached/estranged, but still has normal degree of contact with others
2 = sometimes avoids contact that would normally participate in
3 = definitely and usually avoids people with whom would previously associate
4 = absolutely refuses or actively avoids all social contact since the stress

____

Do you startle easily? Do you have a tendency to jump? Is this a problem after unexpected noise, or if you hear or see something that reminds you of the trauma?
0 = no problem
1 = mild: occasional but not disruptive
2 = moderate: causes definite discomfort or an exaggerated startle response at least every two weeks
3 = severe: happens more than once a week
4 = extremely severe: so bad that patient cannot function at work or socially

____

TOTAL SCORE ____

Davidson Trauma Scale (A representative sample)

Name:________________________ Age: ______ Sex: ❐ Male ❐ Female

Date: _____/_____/_____

Please identify the trauma that is most disturbing to you

____

____

Each of the following questions asks you about a specific symptom. For each question, consider how often in the last week the symptom troubled you and how severe it was. In the two boxes beside each question, write a number from 0–4 to indicate the frequency and severity of the symptom.

FREQUENCY	SEVERITY
0 = Not at all	0 = Not at all distressing
1 = Once only	1 = Minimally distressing
2 = 2–3 times	2 = Moderately distressing
3 = 4–6 times	3 = Markedly distressing
4 = Every day	4 = Extremely distressing

	Frequency	Severity
Have you ever had distressing dreams of the event?	☐	☐
Have you been upset by something that reminded you of the event?	☐	☐
Have you been avoiding any thoughts or feelings about the event?	☐	☐
Have you found yourself unable to recall important parts of the event?	☐	☐

	FREQUENCY 0 = Not at all 1 = Once only 2 = 2–3 times 3 = 4–6 times 4 = Every day	SEVERITY 0 = Not at all distressing 1 = Minimally distressing 2 = Moderately distressing 3 = Markedly distressing 4 = Extremely distressing
Have you felt distant or cut off from other people?	☐	☐
Have you found it hard to imagine having a long life span and fulfilling your goals?	☐	☐
Have you been irritable or had outbursts of anger?	☐	☐
Have you been jumpy or easily startled?	☐	☐

Structured Interview for PTSD (SIP)

Initials______ ID # ______ Date ______ Visit # ______ Age ______ Sex ______

Race ______________

Introduction (if this is the first encounter with subject)

I should like to ask about the difficulties or problems that caused you to come for help.

First would you please tell me your age?______ Where do you live? ______________

Are you employed? If yes: What is your job? ________________________________

If no: When did you last work? ____

What did you do? ________________ Why did you stop work? ____________

With whom do you live? ____

Please tell me about your family, friends, and social activities.

____

____

A. Experience of trauma

A1 Did you ever experience, witness or have to confront an extremely stressful event which involved actual or threatened death or serious injury, or a threat to the physical integrity of yourself or others?

No____ Yes____

A2 Did you react to the event(s) with intense fear, helplessness or horror?

No ____ Yes ____

How long were you in that situation? _____ What was the worst thing about it for you?

A3 Define the event(s). Identify by numbers below. Narrative comment may be added.

Event	Age at event
1 = combat	______
2 = rape	______
3 = incest	______
4 = other physical assault/attack	______
5 = seeing someone killed or hurt	______
6 = natural disaster	______
7 = accident	______
8= complicated bereavement	______
9 = threat of close call	______
10 = life-threatening illness	______
11 = other (identify	______

A4 Identify which event was the worst, and focus on this for the interview. ____________

B. Reexperiencing the traumatic event

After it was over, did you find yourself persistently remembering or dreaming about the events over and over again for at least one month?

No ____ Yes ____

Did this happen even when you were not trying to remember?

No ____ Yes ____

THE TIME PERIOD WILL USUALLY BE THE PAST WEEK, IT CAN BE ADJUSTED IF THE PURPOSE OF THE INTERVIEW IS FOR WORST EVER OR TO ASSESS DIAGNOSIS, FOR WHICH A FOUR-WEEK PERIOD OF SIMULTANEOUS SYMPTOMS IS REQUIRED.

B. Trauma

B1 Have you experienced painful images, thoughts or memories of the trauma which you could not get out of your mind even though you may have wanted to?
Have these been recurrent?

0 = not at all
1 = mild: rarely and/or not bothersome
2 = moderate: at least once a week and/or produces some distress
3 = severe: at least four times per week or moderately distressing
4 = extremely severe: daily or produces so much distress that patient cannot work or function socially

Rate past week ______

B2 Dreams

I would like to ask you about your dreams. Have you had repeated dreams of violence, injury, danger, combat, death or other theme related to trauma? Were these of actual scenes you were involved in? Do you recognize people in the dream? Are these dreams of the event? How frequent are these dreams? Do you wake up sweating or shouting? Trembling? Palpitations? Trouble breathing? Are the nightmares so bad that your spouse (partner) does not sleep in the same bed, or in the same room?

0 = no problems
1 = mild: infrequent or not disruptive
2 = moderate: at least once a week/somewhat distressing
3 = severe: at least four times a week/moderately distressing
4 = extremely severe: six to seven times a week/extremely distressing

Rate past week ______

B3 Acting or feeling as if event was currently happening

At times have you reacted to something as if you were back in the event? Has it seemed that the event was recurring or that you were living through it again? Did you have hallucinations of the event?

0 = not at all
1 = rarely/once a week

2 = sometimes/two to four times a week
3 = often/five to six times a week
4 = every day

Rate past week ______

B4 Psychological distress at exposure to reminders of event(s)
Do any of the symptoms occur or get worse if something reminds you of the stressful event? (Ask about TV programs, weather conditions, news, Veterans' Day, recent disaster involving loss of life, loss of good friends, being in places which remind person of the event.) (Feel angry, sad, irritable, anxious, or frightened?)

0 = not at all
1 = a little bit: infrequent or of questionable significance
2 = somewhat
3 = significantly: several symptoms occur or one symptom with much distress
4 = marked: very distressing, may have activated an episode of the illness, resulting in hospitalization, different treatment, etc.

Rate past week ______

B5 Does exposure to an event that reminds you of, or resembles, the event cause you to have any physical response? (Sweating, trembling, heart racing, nausea, hyperventilating, dizziness, etc.)

0 = not at all
1 = a little bit: infrequent or questionable
2 = somewhat: mildly distressing
3 = significantly: causes much distress
4 = marked: very distressing, or has sought help from doctors because of the physical response (e.g., chest pain so severe that patient was sure he or she was having a heart attack)

Rate past week ________

C. Avoidance of stimuli associated with trauma

C1 Have you tried to avoid thoughts or feelings about the trauma?

0 = no avoidance
1 = mild: of doubtful significance
2 = moderate: definite effort is made, but is able to function at work and socially

3 = severe: definite avoidance which affects life in some way (keeps moving from place to place/cannot work/works excessively/or episodic substance abuse because of need to avoid thoughts or feelings)
4 = very severe: dramatic effect on life

Rate past week ______

C2 Avoidance of activities that arouse recollection of the event
Have you avoided places, people, conversations or activities that remind you of the event?

0 = no avoidance
1 = mild: of doubtful significance
2 = moderate: definite avoidance of situations
3 = severe: very uncomfortable and avoidance affects life in some way
4 = extremely severe: house-bound, cannot go out to shops and restaurants, major functional restrictions

Rate past week ______

C3 Psychogenic amnesia
Is there an important part of the event that you cannot remember?

0 = no problem: remembers everything
1 = mild: remembers most details
2 = moderate: some difficulty remembering significant details
3 = severe: remembers only a few details
4 = very severe: claims total amnesia for the trauma

Rate past week ______

C4 Loss of interest. Have you experienced less interest (pleasure) in things that you used to enjoy?
What things have you lost interest in? What do you still enjoy?

0 = no loss of interest
1 = one or two activities less pleasurable
2 = several activities less pleasurable
3 = most activities less pleasurable
4 = almost all activities less pleasurable

Rate past week ______

C5 Detachment/estrangement

Do you have less to do with other people than you used to? Do you feel estranged from other people?

0 = no problem
1 = feel detached/estranged, but still has normal degree of contact with others
2 = sometimes avoids contact that you would normally participate in
3 = definitely and usually avoids people with whom would previously associate
4 = absolutely refuses or actively avoids all social contact

Rate past week ______

C6 Restricted range of affect

Can you have warm feelings/feel close to others? Do you feel numb?

0 = no problem
1 = mild: of questionable significance
2 = moderate: some difficulty expressing feelings
3 = severe: definite problems with expressing feelings
4 = very severe: has no feelings, feels numb most of the time

Rate past week ______

C7 Foreshortened future

What do you see happening in your future? What do you visualize as you grow old? What are your expectations of the future?

0 = describes positive or realistic future
1 = mild: describes pessimistic outlook at times, but varies from day to day depending on events
2 = moderate: pessimistic much of the time
3 = severe: constantly pessimistic
4 = can see no future/views early death as likely (but without adequate medical basis)

Rate past week ______

D. Increased arousal

D1 Sleep disturbance

We spoke earlier about nightmares. What about other aspects of sleeping? Have you had any trouble falling asleep? Do you wake in the middle of the night? Are you able to go back to sleep after waking?

0 = no loss of sleep
1 = mild: occasional difficulty but no more than two nights/week
2 = moderate: difficulty sleeping at least three nights/week
3 = severe: difficulty sleeping every night
4 = extremely severe: less than 3 hours sleep/night

Rate past week ______

D2 Have you been more irritable or more easily annoyed than usual?

How did you show your feelings? Have you had angry outbursts?

0 = not at all
1 = mild: occasional feelings of annoyance or anger which may go unnoticed by others
2 = moderate: increased feelings of annoyance, becomes snappy or argumentative (at least once every two weeks); others may have commented
3 = severe: almost constantly irritable or angry/often loses temper or has significant impairment in ability to relate to others as a result of this
4 = very severe: preoccupied with anger or feelings of retaliation, overtly aggressive or assaultive/marked impairment in function

Rate past week ______

D3 Impairment in concentration

Have you noticed any trouble concentrating? Is it hard to keep your mind on things? Can you pay attention easily? What about reading or watching TV?

0 = no difficulty
1 = patient acknowledges slight problem
2 = patient describes difficulty
3 = interferes with daily activities, job, etc.
4 = constant problems: unable to do simple tasks

Rate past week ______

D4 Hypervigilance

Do you have to stay on guard? Are you watchful? Do you feel on edge? Do you have to sit with your back to the wall?

0 = no problem
1 = mild: occasional/not disruptive
2 = moderate: causes discomfort/feels on edge or watchful in some situations
3 = severe: causes discomfort/feels on edge or watchful in most situations
4 = very severe: causes extreme discomfort and alters life (feels constantly on guard/must keep back to wall/socially impaired because of feeling on edge

Rate past week ______

D5 Startle

Do you startle easily? Do you have a tendency to jump? Is this a problem after unexpected noise, or if you hear or see something that reminds you of the original trauma?

0 = no problem
1 = mild: occasional/not disruptive
2 = moderate: causes definite discomfort or an exaggerated startle response at least every two weeks
3 = severe: happens more than once a week
4 = extremely severe: so bad that patient cannot function at work or socially

Rate past week ______

E. How long has this condition lasted?

E1 Did the symptoms which you have described last for at least four weeks? ______

E2 How many months after the trauma did these symptoms first develop? ____

E3 Age at the time symptoms began. ____

F. In the interviewer's judgment, and taking into account the subject responses, has the disturbance caused clinically significant distress or impairment in social, occupational or other important areas of functioning?

No ____ Yes ____

SCORESHEET: SIP

Initials______ ID #______ Date:______ Visit #______

B	1	______
	2	______
	3	______
	4	______
	5	______
(Subtotal)		______
C	1	______
	2	______
	3	______
	4	______
	5	______
	6	______
	7	______
(Subtotal)		______
D	1	______
	2	______
	3	______
	4	______
	5	______
(Subtotal)		______
Total (B, C, D)		

SCORESHEET FOR STRUCTURED PTSD INTERVIEW

Total (past week or other designated period) score for all B, C, and D items ______ Total

Score No as 1, Yes as 2 to all answers below

DSM-IV Diagnosis

Traumatic event definitely present? ______

At least one item from category B with score of at least 2 ______

At least three items from category C with score of at least 2 (at least one item must be from C1–2 and one must be from C3–7) ______

At least two items from category D1–5 (each must score at least 2) ______

Diagnosis? ____

Index

Page references in *italics* refer to tables or boxed material; those in **bold** to figures